T0252157

The Chest X-Ray

A Systematic Teaching Atlas

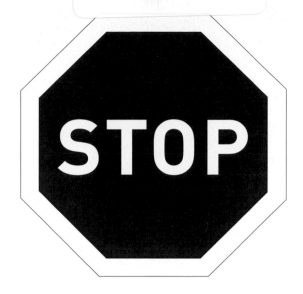

STOP

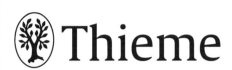

Thieme

Getting the Most out of this Book

This workbook has several features that will help you learn the systematic viewing and interpretation of chest radiographs in the most efficient way:

To save time, the figure numbers are based on page numbers
While many textbooks require readers to leaf through numerous pages to find, say, "Figure 2.23" (i.e., the 23rd figure in Chapter 2), the figures in this workbook are easy to locate because they are based on page numbers. For example, if you are looking for Figure 121.2a, you can find it quickly and easily by turning to page 121.

Additional time is saved by presenting topics on facing pages
The running text that describes abnormalities and their imaging features is generally placed close to the corresponding images – usually on the same page or on two facing pages. This makes it easy to compare posteroanterior (PA) and lateral radiographs or ultrasound images and computed tomography (CT) scans without having to hunt through the book.

Numerical labels and colors
Many structures in the illustrative images are labeled with numbers rather than abbreviations. These **black numerical labels** appear in **boldface type** and parentheses when they are cited in the text. This allows you to view every image with a detective's eye and identify structures on your own, **without** being prompted by a label that gives you the answer. This active problem-solving approach is an excellent way to learn, even though it may seem "inconvenient" at first. The [numbers in brackets refer to the list of references on the back flap of the book.

Direction of the blue arrows
Many critical findings in images are indicated by green arrows. Notice which direction the arrows are pointing when you want to find the arrow reference quickly in the text. The direction in which a particular arrow is pointing in an image corresponds precisely to the direction the arrow in the accompanying text on that page is pointing. This makes it easy to locate the text passage that describes the finding of interest.

Repetition
In some cases the same finding may appear at different places in the book. Firstly, this repetition is based on discoveries from research on learning and memory, which confirm the value of repeating information at intervals (this principle is reinforced by the quiz sections). Also, some findings may have a patchy, focal, or reticular appearance on images and are therefore listed as a possible differential diagnosis in more than one chapter.

Matthias Hofer, MD, MPH, MME
Diagnostic Radiologist
University Hospital Duesseldorf
Heinrich-Heine University
Duesseldorf, Germany

Nadine Abanador, MD
Department of Cardiology
Helios Clinic Wuppertal
Wuppertal, Germany

Lars Kamper, MD
Clinic for Internal Medicine and Cardiology
Alfried-Krupp Hospital
Essen, Germany

Henning Rattunde, MD
Institute for Diagnostic, Interventional,
and Pediatric Radiology
Inselspital, University Hospital Bern
Bern, Switzerland

Christian Zentai
University Hospital Aachen
Clinic for Anesthesiology
Aachen, Germany

Important Note: Medicine is an ever-changing science undergoing continual development. Research and clinical experience are continually expanding our knowledge, in particular our knowledge of proper treatment and drug therapy. Insofar as this book mentions any dosage or application, readers may rest assured that the authors, editors, and publishers have made every effort to ensure that such references are in accordance with *the state of knowledge at the time of production of the book.*

Nevertheless this does not involve, imply, or express any guarantee or responsibility on the part of the publishers in respect of any dosage instructions and forms of application stated in the book. *Every user is requested to examine carefully* the manufacturers' leaflets accompanying each drug and to check, if necessary in consultation with a physician or specialist, whether the dosage schedules mentioned therein or the contraindications stated by the manufacturers differ from the statements made in the present book. Such examination is particularly important with drugs that are either rarely used or have been newly released on the market. Every dosage schedule or every form of application used is entirely at the user's own risk and responsibility. The authors and publishers request every user to report to the publishers any discrepancies or inaccuracies noticed.

Library of Congress Cataloging-in-Publication Data is available from the publisher.

© 2007 (english edition), Georg Thieme Verlag,
Rüdigerstraße 14, 70649 Stuttgart, Germany
Thieme New York, 333 Seventh Avenue,
New York, N.Y. 10001, U.S.A.

Design and Typesetting by:
Dipl. Des. Inger Jürgens, Cologne: www.ingerj.de

Printed in Germany by: WAZ-Druck, Duisburg

If errors in this work are found after publication, errata will be posted at www.thieme.com on the product description page.

ISBN 978-3-13-144211-6 (GTV)
ISBN 978-1-58890-554-3 (TNY)
ISBN 978-3-13-144971-9 (Asia)

Contents Overview

Detailed information on chapter contents can be found at the beginning of each chapter and in the Table of Contents on pages 4 and 5.

Foreword

Radiography of the heart and lung is still the most widely practiced imaging procedure. Chest radiographs are an indispensable part of the basic diagnostic workup in major medical disciplines such as internal medicine, the surgical specialties, anesthesiology, and occupational medicine.

For that reason, students, residents and beginning practitioners have need for a practical reference guide that can lead them on the path from radiographic features to diagnostic interpretation in a systematic way. The analytical format of this book should enable you to recognize the most important and most common findings while giving you greater confidence in reading and interpreting radiographs.

This book contains numerous illustrative radiographs, all vividly instructive and many accompanied by examples from other imaging modalities. Text and illustrations are presented side-by-side to facilitate learning, and structures of key interest are clearly indicated by arrows and numerical labels. A fold-out number key underscores the practice-oriented and user-friendly format in which the material is presented. The numerous quiz sections allow you to check your progress and see how well you have mastered the essentials. The book is characterized by a high density of information within a small space – even including step-by-step instructions on thoracentesis, chest tube insertion, and the insertion of central venous catheters (CVCs).

The superb image quality, concise text, and extremely favorable cost-to-value ratio make it easy to recommend "Chest X-Ray"-Atlas for all students and residents who are embarking on their professional career.

Prof. U. Mödder, M.D.
Director, Department of Diagnostic Radiology
Düsseldorf University Medical Center
Düsseldorf, Germany

Preface by the Authors

What makes this book different from comparable titles?
Most radiology textbooks are organized according to disease groups or pathophysiological categories. But in the everyday practice of chest radiography, we do **not** address the question of, say, which "pneumoconiosis" should be considered in the differential diagnosis. Instead, the interpreting physician is confronted with patchy, streaky, reticular, or nodular opacities in the pulmonary interstitium or parenchyma that he or she must fit into a differential diagnostic framework. Accordingly, this workbook is organized according to the morphological patterns that are actually seen on chest radiographs. There are also chapters that teach readers how to interpret the widening of the mediastinum and how to address specific clinical problems in ventilated intensive care unit (ICU) patients and trauma patients.

In using this book, you will come upon quiz sections that present illustrative cases and ask questions about them. These questions are designed to help you learn through the repetition and practical application of key points – points that might be missed or quickly forgotten by just skimming through the material. As a result, you may find this workbook somewhat "unpleasant" at first, but on closer scrutiny you will see how effective it is in reinforcing long-term learning.

We hope you will enjoy using this book and we wish you much success in applying what you have learned.

On behalf of the authors: Matthias Hofer, M.D., MPH, MME (ed.)
October 2006

Matthias Hofer

Thoracic Anatomy

Chapter Goals:

We begin this workbook by familiarizing you with thoracic anatomy as it normally appears on chest radiographs. The positive identification of anatomical structures is essential for accurate image analysis and will prevent many potential errors of interpretation.

A major goal of this chapter is to acquaint you with the appearance of pulmonary vessels, bronchi, thoracic skeletal structures, and the mediastinal contours. On completing this chapter, you should be able to:

- correctly identify (step 1) and draw (step 2) the structures of thoracic topographical anatomy as they appear on chest radiographs;

- localize focal abnormalities to specific pulmonary lobes and segments;

- draw and correctly label from memory the mediastinal borders as they appear on postero-anterior (PA) and lateral radiographs;

- detect any abnormalities in the mediastinal silhouette and relate them to the most likely causes;

- correctly describe the basic anatomical structure of the lung, its tracheobronchial tree, and the pulmonary vessels;

- describe the basic physiological principles of respiration, gas exchange, and lung perfusion.

Please take the self-quiz at the end of Chapter 2 (p. 32-34) to see how well you have achieved these goals. To avoid the false sense of security that short-term memory gives, we suggest that you wait several hours before taking the quiz. Working through these first two introductory chapters can be a valuable exercise for physicians as well as medical students, because we know from experience that many details of topographical anatomy can fade over time, often to an unexpected degree. We wish you much success!

1

Thoracic Skeleton

The bony structures of the chest absorb and scatter roentgen rays, thus causing greater attenuation (weakening) of the roentgen ray beam than the lung tissue and other thoracic soft tissues. Because of this, less radiation reaches the roentgen ray intensifying screen behind vertebral bodies (26), ribs (2), clavicles (23), and scapulae (27), and less film blackening occurs in those areas. This is why bony structures appear lighter on radiographs than the darker lung parenchyma, for example. These areas of increased attenuation are called "opacities" in radiology, despite their greater brightness (Fig. 8.1).

Conversely, areas that are more easily penetrated by the roentgen ray beam are called "lucencies" because of their **hyper**lucent (= darker than normal) appearance. Examples are hyperinflated lung areas and emphysematous bullae. The posterior rib segments (22a) are directed more or less horizontally, while the anterior segments (22b) pass obliquely forward and downward. Occasionally, beginners will misinterpret the apical lung region enclosed by the first rib (★) as an emphysematous bulla (see p. 119) or apical pneumothorax (see p. 120) because of its hyperlucent appearance. Actually this is an optical illusion created by the strong contrast between the low radiographic density of the apical lung and the high radiographic density of the first rib.

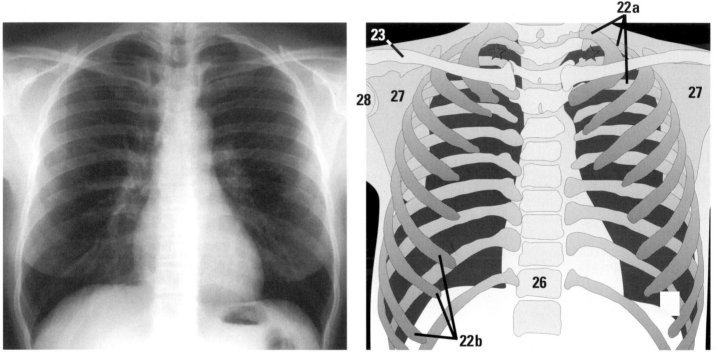

Fig. 8.1a

Fig. 8.1b

Thus, the radiographic appearance of thoracic structures depends mainly on their density. While areas with a high density per unit volume (e.g., cortical bone) appear light or white, areas with a lower density that are more transparent to roentgen rays (e.g., air in the alveoli) appear dark (Fig. 8.2).

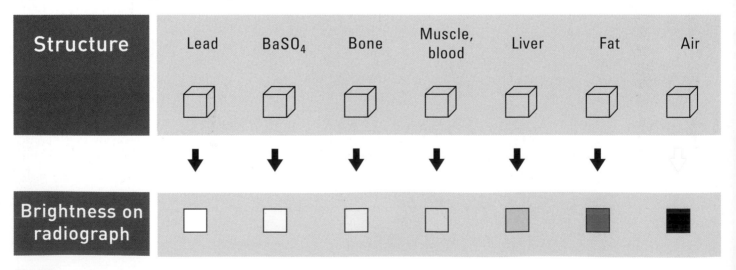

Fig. 8.2

Moreover, the interface between tissues of different density must be struck tangentially by the roentgen ray beam in order to appear as a well-defined boundary line on radiographs **(Fig. 9.1)**. For example, the horizontal fissure of the lung **(30)** is directed parallel to the beam axis in lateral and PA radiographs, and therefore it appears as a thin, white boundary line in both projections (**Fig. 8.1a** and **Fig. 9.2**). The same phenomenon occurs with the ribs. Normally only the superior and inferior cortical rib margins bounded by the intercostal spaces are displayed as boundary lines. The density difference between the center of the ribs and the adjacent lung or adjacent soft-tissue envelope is not visualized **(Fig. 9.1)**.

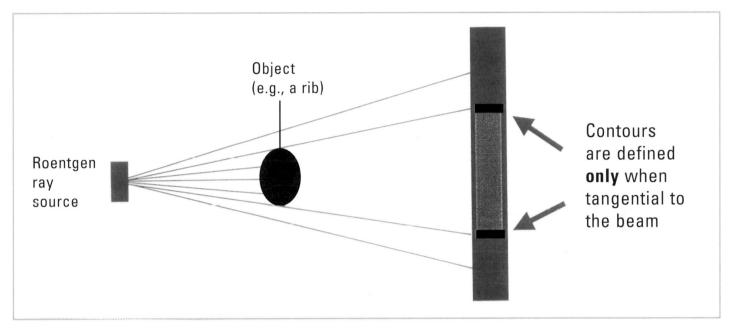

Fig. 9.1 **Note:** Only interfaces that are struck tangentially by the roentgen ray beam appear as boundary lines on the radiograph

In the lateral projection, the roentgen ray beam is tangential to the upper and lower endplates of the thoracic vertebral bodies **(26)**, to the sternum **(24)**, and to the cortical lines of the scapulae **(27)**. As a result, these structures are prominently displayed as white boundary lines **(Fig. 9.2)**. The clavicles **(23)** are usually obscured by a summation effect from the soft tissues of the superior thoracic aperture and the neck.

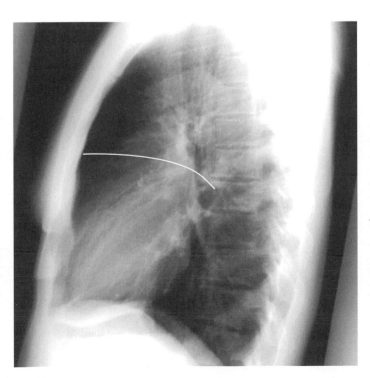

Fig. 9.2a

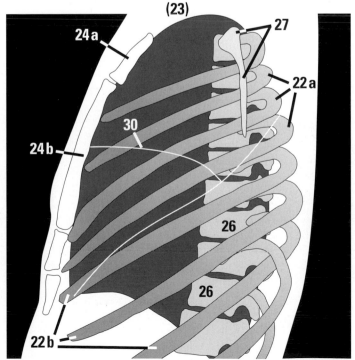

Fig. 9.2b

1

Principal Divisions of the Lung

The upper portion of the lung in the PA radiograph can generally be divided into an apical zone **(AZ)** located above the clavicle **(23)** and an upper zone **(UZ)** extending from the inferior border of the clavicle to the superior border of the pulmonary hilum **(Fig. 10.1)**. Just below the UZ is the middle zone **(MZ)**, which extends down to a line separating the middle and lower thirds of the lung, approximately at the lower end of the pulmonary hilum. The lower zone **(LZ)** of the lung extends from that line down to the diaphragm leaflet **(17)**. Additionally, distinguishing the perihilar **root of the lung** from the central lung and the peripheral lung **(Fig. 10.2)** can be helpful in the pathophysiological classification of some diseases. For example, these regions are drained by different lymphatic channels, and this has a bearing on the potential routes of lymphogenous metastasis.

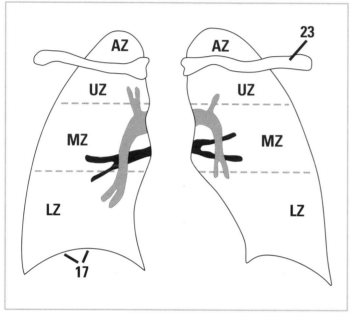

Fig. 10.1

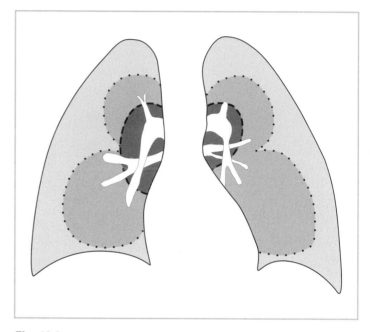

Fig. 10.2

Lobar Anatomy

The divisions described above do not conform to the lobar boundaries of the lung. It is interesting to note that each of the lower lobes (LLs) **(34)** extends to a much higher level, especially posteriorly, than the beginner might think **(Fig. 10.3)**. The superior segment of the LL (segment no.6, see p. 12) usually extends slightly higher on the left side than on the right, and on both sides it occupies a higher level than the typical extent of the right middle lobe (ML) **(33)**.

This may be clinically important in localizing a finding to a particular lobe, as when planning the bronchoscopic extraction of a radiopaque foreign body or a bronchoscopic biopsy.

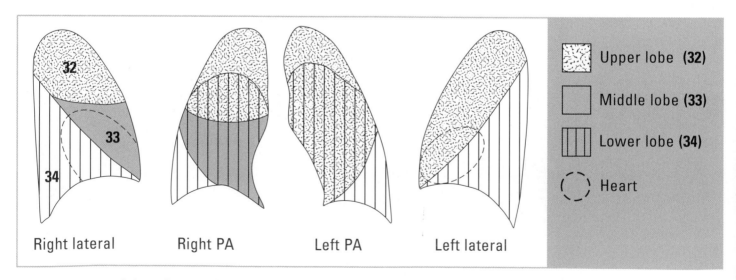

	Upper lobe **(32)**
	Middle lobe **(33)**
	Lower lobe **(34)**
	Heart

Right lateral   Right PA   Left PA   Left lateral

Fig. 10.3 Extent of the pulmonary lobes on radiographs. Summation views in various projections

Lobar Anatomy

Figure 11.1 shows the typical course of the interlobar fissures. The course of the oblique fissure **(30)** between the upper lobe (UL) **(32)** and LL **(34)** resembles a propeller blade. The dotted lines indicate the course of the oblique fissure along the mediastinum, and the solid lines indicate its course along the ribs **(Fig. 11.1)**. The horizontal fissure **(31)** and ML **(33)** exist only in the right lung.

Figures 11.2 and **11.3** show the radiographic projections of the pulmonary lobes as they appear in the right and left lateral views.

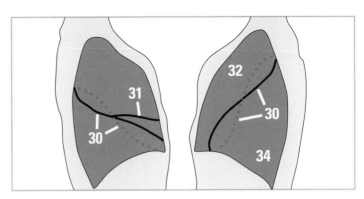

Fig. 11.1   Course of the fissures in the lateral projections

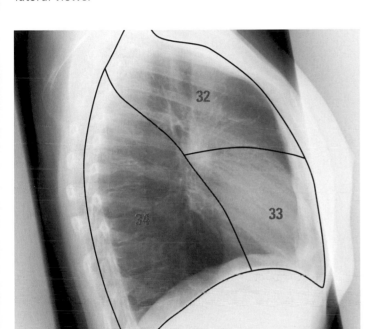

Fig. 11.2   Right lateral view

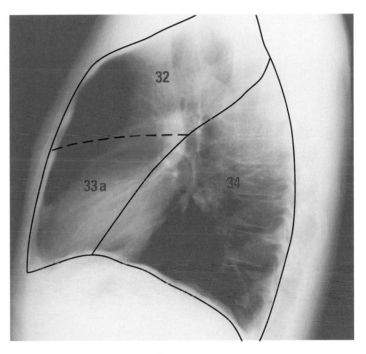

Fig. 11.3   Left lateral view

The inflammatory infiltration of an entire lobe ("lobar pneumonia") appears as a homogeneous lobar opacity that displays a typical configuration and extent in the lateral and frontal radiographs **(Fig. 11.4)**. The lobar volume, and thus the course of the lobar boundaries, usually remains constant in lobar pneumonia, or the volume of the affected lobe may be slightly increased.

A different pattern is produced by decreased ventilation (dyselectasis) or atelectasis in which a lobe is no longer ventilated due, for example, to mucus plugging or neoplastic bronchial obstruction. After a certain latent period, the loss of ventilation causes a decrease in the volume of the affected lobe, which usually shows homogeneous opacity on radiographs (see also p. 111-114).

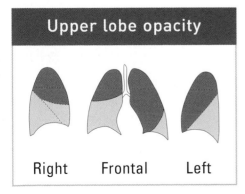
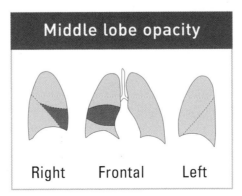
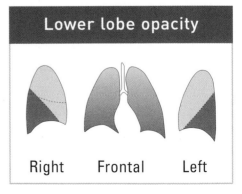

Upper lobe opacity	Middle lobe opacity	Lower lobe opacity
Right Frontal Left	Right Frontal Left	Right Frontal Left

Fig. 11.4

Segmental Anatomy

It is important to have a thorough knowledge of segmental anatomy, as this will enable you to state the precise location of a focal abnormality. The following sports-inspired mnemonic may assist you in learning the names of the various segments (**Fig. 12.1**):

To reach the top, you have to fight your way from back to front, often taking a side route past the middle. Now you're at the top, and the rest are at the bottom. Many are on the sideline, poor souls!

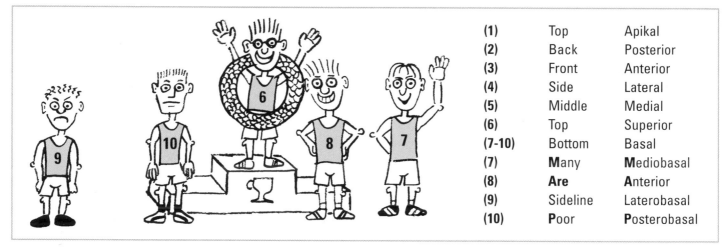

(1)	Top	Apikal
(2)	Back	Posterior
(3)	Front	Anterior
(4)	Side	Lateral
(5)	Middle	Medial
(6)	Top	Superior
(7-10)	Bottom	Basal
(7)	**M**any	**M**ediobasal
(8)	**Are**	**A**nterior
(9)	Sideline	Laterobasal
(10)	**P**oor	**P**osterobasal

Fig. 12.1

It is common to find a variant in the left lung in which segments 1 and 2 arise from the same bronchus and are known collectively as the apicoposterior segment of the UL. Please memorize the location of the individual segments with the aid of these diagrams (**Fig. 12.2**). When you have done this, cover the page and draw the typical segmental arrangement from memory on a separate sheet of paper. Finally, refer back to the diagrams to check the accuracy of your drawing.

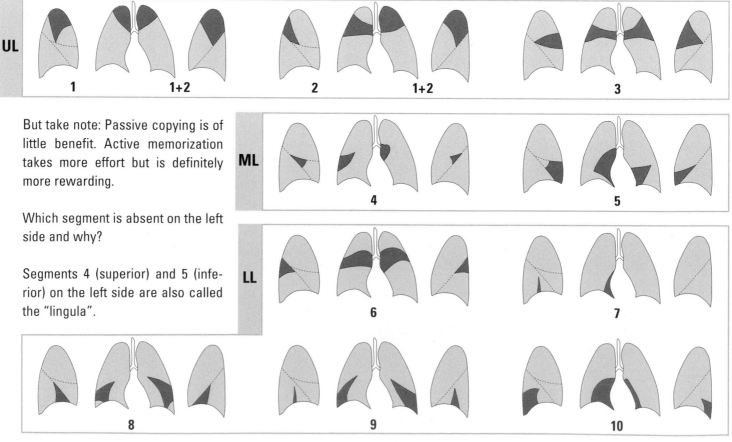

But take note: Passive copying is of little benefit. Active memorization takes more effort but is definitely more rewarding.

Which segment is absent on the left side and why?

Segments 4 (superior) and 5 (inferior) on the left side are also called the "lingula".

Fig. 12.2   Typical arrangement and extent of the pulmonary segments

Tracheobronchial Tree

The trachea **(14)** contains 15-20 horseshoe-shaped cartilage rings that protect it and stabilize it against negative pressures during inspiration. The rings are incomplete posteriorly, sparing the membranous posterior wall of the trachea. The cross section of the trachea is slightly flattened posteriorly during inspiration and reexpands during inspiration to a circular diameter of approximately 26 mm in men and 22 mm in women. The trachea begins at the level of the sixth or seventh cervical vertebrae and descends for approximately 10-12 cm to its bifurcation **(14c)** at the level of the fourth to sixth thoracic vertebrae. There it splits into the two main bronchi, forming a normal bifurcation angle in the PA projection of 55-70° in adults and up to 70-80° in children. The tracheal bifurcation is symmetrical until about 15 years of age, and thereafter the right main bronchus generally runs more vertically than the left. Because of this asymmetry, foreign bodies are more likely to be aspirated into the right main bronchus than the left. A bifurcation angle greater than 90° suggests the presence of a mass lesion near the carina.

The right main bronchus **(14a)** runs more sharply downward than the left, dividing after only about 3 cm into the laterally directed UL bronchus and the 2- to 3-cm-long intermediate bronchus. The ML bronchus arises from the anterolateral aspect of the intermediate bronchus at the same level where the posteriorly directed segmental bronchus branches to the superior LL segment no. **6**. (This is the only segmental bronchus that divides into three subsegmental bronchi; the other segmental bronchi each divide into only two.)

The left main bronchus **(14b)** runs laterally downward for approximately 5 cm before dividing into the upper and LL bronchi. The left UL bronchus also runs laterally. In approximately 80% of cases, the first two segmental bronchi arise from the UL bronchus by a common trunk, which is why segments **1** and **2** on the left side are known collectively as the "apicoposterior segment." Anterior UL segment **3** runs forward, while the lingular segments **4** (superior) and **5** (inferior) run more anterolaterally. The LL bronchi descend sharply to supply the basal segments **7-10** or **8-10** (**Fig. 13.1**).

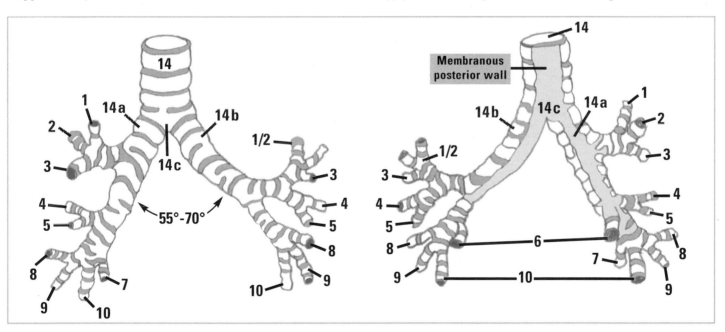

Fig. 13.1 Anterior view   Posterior view

Because both UL bronchi have a relatively horizontal orientation, they are viewed end-on in the lateral radiograph, appearing as round or elliptical radiolucent "holes" below the tracheal column. The right UL bronchus generally occupies a slightly higher level than the left UL bronchus (**Fig. 13.2**). When viewed in the PA radiograph, the anterior segmental bronchus no. **3** of the left lung (✎) is projected as a rounded lucency just lateral to the accompanying artery.

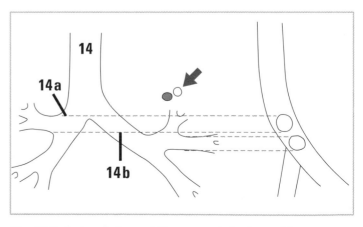

Fig. 13.2 Lateral view of the upper lobe bronchi

Segmental Anatomy on CT Scans

The pulmonary vessels and interlobar fissures can be accurately identified on thin computed tomography (CT) slices (HRCT = high-resolution computed tomography). The horizontal and oblique fissures (solid **blue lines**) can be positively identified by the presence of adjacent hypovascular areas **(Figs. 14.1 to 15.3)**.

Normally, however, the **boundaries between the lung segments** cannot be identified. They are indicated here by **broken blue lines**.

The blue Arabic numbers represent the bronchial segments and do <u>not</u> correspond to the number key at the end of the book.

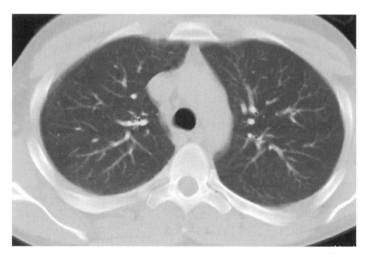

Fig. 14.1 a

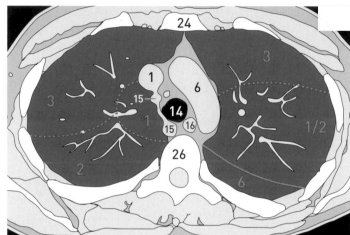

Fig. 14.1 b

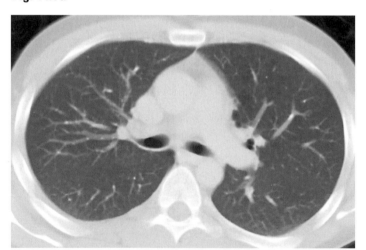

Fig. 14.2 a

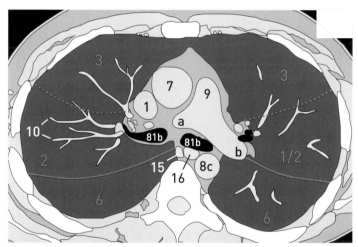

Fig. 14.2 b

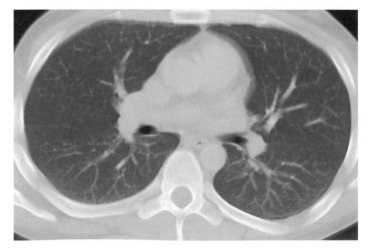

Fig. 14.3 a

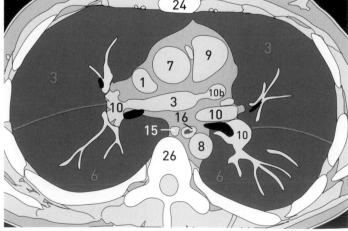

Fig. 14.3 b

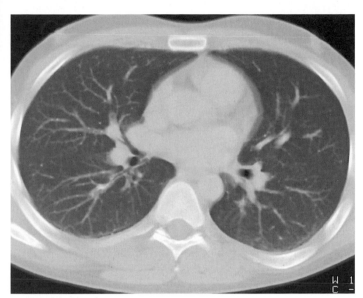

Fig. 15.1 a

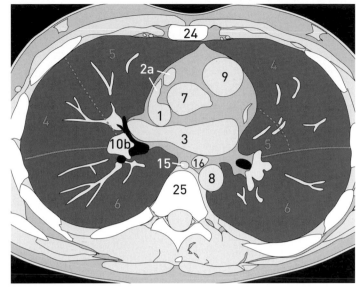

Fig. 15.1 b

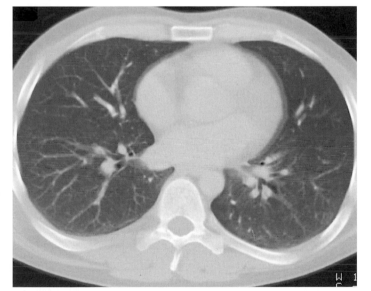

Fig. 15.2 a

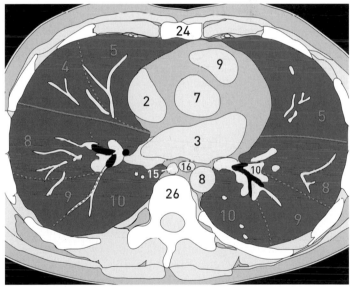

Fig. 15.2 b

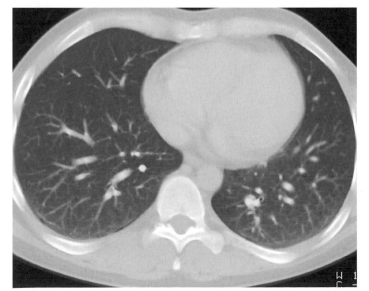

Fig. 15.3 a

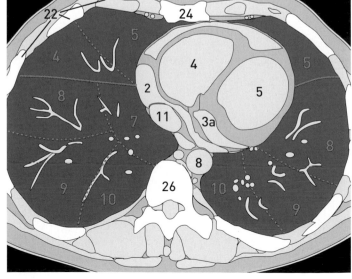

Fig. 15.3 b

Fine Structural Divisions of the Lung

The air passages past the subsegmental bronchi continue to branch in a dichotomous pattern, dividing in approximately seven generations into the lobular bronchioles (1.2 - 2.5 mm in diameter) and terminal bronchioles (1.0 - 1.5 mm in diameter). After entering the secondary lobules (10 - 25 mm in diameter), the passages divide further into multiple acini. Alveoli bud from the walls of the respiratory bronchioles, marking the level at which gas exchange begins **(Fig. 16.1)**. Because the cross section of the air passages expands abruptly at this level, the velocity of the laminar air flow decreases, creating conditions that are favorable for gas exchange. The respiratory bronchioles finally gives rise to 2 - 11 alveolar ducts, which open at numerous sites into the alveolar saccules.

The acini represent the next subunit of a secondary lobule and measure approximately 4 - 8 mm in size. One acinus generally contains approximately 400 alveoli ranging from 0.1 - 0.3 mm in diameter **(Fig. 16.2)**. The acini are the sites where ventilation and perfusion are coordinated in the lung (see p. 29). It is estimated that adults have a total of approximately 300 million alveoli, 90% of which have capillaries available for gas exchange. This is equivalent to a surface area of about 80 m², or the approximate area of a badminton court.

The primary lobules are too small to be resolved on radiograph films. Acinar shadows are larger than the smallest interstitial linear opacities, but they represent the smallest alveolar opacities that can still be seen on radiographs.

Approximately 95% of the alveolar epithelium consists of membranous type I pneumatocytes on a basement membrane. The diffusion pathway to the capillaries in the adjacent interstitium measures only 1 μm or less at many sites. The less numerous, granular type II pneumatocytes are involved in reparative functions and form the surfactant that lowers the surface tension in the lung to prevent alveolar collapse. Various shunts are available for collateral ventilation: Adjacent alveoli are interconnected by pores approximately 5 - 15 μm in size, similar to the Lambert canals between the alveolar ducts and saccules.

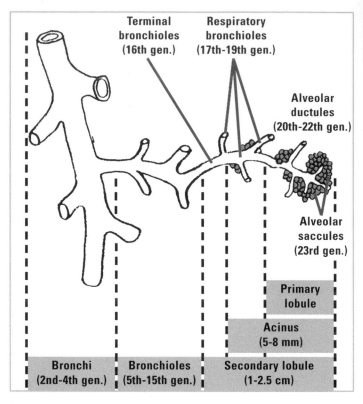

Fig. 16.1

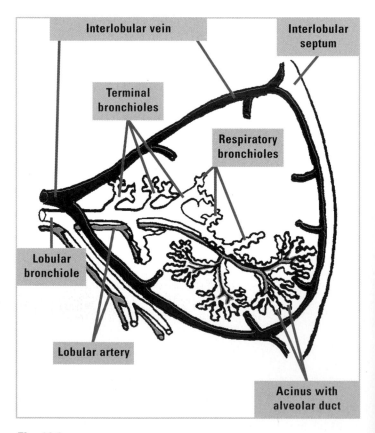

Fig. 16.2

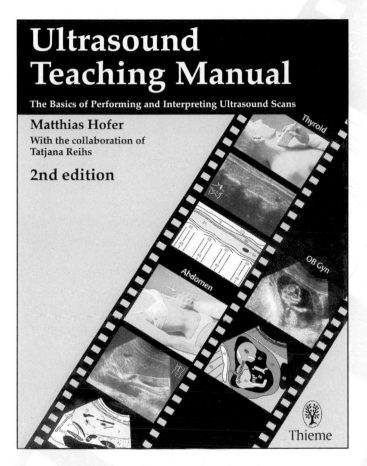
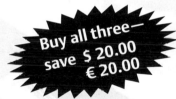
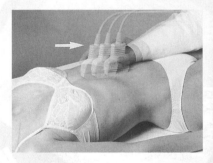
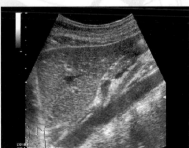

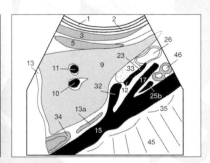
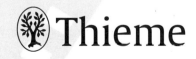

Pulmonary Vessels

The linear opacities in the lung parenchyma are caused by the "shadows" of the pulmonary vessels **(10)**. As these vessels undergo repeated branching, normally their calibers taper smoothly from the central pulmonary hilum to the outer, peripheral region of the lung. Because the pulmonary arteries accompany the bronchi, the direct proximity of a relatively large pulmonary artery to a bronchus in cross section is a good differentiating criterion from pulmonary veins, which run between the segments and not along their centers. Smaller arterial branches are virtually indistinguishable from venous branches in the periphery of the lung. Close to the hilum, however, they can be differentiated by their course.

Course of the vessels in the PA projection

In the LZ, the pulmonary veins **(10b)** run transversely to enter the left atrium, passing horizontally or at a slightly oblique angle through the lung parenchyma. This differs from the course of the pulmonary arteries **(9a, 10a)**, which run sharply upward in the LZ **(Fig. 18.1a)**. Conversely, the veins occupy a somewhat more vertical and more lateral position in the UZ than the medial arteries at the mediastinal border.

Course of the vessels in the lateral projection

In the upper part of the lateral projection **(Fig. 18.1b)**, the brachiocephalic veins **(53)**, the brachiocephalic trunk **(58)**, the left CCA **(57)**, and the left subclavian artery **(56)** run just anterior to the trachea in the pretracheal vascular band. Just below that are the right pulmonary artery **(9a)** and the confluence of the UL veins **(10b)**. The pulmonary veins **(10b)** descend more anteriorly than the arteries **(10a)** in the retrocardiac vascular bundle of the LZ.

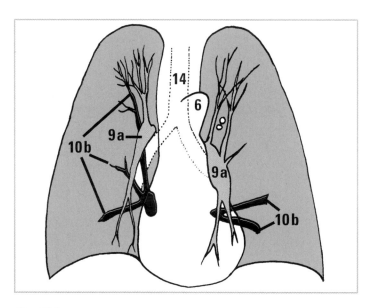

Fig. 18.1 a

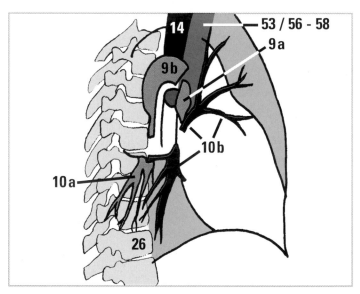

Fig. 18.1 b

The right LL artery is useful in the assessment of lung perfusion, as a longitudinal view of that vessel is consistently displayed in the PA radiograph. It is clearly delineated on its medial side by the intermediate bronchus.

The diameter of the right LL artery is measured at right angles to its long axis (⊢─┤ in **Fig. 18.2**). Values of 16 mm or more in women and 18 mm or more in men are considered abnormal and are suggestive of pulmonary arterial hypertension.

Other imaging signs of pulmonary venous congestion and pulmonary edema are illustrated on p. 141-143.

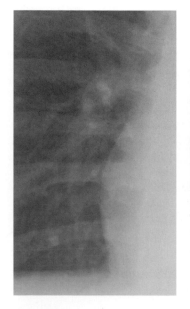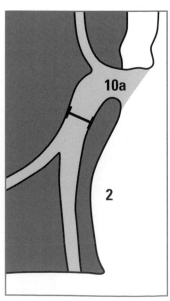

Fig. 18.2

Angiographic visualization of the pulmonary vessels is generally accomplished by infusing contrast medium through a catheter **(59)** advanced into the vena cava, right atrium, or pulmonary circuit. In the radiographs below, the arterial perfusion phase **(Fig. 19.1)** is easily distinguished from the venous phase **(Fig. 19.2)** based on the times at which the films were taken.

Please note the basic agreement between these images and the diagrams on the previous page. Comparing a normal angiogram **(Fig. 19.1)** with a CT scan in a patient with pulmonary embolism **(Fig. 19.3)**, we observe abnormal filling defects caused by embolized thrombi **(51)** secondary to ascending pelvic venous thrombosis.

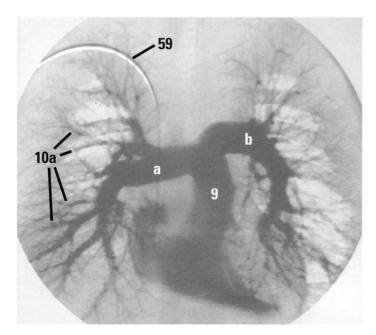

Fig. 19.1

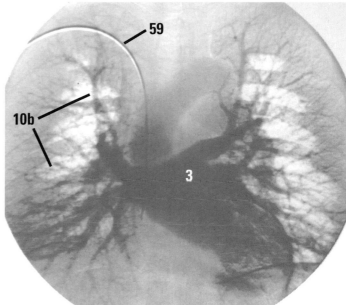

Fig. 19.2

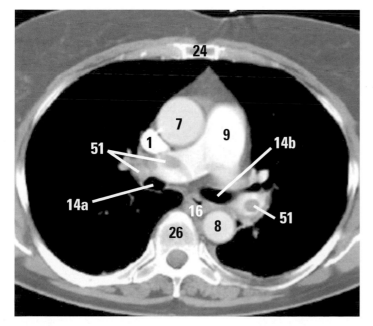

Fig. 19.3

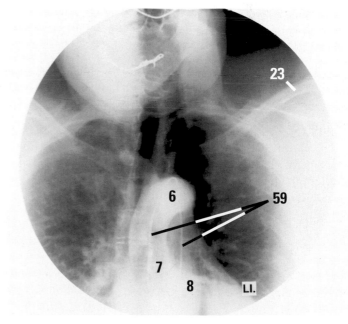

Fig. 19.4

If the catheter **(59)** is advanced in a retrograde fashion from the femoral artery or brachial artery into the ascending aorta counter to the direction of arterial blood flow, the injected contrast medium will opacify the aortic arch and its branches **(Fig. 19.4)**. This film clearly shows how the oblique, antero-

medial-to-posterolateral course of the aortic arch **(6)** defines the left radiographic border of the superior mediastinum (the "aortic knob"). This brings us to the question of what anatomical structures form the mediastinal silhouette on radiographs (see p. 20).

Mediastinal Borders

The radiographic contours of the mediastinum should be scrutinized downward in the PA projection (**Fig. 20.1**), examining the right side first and then the left side.

Right mediastinal border	Left mediastinal border
Superior vena cava (**1**) Azygos vein (**15**) Right atrium (**2**) Inferior vena cava (**11**) (may not be visible in the PA view)	Aortic arch (**6**) Pulmonary artery: Trunk (**9**) and left pulmonary artery (**9b**) Left atrial appendage (**3a**) Left ventricle (**5**) Fat pads

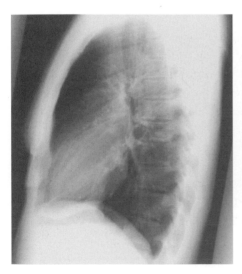

Fig. 20.1 a

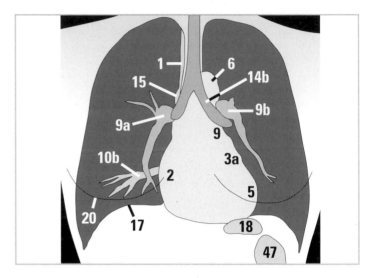

Fig. 20.1 b

The right ventricle (**4**) is located directly behind the sternum (**24**) in the lateral projection. A heart of normal size leaves a clear triangular space behind the sternum called the retrosternal space (RSS, **12**). If the right ventricle is abnormally enlarged, the RSS will be narrowed or opacified. The anterior cardiac silhouette continues upward as the ascending aorta (**7**), which is continuous posteriorly with the aortic arch (**6**) (**Fig. 20.2**). The left atrium (**3**) forms the upper portion of the posterior cardiac silhouette. Just behind it is the esophagus (**16**), which descends in the retrocardiac space (RCS, **13**). A dilated left atrium (**3**) may narrow the RCS or cause posterior bowing of the esophagus (➡ in **Fig. 20.3**), which is clearly demonstrated by oral contrast examination (see p. 85). When the left ventricle (**5**) is viewed in the lateral projection, it forms only the lower part of the posterior heart wall or its inferior margin. On close inspection, the termination of the inferior vena cava (**11**) can be identified as a small, triangular area of decreased lucency. If the left ventricle is enlarged, this "vena cava triangle" cannot be seen.

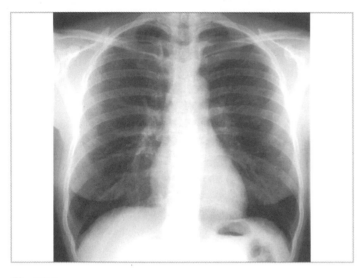

Fig. 20.2 a

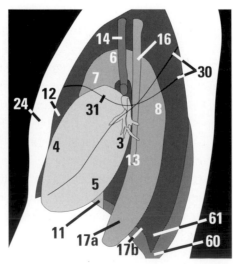

Fig. 20.2 b

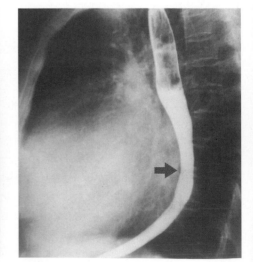

Fig. 20.3

Interstitium and Lymphatic Drainage

The interstitium of the lung consists of septa, connective tissue fibers, and lymphatics. It is divided into two compartments: The peripheral interstitium consists of the subpleural connective tissue and peripheral interlobular septa along with the peripheral veins and lymphatics. Lymphatic drainage, especially from the right UL, may be directed across the pleura to lymph nodes surrounding the (hemi)azygos vein. One fourth of the segments, then, drain directly to the mediastinum. Another distinctive feature of this subserous lymphatic network is found on the basal lung surface abutting the diaphragm. Lymph at that level drains across the pulmonary ligament to subdiaphragmatic and paraesophageal lymph nodes.

The other compartment, the central interstitium, surrounds the bronchovascular bundles and accompanies them from the hilum into the parenchyma of the lung. The lymphatics in this compartment run directly to the central hilum. Within the parenchyma, the central interstitium stabilizes the lobules and has connections with the superficial system. Lymph is propelled toward the hilum by respiratory movements, valves, and active contractions of the larger lymph vessels. The volume of lymphatic drainage is much greater anterobasally than apically. While most of the lymphatic drainage from both lungs is directed toward the ipsilateral hilum, some contralateral drainage may also occur. The mediastinal lymph node stations are described more fully on the page 22 and on pages 72-75.

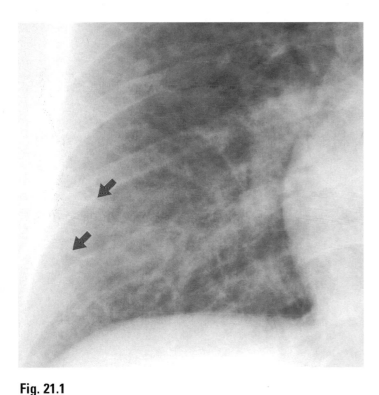

Fig. 21.1

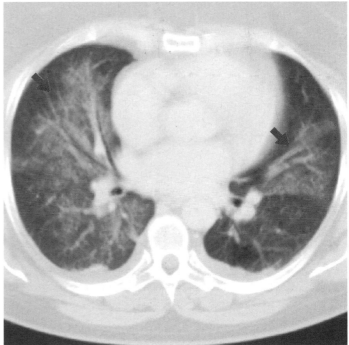

Fig. 21.2

Interstitial Infiltration Pattern

The superficial lymphatics are most clearly visible in the LL, where they border the lobules. If the interlobular septa become thickened or edematous, they may become visible as fine Kerley B lines. These lines typically appear as short, 1- to 2-cm linear opacities (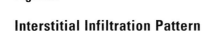) in the subpleural region **(Fig. 21.1)** of the LZ or MZ.

Kerley A lines are somewhat longer lines (5 cm or less) that course from the hila into the ULs. Interstitial lung diseases typically produce a reticulonodular pattern of weblike linear opacities (superimposed interlobular septa) accompanied by small, sharply circumscribed focal opacities (see p. 144-147).

In chronic progressive diseases where tissue contraction occurs due to scarring, the mobility (ventilation) of the lung may be decreased to the point of pulmonary fibrosis, resulting in elevation of the hemidiaphragm, cystic honeycomb changes, and the development of pulmonary emphysema.
Spirometry in the early stages may demonstrate a restrictive ventilatory defect at a time when conventional radiographs still show no interstitial changes. Frequently, however, HRCT will demonstrate ground-glass opacity (↘) of the affected lung regions **(Fig. 21.2)** like that produced by inflammatory exudates or neoplastic infiltration.

The original system of the American Thoracic Society for staging bronchial carcinoma (BC) has been modified several times. Among the most widely used staging systems at present are the TNM classification of the American Joint Committee on Cancer (AJCC) and the Union Internationale Contre le Cancer (UICC) [1.1]. The current staging system (at this writing) for the lymphogenous spread of BC is outlined in **Table 22.1**.

Lymphogenous spread of bronchial carcinoma [1.2]:	
N1	Ipsilateral peribronchial or hilar lymph nodes involved
N2	Ipsilateral mediastinal or subcarinal lymph nodes involved
N3	Contralateral mediastinal or hilar lymph nodes involved Ipsilateral or contralateral scalene or supraclavicular lymph nodes involved

Table 22.1

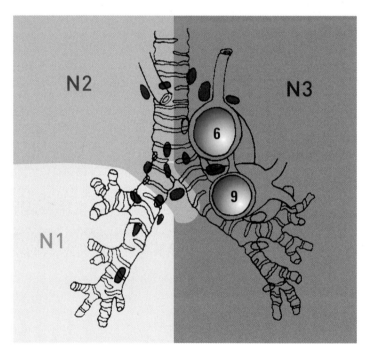

Fig. 22.2 Stages of regional lymph node involvement by bronchial carcinoma in the right lung

Figure 22.2 illustrates the lymph node stations that are relevant in the above TNM classification of non-small-cell BC.
Small-cell BC is usually staged as VLD (very limited disease), LD (limited disease), or ED I to ED IIb (extensive disease).

Bronchial Vessels

The bronchial arteries are the nutrient vessels for the bronchial tree. Approximately 90% of them arise from the anterior side of the descending aorta, pass through the mediastinal fat to the pulmonary hilum, and accompany the bronchi down to the level of the terminal bronchioles. There they establish connections with the network of pulmonary vessels (see p. 18) via the perialveolar capillary network. Many possible variants may be encountered, including common origins from intercostal arteries and branches of the subclavian artery.

The bronchial veins arise from peribronchiolar venous plexuses and drain either to the left atrium via the pulmonary veins or to the right atrium via the (hemi)azygos veins.

Innervation

The vagus nerve supplies the lung with afferent autonomic innervation, which is mediated by stretch receptors in the alveoli and receptors in the bronchioles, bronchi, trachea, and larynx. Additionally, there are pressor receptors in the aortic arch and carotid sinus and chemoreceptors on the para-aortic body and carotid body.

Efferent vagus fibers supply the smooth muscle and glands of the trachea and bronchi. Stimulation of these fibers increases glandular secretions and evokes bronchial constriction. Their counterparts are efferent sympathetic fibers, which induce bronchodilation and inhibit glandular secretions.

Matthias Hofer

Image Interpretation

Chapter Goals:

Building on radiographic anatomy, this chapter will explore some basic rules of image interpretation that are essential for the systematic and proficient reading of chest radiographs. They include physiological relationships, an overview of how chest radiographs are obtained, and the influence of technical parameters on image interpretation. On completing this chapter, you should be able to:

- describe the various methods of obtaining PA and supine radiographs;

- name four factors that may influence cardiac size and the caliber of the pulmonary vessels;

- correctly determine the cardiothoracic ratio (CTR) on chest radiographs;

- explain to a classmate or colleague, with the aid of a sketch pad, how a scatter-reduction grid works;

- correctly describe the Euler-Liljestrand reflex and its importance in lung perfusion;

- make a schematic drawing to explain how the "silhouette sign" is produced.

2

Check Your Progress:

After you have worked through this second chapter, take the quiz at the end to see how much material you can spontaneously reproduce from the first two chapters. This will show you what concepts and principles you have actually understood. We suggest that you retake this quiz at progressively longer intervals (e.g., the next day, three to five days later, and two to four weeks later) to anchor the material in your long-term memory. We know from experience that the active learning elements in particular (drawing exercises, verbal explanations to a colleague) can yield rapid, impressive results when you do these active exercises with a spirit of enthusiasm and then refer back to the book to check your work.

2

Anteroposterior versus Posteroanterior Radiographs

The apparent size of the heart and pulmonary vessels as they appear on radiographs is critically influenced by the object-film distance (or by the object-detector distance in digital imaging systems). For a standard upright PA radiograph, the patient stands with his or her back approximately 180-200 cm from the roentgen ray tube. The backs of the hands are placed on the posterior pelvis and the elbows are drawn forward to rotate the scapulae **(27)** laterally (↶ ↷) and obtain a clear projection of the upper lung zones **(Fig. 24.1)**. The anterior chest wall is placed against the imaging unit so that the heart is very close to the film or detector **(Fig. 24.4 a)**. This results in very little magnification of the projected cardiac image.

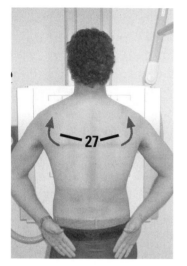
Fig. 24.1

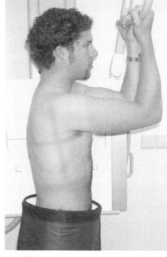
Fig. 24.2

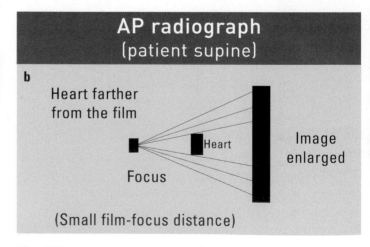
Fig. 24.3

In bedridden or ventilated patients, the film cassette (↖ ↖) must be placed behind the patient's back **(Fig. 24.3)** with the roentgen ray beam passing through the patient in an anteroposterior (AP) direction. As a result, the heart is farther away from the cassette and will appear more magnified **(Fig. 24.4b)**. A smaller film-focus distance is also used, resulting in greater angular divergence of the beam behind the heart and increasing the magnification effect.

Lateral radiographs are generally taken with a right-to-left beam direction. This arrangement places the heart closer to the film cassette **(Fig. 24.2)**, resulting in less magnification of the cardiac image.

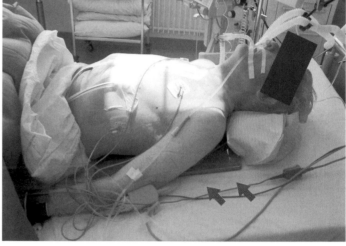

PA radiograph (patient upright)	
a	Heart close to the film ··· Heart ··· True size
	Focus
	(Large film-focus distance)

AP radiograph (patient supine)	
b	Heart farther from the film ··· Heart ··· Image enlarged
	Focus
	(Small film-focus distance)

Fig. 24.4

Physiological factors that may cause cardiac and pulmonary vascular enlargement on AP supine radiographs	
• **Position of the hemidiaphragm**	(higher in the supine position)
• **Upper lobe blood diversion**	(craniocaudal pressure gradient ↓)
• **Possible expiratory position**	(inadequate depth of inspiration)
• **Greater magnification effect**	(shorter film-focus distance on AP films)

Table 24.5

DD of a "White Lung"

Volume increased

- Massive pleural effusion
- Large pulmonary tumors
- Pleural mesothelioma
- Diaphragmatic hernia
- Cardiomegaly

Volume decreased

- Atelectasis (e.g., due to bronchial carcinoma)
- Tuberculosis (contraction due to scarring)
- Previous pneumonectomy
- Aplasia or agenesis of the lung
- Pleural plaques or fibrothorax

Cutoff Values for the Radiographic Detection of Pleural Fluid

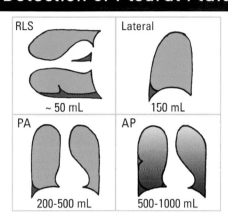

RLS	Lateral
~ 50 mL	150 mL
PA	AP
200-500 mL	500-1000 mL

From the textbook : „The Chest X-Ray", A Systematic Teaching Atlas, Thieme 2007, 224 pages, 865 illustrations + 47 tables. ISBN 987-3-13-144211-6 (GTV), ISBN 987-1-58890-554-3 (TNY), ISBN 987-3-13-144971-9 (Asia), www.thieme.com

DD of Hyperlucent Areas

Bilateral

Normal lung volume:
- Multiple pulmonary emboli
- Pulmonary arterial hypertension
- Stenosis of the pulmonary valve
- Congenital heart disease (with decreased lung perfusion)

Increased lung volume:
- Pulmonary emphysema
- Bronchial asthma, acute attack
- Upper airway stenosis
- Acute bronchiolitis

Unilateral

Due to artifacts or anatomical variants:
- Off-center scatter-reduction grid (in AP projection only!)
- Overexposure (especially in AP projection)
- Rotation (scoliosis, supine, etc.)
- Normal variants of the pectoralis muscle

Due to pathology:
- Prior unilateral mastectomy
- Expiratory check-valve stenosis of a bronchus (e.g., due to foreign body aspiration, see p. 180)
- Compensatory hyperinflation due to contralateral atelectasis, effusion
- Pneumothorax
- Pneumatoceles, large emphysematous bullae
- Decreased perfusion, unilateral pulmonary embolism

From the textbook : „The Chest X-Ray", A Systematic Teaching Atlas, Thieme 2007, 224 pages, 865 illustrations + 47 tables. ISBN 987-3-13-144211-6 (GTV), ISBN 987-1-58890-554-3 (TNY), ISBN 987-3-13-144971-9 (Asia), www.thieme.com

Checklist for Signs of Pulmonary Congestion

a) Direct signs (generally symmetrical)

- Increased pulmonary vascular markings
- Right LL artery > 18 mm (♂) (see p.18)
- Right LL artery > 16 mm (♀)
- Detection of Kerley lines (see p. 21)
- ill-defined vascular outlines and cardiac borders
- ill-defined diaphragm leaflets
- Accentuated and hazy hila
- Thickened interlobar fissures
- Possible upper-lobe blood diversion
- Later, confluent focal opacities (alveolar edema)

b) Additional signs

- Cardiomegaly (particularly, left atrial enlargement in lateral projection)
- Rapid progression of changes
- Pleural effusions: Often right > left

Checklist for Coarctation of the Aorta

- Bilateral notching of the third through ninth ribs
- Prominent, dilated ascending aorta
- Prestenotic and poststenotic widening of the descending aorta ("figure 3 sign")
- Possible widening of the superior mediastinum due to dilatation of the subclavian artery

m the textbook : „The Chest X-Ray", A Systematic Teaching Atlas, Thieme 2007, 224 pages, illustrations + 47 tables. ISBN 987-3-13-144211-6 (GTV), ISBN 987-1-58890-554-3 (TNY), N 987-3-13-144971-9 (Asia), www.thieme.com

Foreign Materials Checklist

Type of Catheter	Correct position	Complications
CVC	SVC at level of azygos termination	• Arrhythmias • Pericardial tamponade • Thrombosis • Vascular injury
Port systems	SVC at level of azygos termination	
Shaldon catheter	SVC at level of azygos termination	
Atrial dialysis catheter	Right atrium	
Pulmonary artery catheter	≤ 2 cm distally in right or left main pulmonary artery trunk	**Same as CVC** • Rupture of pulmonary artery • Pulmonary artery infarction
Pacemaker systems		
VVI	Lead in right ventricle	• Arrhythmias • Pericardial tamponade • Thrombosis • Vascular injury • Pneumothorax • Infections
DDD	Lead in right atrium and right ventricle	
AAI	Lead in right atrium	
VDD	Lead in right ventricle	
Biventricular	Leads in right atrium, right ventricle, and coronary vein	
Intra-aortic balloon pump (IABP)	Aortic arch, **distal** to subclavian artery	• Vascular occlusion with ischemia • Gas embolism due to rupture
Endotracheal tube	5 - 7 cm above carina	• Mucosal injury • Atelectasis • Pneumothorax • Vocal cord lesions
Feeding tubes	Distal to esophageal hiatus	• Reflux • Aspiration pneumonia • Esophageal perforation • Mediastinitis

Segmental Anatomy

Mnemonic:

To reach the **top**, you have to fight your way from **back** to **front**, often taking

a **side** route past the **middle**. Now you're at the **top**, and the rest are at the **bottom**. **Many are** on the **sideline, poor** souls!

(1)	Top	apikal
(2)	Back	posterior
(3)	Front	anterior
(4)	Side	lateral
(5)	Middle	medial
(6)	Top	superior
(7-10)	Bottom	basal:
(7)	**Many**	**m**ediobas**al**
(8)	**a**re	**a**nterior
(9)	Sideline	late<u>ro</u>basal
(10)	**Poor**	**po**sterobasal

Signs of Pneumomediastinum

- Cervical soft-tissue emphysema
- Paracardiac or para-aortic hyperlucency, bounded laterally by parietal pleura
- Subcardiac or retrocardiac air with continuous visualization of the diaphragm
- Thymic sail sign ("spinnaker sign") in children
- Pneumothorax
- Pneumopericardium
- Air around the pulmonary arterial ring (in the lateral projection)

Characteristics of Pleural Thickening

Radiographic features	• Anterior or posterior plaques appear diffuse with ill-defined margins. • Plaques struck tangentially by the roentgen ray beam are sharply delineated.
Frequent causes	• Postinflammatory (postpleuritic) changes; unifocal pleural thickening is most common.
Key cutoff values	• Indeterminate pleural thickening > 3 mm: Order CT scans. • Pleural thickening > 1 cm: Suspicious for tumor.

Mitral Stenosis

Cardiac size
- Normal-sized left ventricle
- Dilated left atrium ⇨
  - PA: Possible double-contour sign
  - Lat: High narrowing of RCS by the left atrium **alone**
- Small aortic knob (compared with aortic stenosis)
- With high-grade stenosis: Possible relative tricuspid insufficiency

Pulmonary vessels
- Marked signs of pulmonary venous congestion (p.77) (constant pressure load in pulm. circulation)
- Signs of pulmonary hypertension (see p. 77)

Aortic Stenosis

Cardiac size
- CTR often normal initially; later CTR (pressure load ⇨ concentric hypertrophy)
- RCS: Initially normal; becomes narrowed later

Aorta
- Possible poststenotic ectasia (does not correlate with degree of stenosis)
- Fluoroscopy may show aortic valve calcification

Mitral Insufficiency

Cardiac size
- Left ventricular dilatation plus
- Left atrial dilatation ⇨
  - PA: Possible double-contour sign
  - Lat: Complete narrowing of RCS by the left atrium **and** ventricle

Pulmonary vessels
- Relatively mild signs of pulmonary venous congestion (periodic pressure load on pulmonary circulation)

Aortic Insufficiency

Cardiac size
- CTR ⇨ (volume load ⇨ eccentric dilatation)
- RCS: Immediate narrowing

Aorta
- Normal luminal size in primary aortic insufficiency
- Secondary insufficiency (e.g., aneurysm) ⇨ signs of aortic dilatation (see p.93)

Signs of Aortic Aneurysm

Lateral	• D_{AO} > 4.5 cm in lateral projection
PA	• D_{TM} > 5.0 cm • Ascending aorta forms upper right border of cardiovascular silhouette • Trachea displaced to the right side • Left main bronchus displaced upward

Common Primary Tumors that Metastasize to the Lung

Breast carcinoma	~20%
Renal carcinoma Head and neck tumors Colorectal carcinoma	~10% each
Uterine and ovarian carcinoma Pancreatic carcinoma Prostatic carcinoma Gastric carcinoma	~5% each

Causes of Pulmonary Nodules

Very common:	Less common:
• Tuberculoma • Bronchial carcinoma • Hamartoma • Metastases	• Pneumonia and abscesses • Bronchial cysts • Bronchial adenoma • Neurofibroma

Mediastinal Shift

Diagnosis

Three reference points:

1. Vertical course of the trachea (junction with the carina is just to the right of the midline)
2. Left paravertebral knob of the aortic arch (approximately at the level of the posterior part of the fifth rib)
3. Right cardiac border is to the right of the vertebral column.

Normal CTR Values in the PA Radiograph

Up to age 1 year:	< 0.65
Up to age 2 years:	< 0.6
Adults:	< 0.5

Causes

Contralateral pressure:
- Tension pneumothorax
- Diaphragmatic hernia
- Asymmetrical emphysema

Ipsilateral traction:
- Atelectasis (bronchial obstruction) or previous lobectomy
- Pleural adhesions
- Unilateral pulmonary hypoplasia (rare)

From the textbook : „**The Chest X-Ray**", A Systematic Teaching Atlas, Thieme 2007, 224 pages, 865 illustrations + 47 tables. ISBN 987-3-13-144211-6 (GTV), ISBN 987-1-58890-554-3 (TNY), ISBN 987-3-13-144971-9 (Asia), www.thieme.com

Calibers of Pulmonary Vessels

The pulmonary vessels are not equally perfused in the upper and lower lung zones in upright stance. The degree of perfusion increases toward the lower zones (LZs) because of the hydrostatic pressure gradient. A colleague demonstrated this principle by standing on his head. A normal standing PA radiograph **(Fig. 25.1)** shows a "LZ predominance" of blood flow, i.e., the vessels are considerably more prominent in the basal lung zones (↘ ↘) than in the upper and apical zones (see also p. 10). But when the same individual stood on his head **(Fig. 25.2)**, the upper lobe (UL) vessels in both lungs show a marked increase in caliber (↗ ↖) as a result of UL blood diversion, while the pulmonary vessels in the LZs appear markedly smaller **(Fig. 25.3)**. The headstand also causes a cephalad displacement of the cardiac apex from the diaphragm (↑) with a normal cardiac size.

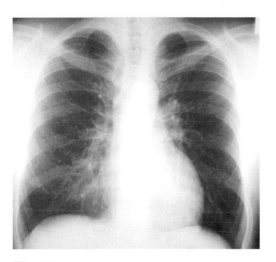

Fig. 25.1

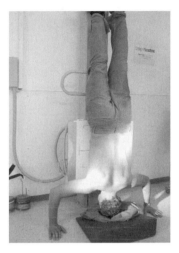

Fig. 25.2

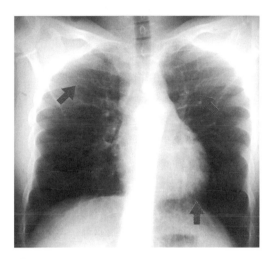

Fig. 25.3

In a patient with pulmonary venous congestion, like that occurring in the setting of congestive heart failure, the chest radiograph shows a similar pattern of UL blood diversion with accentuated vascular markings not only in both hila but particularly in both upper zones (UZs). Other illustrative images of pulmonary congestion are shown on pages 141-143.

The assumption of a supine position, as shown in **Figure 24.3**, is sufficient to cause a similar accentuation of the pulmonary vessels in the upper and apical zones and should not be mistaken for true pathological congestion. Often the differential diagnosis is aided by comparison with previous radiographs, which are frequently available, especially in intensive care unit (ICU) patients.

Often you can tell that a radiograph was taken in the supine position **(Fig. 25.4)** because both apical zones (↓ ↓) above the clavicles **(23)** appear smaller than they do on an upright radiograph due to the more oblique beam angle (see also **Fig. 20.1a**).

Depth of Inspiration

The radiograph shown in **Figure 25.4** is an expiratory film. Due to the relatively high position of the diaphragm leaflets, the heart is elevated and appears broadened. The elevated diaphragm leaflets may also compress the pulmonary vessels, mimicking the appearance of pulmonary venous congestion.

Thus, an adequate depth of inspiration is important in chest radiography. Inspiration is adequate when the posterior segment of the ninth rib is clear and is not obscured by superimposed diaphragm. This distinction is particularly important in evaluating cardiac size on supine radiographs (see p. 27) and interpreting radiographs taken in ICUs (see Chapter 11).

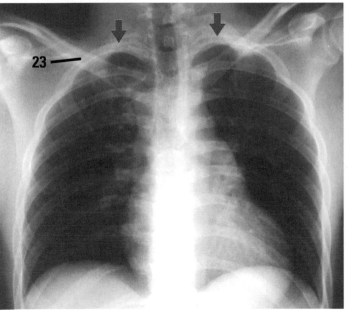

Fig. 25.4   Exspiration in supine position

Scatter-Reduction Grids

It is more difficult to position the roentgen ray tube precisely over the midsagittal plane of supine patients than in patients standing against a wall-mounted cassette holder. To reduce scattered radiation, the film cassettes are combined with a scatter-reduction grid designed to reduce image unsharp-ness caused by randomly scattered radiation from the patient (↘ in **Fig. 26.1**). In the optimum case, the cassette is positioned precisely at right angles to the roentgen ray tube with no obliquity and filters out only scattered radiation (**Fig. 26.2a**), resulting in equal exposure of both lungs (**Fig. 26.3**).

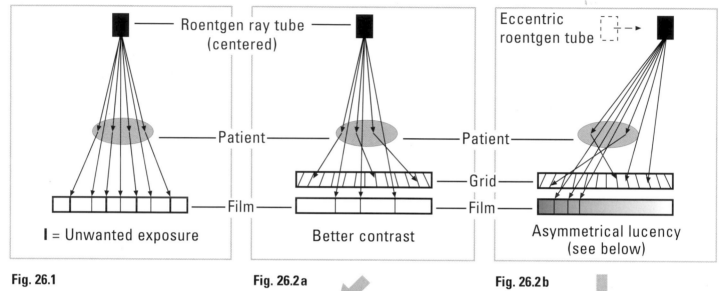

Fig. 26.1   **Fig. 26.2a**   **Fig. 26.2b**

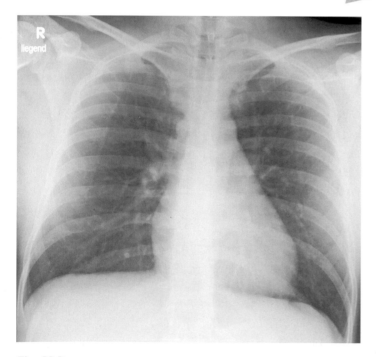

Fig. 26.3

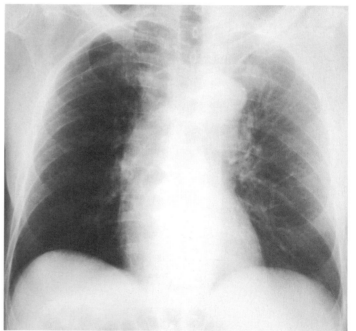

Fig. 26.4

But no matter how carefully the technician positions the cassette, it may still be slightly oblique in relation to the beam axis. In this case more radiation will pass through the filter on one side than the other (**Fig. 26.2b**). This creates the appearance of increased opacity in one lung (**Fig. 26.4**), which can mimic a layered-out pleural effusion or hemothorax on the affected side (see p. 106-108, p. 186). The following tip may assist in the differential diagnosis of such cases: A pleural effusion of this size will usually cause concomitant unsharp-ness of the ipsilateral diaphragm leaflet or costophrenic angle. This sign is absent when the opacity is an artifact caused by an angled cassette.

Determining the CTR

The cardiothoracic ratio (CTR) is determined as a means of assessing cardiac size. It is defined as the ratio of the transverse width of the heart to the width of the thoracic outlet. To determine the CTR, draw a perpendicular line at each lateral border of the cardiac silhouette (**– – –**), dropping the lines at the points where the right and left cardiac borders show their greatest lateral extent (**Fig. 27.1**). This point will usually be somewhat higher on the right cardiac border (right atrium) than on the left border (left ventricle). Now measure the horizontal (nonoblique) distance (**◄·····►**) to determine the cardiac width (**C**).

Next, measure the greatest horizontal distance between the inner margins of the ribs (**◄——►**), measuring from pleural boundary to pleural boundary (**T**). The ratio of $\frac{C}{T}$ should not exceed 0.5 in adults, meaning that the width of the heart should be no more than 50% of the inner thoracic diameter (see also p. 81).

The heart is larger in relation to the thorax in children up to two years of age, and so the CTR in these patients has an upper normal value of 0.65 (less than one year) to 0.60 (one to two years) [2.1].

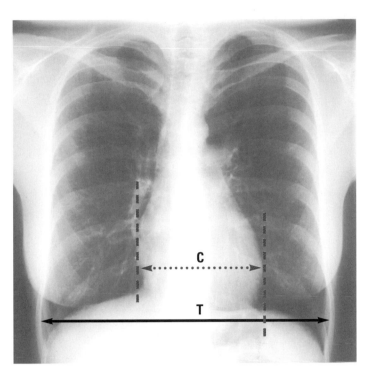

Fig. 27.1

$$CTR = \frac{C}{T} \leq 0.5$$

Effect of Age

The radiographs below were taken in three different patients. Note the continuous increase in the size of the cardiac silhouette from left to right. These differences are not a result of disease but constitute normal findings in a very thin 18-year-old girl (**Fig. 27.2**), a slender woman in her mid-20s

(**Fig. 27.3**), and an older woman (**Fig. 27.4**). This comparison shows that the width of the cardiac silhouette will vary over a certain normal range with increasing age and in different constitutional types. For practice, try to determine the CTR for each of these radiographs and compare your results with the answers at the end of the book.

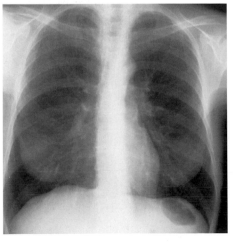

Fig. 27.2

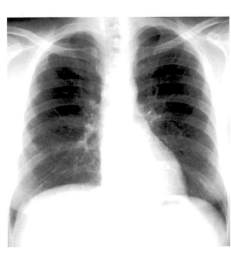

Fig. 27.3

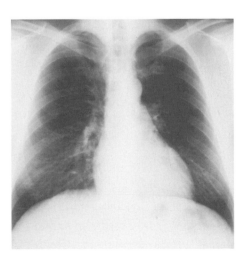

Fig. 27.4

Silhouette Sign

You will recall from page 9 that areas of different density form a visible boundary line on the radiograph only if their interface is tangential to the roentgen ray beam. This fact can be utilized, for example, to help determine the location of an inflammatory infiltrate. Often it is necessary to determine whether an area of increased density in the right lower lung is caused by decreased ventilation or infiltration of the right middle or lower lobe (LL; see p. 112, p. 145).

Look at the two axial computed tomography (CT) scans (**Fig. 28.1**) taken at the level of the right atrium (**2**). The first image (**Fig. 28.1a**) shows an infiltrate (**37**) in the right middle lobe (**33**) that is in contact with the right atrium (**2**). The infiltrate and accompanying edema have increased the density of the affected lung area, causing it to approximate the density (roentgen ray absorption) of the adjacent heart. As a result, the boundary line between the lung parenchyma and right cardiac border is not visualized (**Fig. 28.2**).

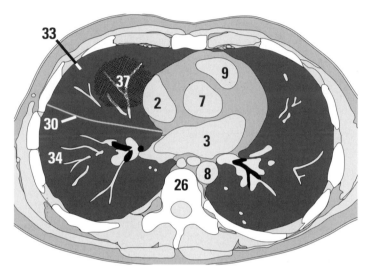

Fig. 28.1 a

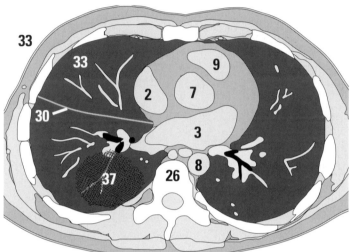

Fig. 28.1 b

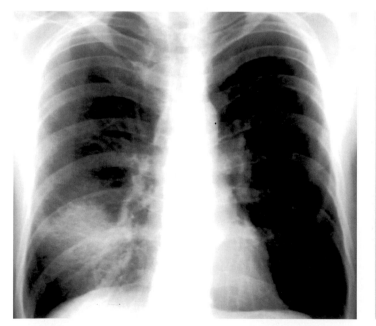

Fig. 28.2

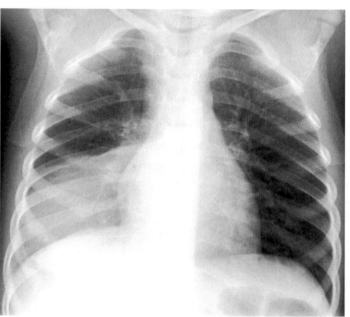

Fig. 28.3

But if the infiltrate is located farther back in the LL (**34**) and is **not** in contact with the heart (**Fig. 28.1b**), the density contrast between the middle lobe (ML) (**33**) and right atrium will be preserved, and a distinct boundary line can be seen between the right cardiac border and the lung (**Fig. 28.3**).

Note the following rule of thumb: If a boundary line can be seen between the lung opacity and the heart, the opacity is located posteriorly in the LL. If a boundary line cannot be identified, the opacity must have a more anterior location in the ML.

Perfusion and Ventilation

Perfusion: Pulmonary blood flow is determined chiefly by gravity. In upright stance and deep inspiration, the apical vessels have very little blood flow or may even be in a collapsed state while the vessels in the lower and basal lung regions are dilated. The calibers of the pulmonary veins are highly variable, and they are roughly equal throughout the lung only in a recumbent position. In the standing position, the veins in the LZ are three times larger than in the apical zone (AZ). The pressure relationships are summarized in **Table 29.1**.

During stance, a pressure gradient of up to 22 mmHg exists from the apical to the basal lung vessels in a normal adult. Thus, the perfusion of the basal lung zone depends mainly on the arteriovenous pressure gradient. The perfusion of the middle zone (MZ) depends chiefly on the relationship of the arterial pressure (P_{art}) to the intra-alveolar pressure (P_{alv}); the arteriovenous pressure gradient is of little importance at this level. Apical and basal lung perfusion are approximately equal in the supine position and during expiration.

Pressure relationships
(during inspiration in upright stance)

UZ:	P_{alv}	>	P_{art}	>	P_{ven}
MZ:	P_{art}	>	P_{alv}	>	P_{ven}
LZ:	P_{art}	>	P_{ven}	>	P_{alv}

Table 29.1

Adaptation to exercise: The mean pressure in the pulmonary vessels is between 5 and 20 mmHg (= 0.7-2.7 kPa), which roughly equals the range of venous pressures in the systemic circulation. At rest, only about 25% of the pulmonary capillaries are perfused and the cardiac output is approximately 5 liters per minute. When the cardiac output is greatly increased during exercise, the remaining capillaries are recruited, with the result that the mean pressure in the pulmonary vessels changes very little despite the increase in perfusion.

Ventilation, on the other hand, increases more basally than apically in response to exercise, because the apical alveoli are already in a more prestretched condition than the basal alveoli, which are more compliant. This is based on the fact that the negative pressure in the interpleural space is lower apically than basally. If now the ventilation of several lung regions were seriously impaired due to thick bronchial secretions or an obstructing tumor or foreign body, constant perfusion of the affected lung areas would be ineffectual because gas exchange could no longer take place in those areas. This problem is solved by the Euler-Liljestrand reflex, in which a baroreceptor system induces vasoconstriction in hypoventilated lung areas to protect the body from hypoxemia (see also p. 141).

Do you remember the effects that different parts of the autonomic nervous system have on the perfusion and ventilation of the lung? Please take a moment to actively refresh your memory, and write your answers here **before** referring back to page 22.

Effects of efferent vagus fibers:

Effects of afferent vagus fibers:

Sequence of Radiographic Interpretation

Various recommendations have been made for a systematic approach to the interpretation of chest radiographs, and all have proved useful in practice. The best approach is probably not to define a single "best" sequence but to follow a consistent routine to ensure that changes are not missed. Sometimes the most important finding will be less conspicuous than a relatively unimportant incidental finding. We therefore recommend that you follow the systematic routine which is outlined below:

Systematic interpretation of chest radiographs

I. Type and quality of the radiograph
II. Chest wall: Soft tissues and bone
III. Diaphragm and pleural boundaries
IV. Mediastinum and hila
V. Lung parenchyma
VI. Foreign material

The table below gives a checklist of the items (→) that should be covered in this six-step routine.

I   Type and quality of the radiograph

• PA or AP projection	→ Marked on the film? Size of the AZ above the clavicles (see p. 24)?
• Rotated view	→ Spinous processes correctly centered (equidistant) between the clavicles?
• Adequate depth of inspiration?	→ Posterior segment of ninth or tenth rib clear of superimposed diaphragm?
• Adequate penetration	→ Vertebral bodies well defined behind the heart and pulmonary vessels?

II   Chest wall: Soft tissues and bone

• Neck	→ Trachea centered and of normal diameter. Thyroid or lymph node calcifications? (DD: intrapulmonary lesions)
• Shoulder girdle	→ Clavicles; scapulae rotated to clear the lungs? (DD: pulmonary opacity)
• Ribs	→ Normal position and course? No discontinuities?
• Thoracic spine	→ Osteolytic lesions? Wedging of vertebrae, endplate fractures? All pedicles visible?
• Breasts	→ Symmetrical breast shadows? Nipples visible? (DD: pulmonary nodules)
• Soft tissues	→ Soft-tissue emphysema, symmetry, skin folds? (DD: pneumothorax)
• Abdomen	→ Free subphrenic air? Air in the gastric fundus: distance from diaphragm < 1 cm? Fluid levels?

III   Diaphragm and pleural boundaries

• Diaphragm leaflets	→ Harmonious curve, smooth contours on both sides? Right leaflet usually slightly higher than the left.
• Costophrenic angle	→ Acute and sharply defined? (DD: effusion, pleural thickening)
• Pleura	→ Calcifications? Subpleural fat? (DD: skin folds, bedsheet folds on supine films)
• Fissures	→ Normal course of the minor and major fissures? Width < 2 mm?

IV   Mediastinum and hila

• Superior mediastinum	→ Width and overall position? Size of the aorta, superior vena cava (SVC), and azygos vein?
	→ Location and width of trachea and main bronchi? Bifurcation angle 55-70°?
• Heart	→ Size: CTR and width of RSS and RCS (see p. 20)?
	→ Position and configuration? (DD: changes suggestive of anomalies, see p. 82-85)?
	→ Coronary or valvular calcifications?
• Hila	→ Configuration and position: usually higher on the left side than on the right. Right LL artery < 16 mm or 18 mm?

V   Lung parenchyma

• Pulmonary vessels	→ Regional caliber in LZs >> than in UZs (on upright inspiratory films)?
	→ Smooth tapering of vascular calibers from hilum to periphery?
• Focal or diffuse changes	→ Close scrutiny (DD: extrapulmonary foci)

VI   Foreign Material

• Central venous catheter (CVC)	→ Correctly positioned at the level of the azygos vein termination (see p. 158)? Coiling?
	→ Pneumothorax due to CVC insertion? (May consist only of a small apical pneumothorax)
• Endotracheal tube	→ Correctly positioned 2-4 cm above the bifurcation (see p. 177)?
• Pleural drains	→ Position? Last hole intrathoracic (see p. 204-206)?
• Pacemaker	→ Lead position, atrial or ventricular lead (see p. 167–179)? Cable intact?

Interpreting the chest radiographs of premature infants poses a special challenge. An assistant may hold the infant upright for a "suspension" film, or the patient may be secured carefully and briefly in a radiolucent positioning shell.

Small children can be held on a seat by an assistant (e.g., the mother / father if available) with the arms raised **(Fig. 31.1)**. Understandably, infants in particular are not always happy with this procedure, and sometimes the film is taken just when the child utters a "cry of protest," resulting in an expiratory view.

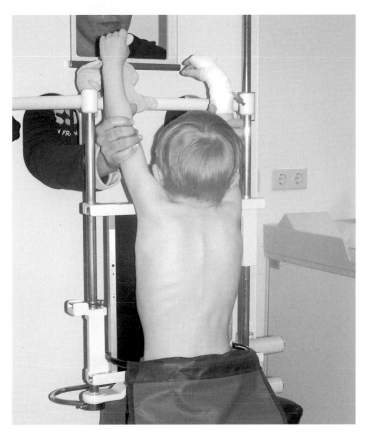

Fig. 31.1

"Crying Lung" (Pediatrics)

When an infant or small child cries, the expiratory effort moves the diaphragm to an elevated position, and portions of the lung may even collapse in some circumstances. This causes the pulmonary vessels to appear accentuated or congested **(Fig. 31.2a)**. The overall appearance of the chest radiograph may be misinterpreted as pneumonic infiltration (see p. 144 et seq.) or meconium aspiration (see p. 133).

So when you read the chest radiographs of infants, make sure to determine the respiratory position in which the films were taken. A follow-up radiograph will show absolutely clear lungs **(Fig. 31.2b)** with no signs of infiltration or congestion, but the air swallowed by the crying child will be clearly visible within the stomach **(18)**.

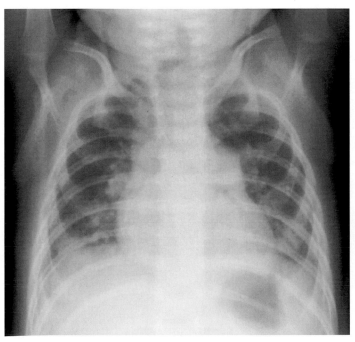

Fig. 31.2a

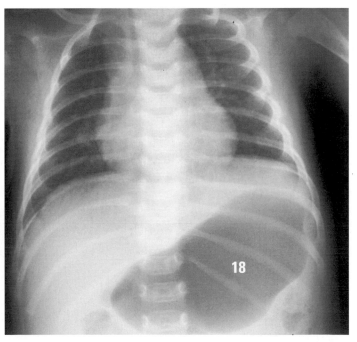

Fig. 31.2b

The following pages are designed to increase the half-life of your knowledge through active, selective repetition. The quiz questions will also give you feedback on how well you can actively and correctly reproduce the contents of the first two chapters. So activate your memory and complete **all** of the quiz questions **before** you look back in the chapters or check the answer key at the end of the book. Looking up the answers before you complete the quiz is just a passive exercise that will do little or nothing to reinforce learning.

1 In the projections below, draw lines indicating the boundaries of the upper, lower, and middle lobes of the lung. (Finish the entire quiz before comparing your drawing with **Fig. 10.3**.

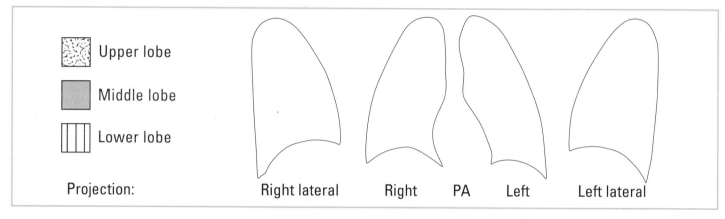

Fig. 32.1

2 Label this tracheobronchial tree with the names and numbers of the pulmonary segments. Do you remember the sports mnemonic that may help you in this task? How does it go? Write it in the box below:
(Answers on p. 12-13)

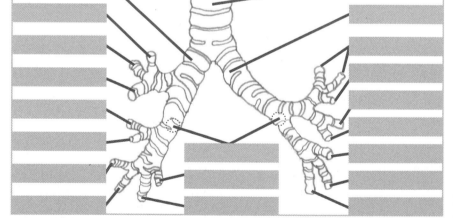

Fig. 32.2

3 What are the differences between the pulmonary arteries and veins with respect to their course and their location in the PA projection? Indicate the differences by writing key words in the table below (Answers on p. 18) :

Pulmonary arteries	Pulmonary veins
UZ	
LZ	

4   Complete these two drawings and label the structures that form the mediastinal borders:

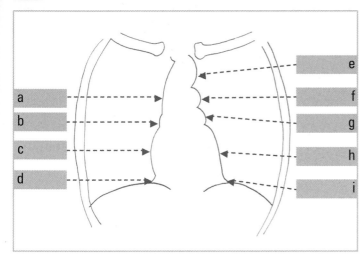

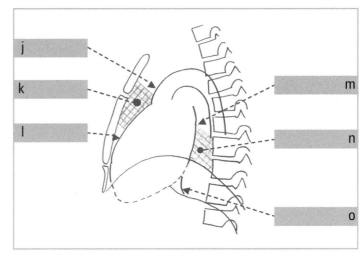

Fig. 33.1a   **Fig. 33.1b**

For each of the structures labeled, name a condition that could produce a bulge or contour change at that location.

a   f   k

b   g   l

c   h   m

d   i   n

e   j   o

5   List four factors that can influence the apparent size of the heart and caliber of the pulmonary vessels in the **supine AP** radiograph versus the **upright PA** radiograph:

-
-
-
-

6   Describe in writing the differences in the perfusion of the upper and lower lung zones in the supine and upright positions. What changes and why?

7 These two radiographs were taken several days apart in the **same patient**. How are they different? Use a ruler to determine the CTR in both images, and write down the measurements that you used in determining the ratio.

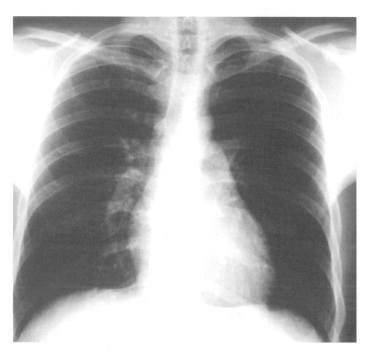

Fig. 34.1 a

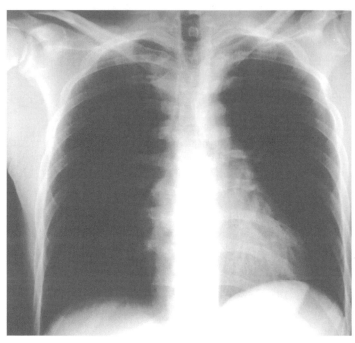

Fig. 34.1 b

8 Look closely at the following supine radiograph, which was taken in an ICU patient who underwent cardiac surgery several days before. First describe **only the morphological features** that you observe in the image. Next make a list of possible differential diagnoses, and then decide on the most likely presumptive diagnosis.

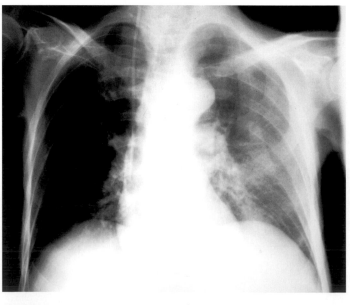

Fig. 34.2

Description:

Differential diagnosis:

Presumptive diagnosis:

Henning Rattunde
Matthias Hofer

Chest Wall: Soft Tissues and Bone

Chapter Goals:

A complete analysis of the chest radiograph should include changes in the thoracic soft tissues and thoracic skeleton. Because the soft tissues appear only as a low-contrast gray background on a normal chest radiograph film, the reader should be on the alert for any changes in their radiographic appearance.

Although many changes in the thoracic skeleton are easily recognized, you should be aware that the hard radiation technique used for chest radiographs is not optimum for skeletal imaging. Thus, if the skeletal findings are equivocal on the chest radiograph or if special information is needed, it may be helpful to obtain special views of the desired region or perform a computed tomography (CT) examination.

On completing this chapter, you should be able to:

- distinguish physiological variations in the soft-tissue mantle from a true abnormality;

- recognize and differentiate abnormal air collections in the tissue;

- recognize changes in the thoracic skeleton and initiate any further diagnostic tests that may be needed;

- detect any abdominal pathology that may be visible on the chest radiograph.

3

Asymmetrical Lucency

A complete thoracic examination includes an evaluation of the soft-tissue mantle of the chest and the thoracic skeleton, including imaged portions of the lower cervical spine. The actual soft-tissue mantle of the chest shows considerable individual variation in its thickness and radiographic density, depending on such factors as sex, level of conditioning, and nutritional state.

A unilateral increase in lucency may have various causes. In patients who have had a mastectomy, you may notice increased lucency in the corresponding lower lung zone (★) and the absence of a breast shadow compared with the intact opposite side (↑ ↑ ↑ in **Fig. 36.1a**). In doubtful cases, look in the axilla for possible metal clips (↘) remaining from an axillary lymph node dissection **(Fig. 36.1b)**. The disparity in the lucency of the lower lung zones may be very pronounced **(Fig. 36.2)**, or it may be more subtle as illustrated by the left mastectomy in **Figure 36.3**. The key point is to avoid mistaking this disparity for an intrapulmonary density or a layered-out effusion (see p. 106-109).

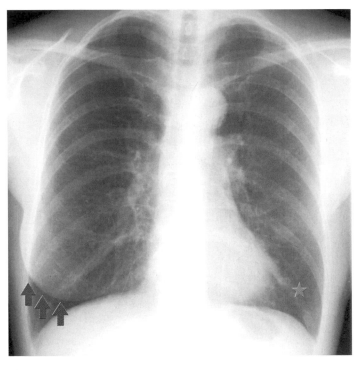

Fig. 36.1 a

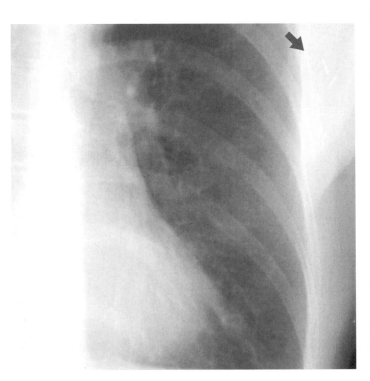

Fig. 36.1 b

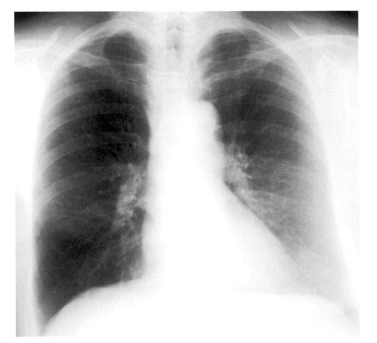

Fig. 36.2

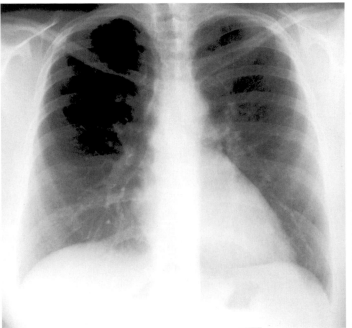

Fig. 36.3

Asymmetrical lucency may also be caused by a previous radical neck dissection, a posttraumatic chest-wall hematoma, or circumscribed areas of muscular hypertrophy or atrophy. Can you think of another possible cause of increased lucency in one lung on a supine radiograph? (If not, refer back to p. 26.)

Other Soft-Tissue Effects

Another potential source of confusion is the nipples (➡), which may be mistaken for intrapulmonary nodules

(Fig. 37.1a). In doubtful cases the radiograph can be repeated after identifying the nipples with metallic skin markers **(Fig. 37.1b)**. A hair braid **(Fig. 37.2)** or strands of hair (↓) may create superimposed figures that mimic cutaneous or ascending mediastinal emphysema (see p. 99). The stump of an amputated arm typically appears in the lateral radiograph as a paddle-shaped opacity (▶) projected over the superior mediastinum **(Fig. 37.3)**. It may be mistaken for a mediastinal mass.

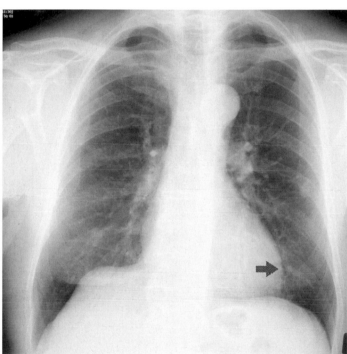

Fig. 37.1 a

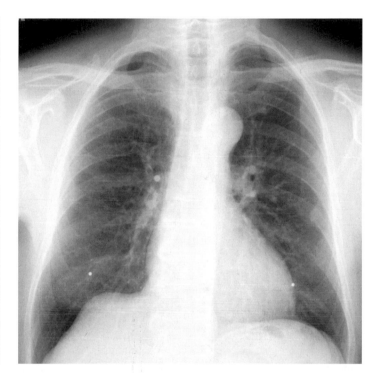

Fig. 37.1 b

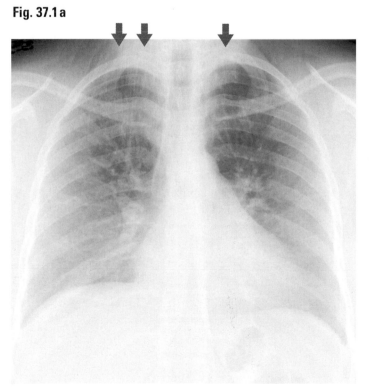

Fig. 37.2

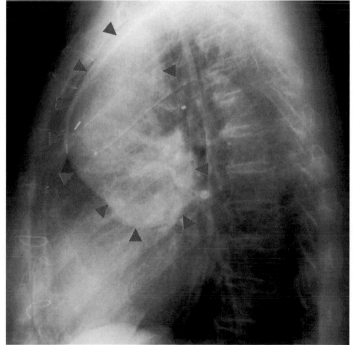

Fig. 37.3

Air Collections in Soft Tissues

Attention should be paid to the possible occurrence of abnormal air collections within the soft tissues. The most frequent cause of air in the mediastinum is a spontaneous pneumomediastinum [3.1]. But a variety of other causes are listed in **Table 38.1**. The diagnosis of traumatic soft-tissue emphysema is described more fully in Chapter 10 (p. 193).

Possible Causes of Pneumomediastinum

Spontaneous:	Crying, vomiting, hyperventilation, Valsalva maneuver, vigorous phonation in singers
Posttraumatic:	Rib fracture, tracheal rupture, barotrauma, foreign bodies
Neoplastic:	Esophageal perforation, erosive airway lesions
Iatrogenic:	Ventilation, endoscopy
Inflammatory:	Descending retropharyngeal abscess

Table 38.1

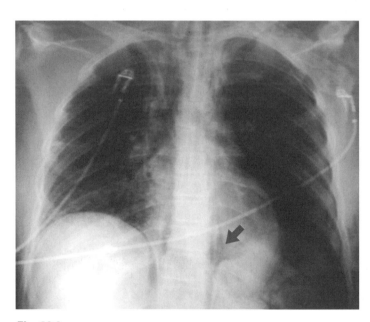

Fig. 38.2

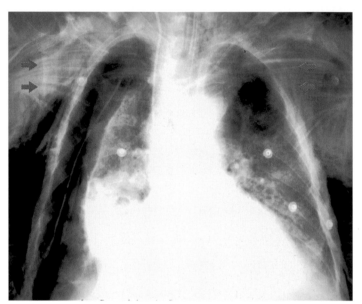

Fig. 38.3

Hyperlucencies in the posteroanterior (PA) projection are most commonly found along the cardiac border and/or along the aorta (✎) with associated elevation of the mediastinal part of the parietal pleura (**Fig. 38.2**). In severe cases the air also spreads into the pectoral muscles, accentuating their pennate pattern (➡ ⬅) on the radiograph (**Fig. 38.3**). The typical radiographic signs of pneumomediastinum are listed in **Table 38.4**. Approximately one half of pneumomediastinum cases are not diagnosed in the PA radiograph, and therefore a lateral projection is often indicated.

The most sensitive modality is CT, which can demonstrate even very small mediastinal air collections (**38**) (**Fig. 38.5**) [3.2].

Radiographic Signs of Pneumomediastinum

- Cervical soft-tissue emphysema
- Paracardiac or para-aortic hyperlucency bounded laterally by the parietal pleura
- Subcardiac or retrocardiac air with continuous visualization of the diaphragm
- Thymic sail sign ("spinnaker sign") in children
- Pneumothorax
- Pneumopericardium
- Air around the pulmonary arterial ring (in the lateral projection)

Table 38.4

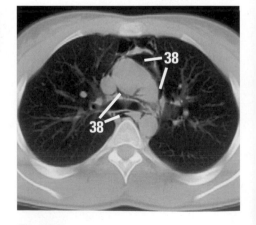

Fig. 38.5

Variants of the Thoracic Skeleton

The superior and inferior rib margins are sharply defined in the PA projection, although it is quite normal to find slight unsharpness of the rib margins in the middle and lower thoracic regions. In patients over 15 years of age, varying degrees of calcification are found at the chondro-osseous junctions (←) of the ribs. They are usually symmetrical and are more common in females than in males **(Figs. 39.1, 39.2)**.

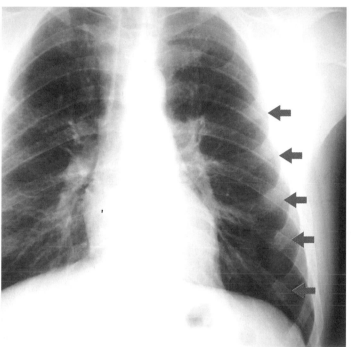

Fig. 39.1

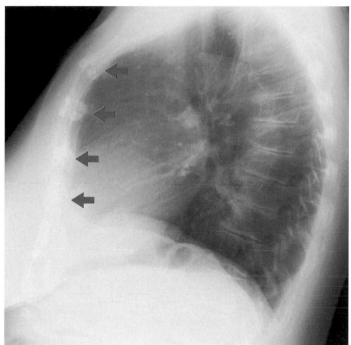

Fig. 39.2

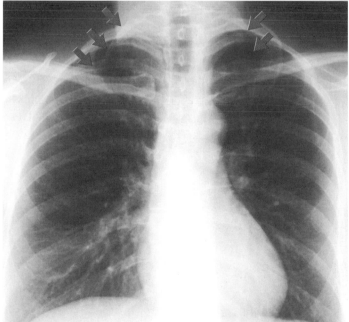

Fig. 39.3

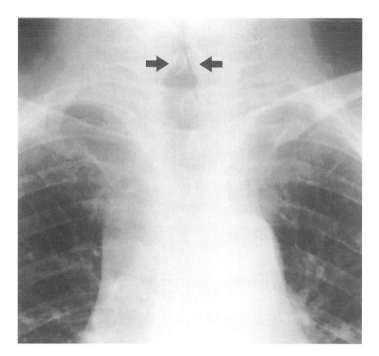

Fig. 39.4

Cervical ribs are most commonly found on the seventh cervical vertebra. Most are asymptomatic and are detected incidentally on the PA chest radiograph. They are not always as conspicuous (⬎) as the right-sided rib in **Figure 39.3**; they may be shorter and more subtle (⬏). But cervical ribs may also give rise to a thoracic outlet syndrome, and so their presence should be documented in the written report [3.3, 3.4].

Another possible incidental finding is incomplete closure of the vertebral arch (→ ←), **(Fig. 39.4)** which may occur as an isolated defect at the cervicothoracic or thoracolumbar junction.

Clavicle

Clavicular fractures (➘) are among the most common injuries of the thoracic skeleton and generally heal without complications. They may be caused by a direct impact in vehicular or sports-related injuries, or they may occur indirectly from a fall onto the shoulder or arm **(Fig. 40.1a)**. A typical pattern is an oblique or wedge fracture in the middle third of the bone. The medial fragment is displaced upward by the pull of the sternocleidomastoid muscle (⬆ in Fig. 40.1a and **Fig. 41.2**). Most clavicular fractures are treated conservatively with a figure-of-eight bandage. The desired downward pressure on the medial fragment (➚) is produced by tightening the loop of the bandage (◠◡ in **Fig. 40.1b**). Rigid internal fixation is necessary only in rare cases. Caution is advised in dealing with fractures of the first three ribs or first two ribs plus the clavicle, as this pattern may be associated with injuries of the brachial plexus and nearby vessels [3.5].

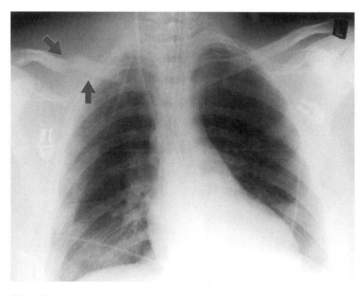

Fig. 40.1 a

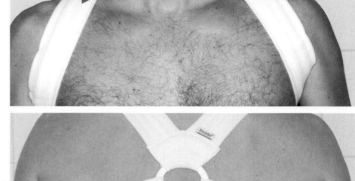

Fig. 40.1 b

Acromioclavicular Joint

The laterally situated acromioclavicular (AC) joint is vulnerable to isolated tears of the joint-stabilizing ligaments between the clavicle and acromion, and between the clavicle and coracoid process (see **Fig. 41.2**). Traction from the sternocleidomastoid muscle pulls the clavicle past the acromion **(Fig. 40.2a)**, creating a visible step-off where the clavicle can be pushed down but will spring back when pressure is released (the "piano key sign").

Tossy classified acromioclavicular joint separation into three grades of severity. With the expanded classification of Rockwood, other less common types can also be classified (see **Table 41.1** [3.6, 3.7]). The step-off is assessed by having the patient hold a 5-kg weight in each hand to pull the acromion downward (⬇ in **Fig. 40.2c**). The fracture can be operatively stabilized with a hook plate, for example **(Fig. 40.2b)**.

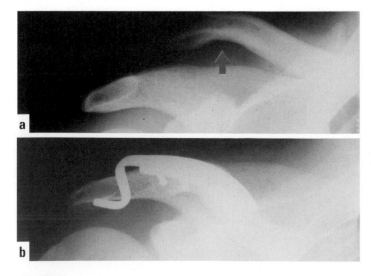

Fig. 40.2

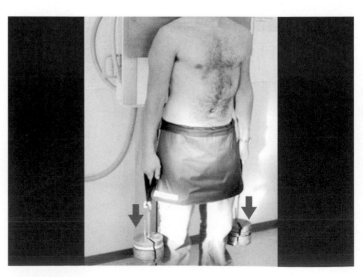

Fig. 40.2 c

Classification of Acromioclavicular Separation
(Tossy Grades I–III and Rockwood Grades IV–VI)

Grade	Affected ligaments	Radiographic signs with a 5-kg traction weight
I	Stretching of the acromioclavicular and coracoclavicular ligaments	None
II	Rupture of the acromioclavicular ligament Stretching of the coracoclavicular ligament	Displacement of the clavicle by one half the joint height
III	Rupture of both ligaments	Displacement by one shaft width
IV	Like Tossi III, but with posterior displacement of the lateral end of the clavicle	
V	Like Tossi III, but with extreme displacement	
VI	Dislocation of the clavicle beneath the acromion (rare)	

Table 41.1

Humerus

Subcapital fractures of the humerus are generally caused indirectly by a fall onto the hand or elbow and less commonly by a direct blow to the arm. They are easily recognized on ordinary chest radiographs and should not be missed due to carelessness. In the PA projection in our example (**Fig. 41.3a**), note that the proximal humeral shaft is not centered normally below the humeral head (**28**) but has been displaced medially (→). The proximal stump of the humeral shaft (←) can be seen in the lateral projection (**Fig. 41.3b**). Subcapital humeral fractures most commonly occur in elderly women (with osteoporosis) due to a fall onto the outstretched arm.

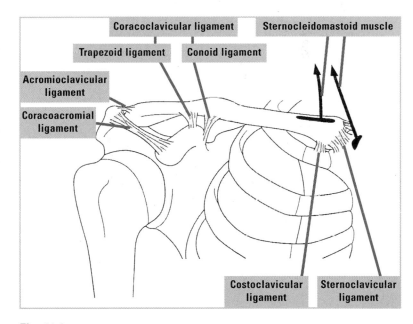

Fig. 41.2

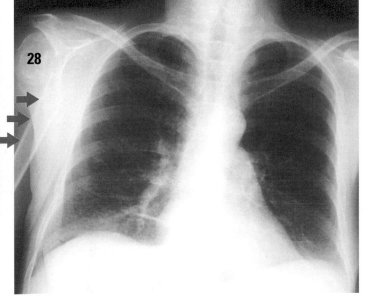

Fig. 41.3a

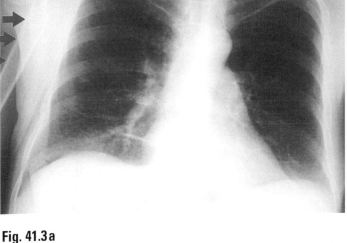

Fig. 41.3b

3

Ribs

A rib fracture presents radiographically as a step-off or discontinuity (↖) in the radiographically dense cortical line of an otherwise intact rib. The radiographic diagnosis generally presents no difficulties in patients with complete, displaced fractures **(Fig. 42.1)**.

More detailed information on these injuries can be found in the chapter dealing with thoracic trauma (see p. 184-186).

"Rib notches" are peripheral, sharply circumscribed osteolytic lesions (↑) 2-4 mm wide that are typically seen in the inferior margin of a lateral or posterolateral rib segment **(Fig. 42.2)**. Rib notching is caused by the mechanical pressure that is exerted by dilated intercostal arteries. It may occur in coarctation of the aorta, for example, when the intercostal arteries function as collateral channels (see p. 88).

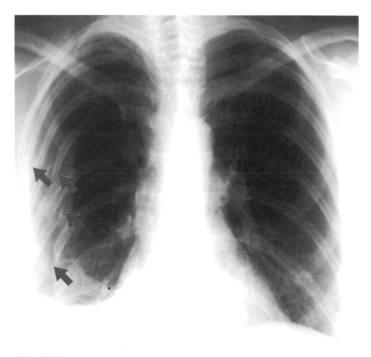

Fig. 42.1

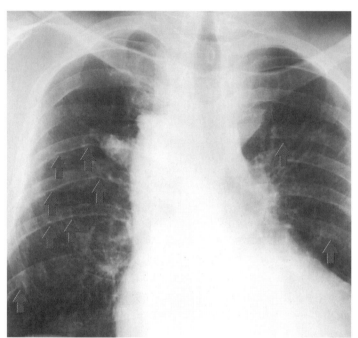

Fig. 42.2

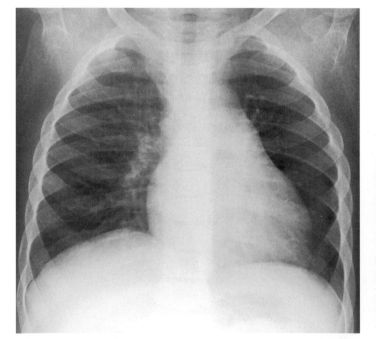

Fig. 42.3

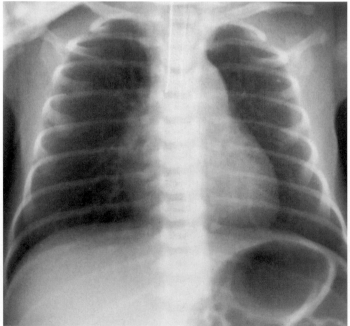

Fig. 42.4

Note also the caliber of the ribs themselves. The ribs may be thickened, for example, as a result of extramedullary hematopoiesis ↖ in patients with thalassemia **(Fig. 42.3)**.

By contrast, marked thinning of all the ribs may be noted in certain forms of congenital skeletal dysplasia in children **(Fig. 42.4)**.

Skeletal Metastases

Hematogenous metastases are the most common tumors of the thoracic skeleton in older patients. Bones that contain red marrow (ribs, sternum, vertebrae) are particularly suspectible. Note the discontinuities (↖) and clublike expansion of the ribs shown in **Figure 43.1**. A spot film taken three months later **(Fig. 43.1b)** shows definite progression of the cortical defect and metastatic rib expansion compared with the previous radiograph **(Fig. 43.1a)**. Do not confuse this finding with the fusiform thickening caused by old rib fractures that have healed with callus formation (↑ in **Fig. 43.2**). This benign type of thickening is not accompanied by osteolytic changes.

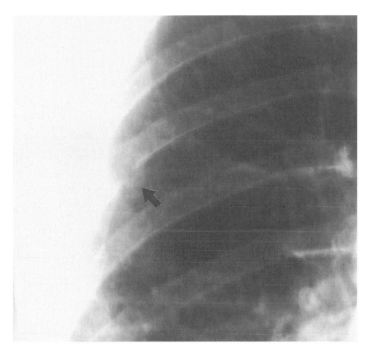

Fig. 43.1 a

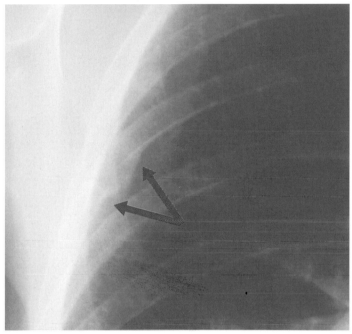

Fig. 43.1 b

When examining tumor patients, you should also watch for osteolysis or decreased height (↓) of thoracic vertebral bodies as shown in **Figure 43.3**. These changes are often missed in the PA projection **(Fig. 43.3a)** but are usually well displayed in the lateral projection **(Fig. 43.3b)**.

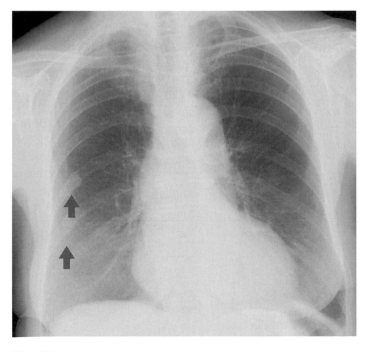

Fig. 43.2

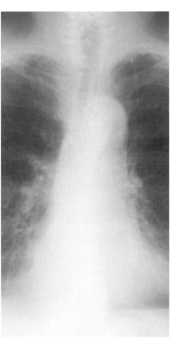

Fig. 43.3 a

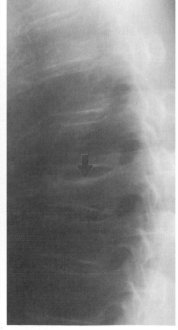

Fig. 43.3 b

In the search for possible primary tumors, it is helpful to draw a distinction between osteolytic and osteoblastic metastases. Osteolytic metastases occur in association with multiple myeloma, as well as carcinoma of the lung, breast, thyroid gland, or kidney (renal metastases are always osteolytic). Osteoblastic metastases most commonly arise from the tumors listed in **Table 44.1**.

Primary Tumors with Osteoblastic Metastases: "Five Bees Like Pollen"

1. **B**	**B**reast (breast carcinoma)
2. **B**	**B**rain (medulloblastoma)
3. **B**	**B**ronchi (bronchial carcinoma)
4. **B**	**B**elly (GI tumor, carcinoid)
5. **B**	**B**ladder (bladder carcinoma)
Like	**L**ymphoma
Pollen	**P**rostatic carcinoma

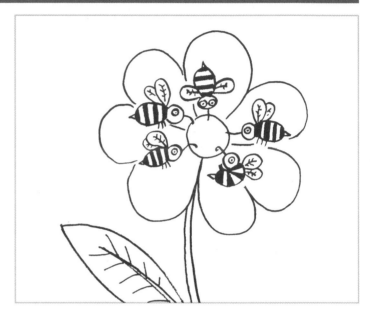

Table 44.1

Figure 44.2 shows an example of extensive skeletal metastases from advanced prostatic carcinoma. When you compare this image with other images, you will notice a diffuse, generalized increase in skeletal density. Spinal involvement by this process is called "ivory vertebrae." In addition to the predominant osteoblastic metastases, we also find isolated lytic lesions (➡). This is called a mixed lytic-blastic type of metastasis, which is typical of prostatic carcinoma, as well as of breast cancer and gastrointestinal tumors. A malignant pleural effusion (★) has also developed at this stage and has spread into the horizontal interlobar fissure on the right side (see also p. 106–107).

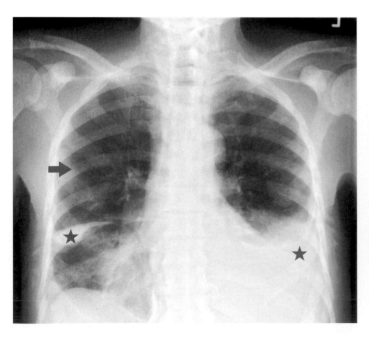

Fig. 44.2a

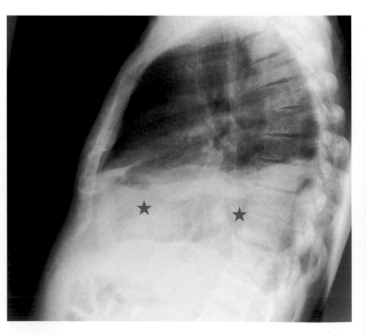

Fig. 44.2b

Spinal Degenerative Changes

Past a certain age, virtually every chest radiograph will show degenerative changes in the vertebral column **(Figs. 45.1, 45.2)**. It is normal for the nucleus pulposus inside the intervertebral disks to lose elasticity with advancing age. Radiographs show joint space narrowing (= chondrosis), as well as bony changes adjacent to the intervertebral disks, consisting of osteochondrosis with bandlike sclerosis (⬇ ⬇ ⬇) and contour irregularities (⬆ ⬆ ⬆) of the adjacent vertebral endplates. This results in reactive new bone formation (⬊), known technically as spondylosis deformans, which represents an attempt to stabilize the aging spine.

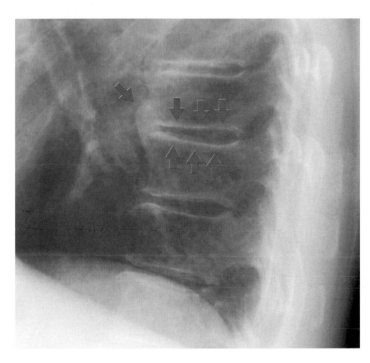

Fig. 45.1

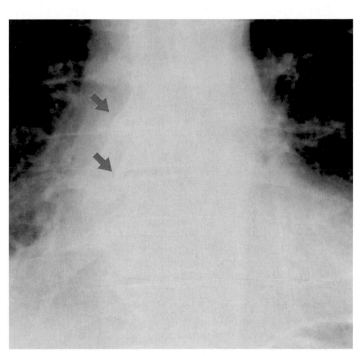

Fig. 45.2

Space For Your Notes

On the anterior side of the vertebral column, it is common to find calcification and ossification of the anterior longitudinal ligament with flowing hyperostosis (➡ in **Fig. 46.1**). If these changes span at least four vertebral bodies and are not associated with other degenerative changes in the intervertebral disks (osteochondrosis, prolapse), they warrant a diagnosis of diffuse idiopathic skeletal hyperostosis (DISH), known also as Forestier disease. The thoracolumbar junction and lower cervical spine are sites of predilection for DISH.

Scoliosis (**Fig. 46.2**) is defined as a fixed lateral curvature of the spine (➡ ←). The individual vertebral bodies in this condition are rotated in relation to one another and are less mobile in the affected segment. Besides the idiopathic form, which may occur at any age, there are a number of secondary forms that may be caused by infections, rheumatoid disease, trauma, or metastatic vertebral deformities.

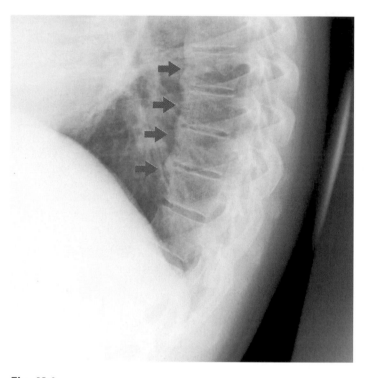

Fig. 46.1

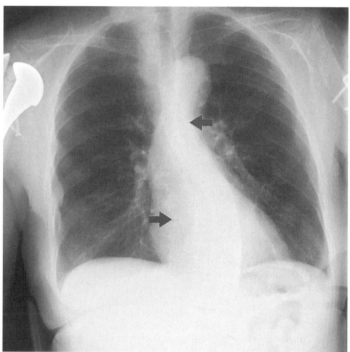

Fig. 46.2

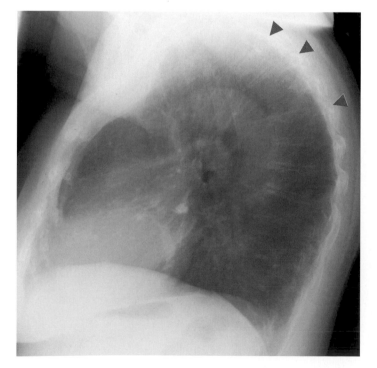

Fig. 46.3

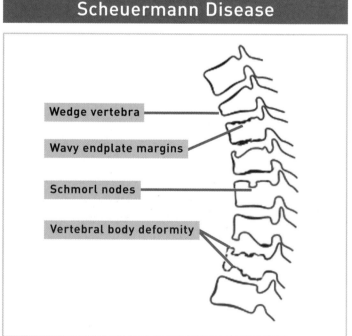

Scheuermann Disease

Wedge vertebra

Wavy endplate margins

Schmorl nodes

Vertebral body deformity

Fig. 46.4

An abnormally increased dorsal convexity of the thoracic spine (◄) is called hyperkyphosis **(Fig. 46.3)**. It may be congenital, age-related, or secondary to a variety of diseases (rickets, ankylosing spondylitis, tuberculous spondylitis). The kyphosis shown in our illustrative case is accompanied by two other age-related changes. Can you find them? (The answers are at the end of the book.) When hyperkyphosis is discovered in a young patient, the differential diagnosis should include adolescent kyphosis (Scheuermann disease),

in which thoracic kyphosis is a cardinal symptom. Later signs include wavy margins of the vertebral endplates and the presence of Schmorl nodes. Located in the middle or anterior margin of the upper and lower vertebral endplates, Schmorl nodes represent intervertebral disk ruptures that have undergone cartilaginous transformation. The disease may eventually progress to an end stage marked by severe deformity of the vertebral bodies. The radiographic signs of Scheuermann disease are illustrated in **Figure 46.4**

Intra-abdominal Findings

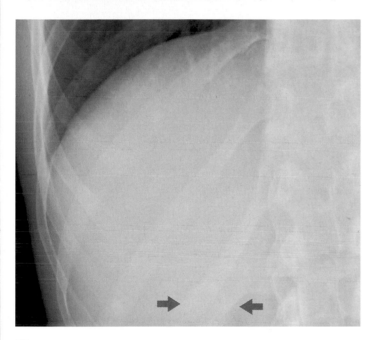

Fig. 47.1

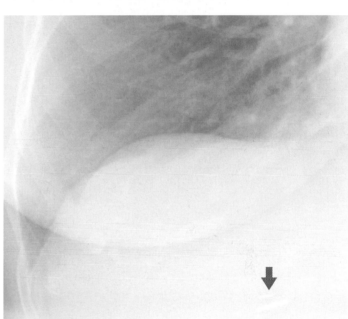

Fig. 47.2

Besides changes in the heart, lung, soft tissues, and bones, there are also intra-abdominal findings that you should mention when reading a chest radiograph. Only radiopaque stones (➡ ⬅) can be seen in patients with cholecystolithiasis **(Fig. 47.1**, ultrasound is a much more sensitive study), but usually it is easy to identify clip material (⬇ in **Fig. 47.2**) following surgical intervention.

As an example of an intra-abdominal foreign body, **Figure 47.3** shows a patient who underwent surgical reduction of the gastric inlet (gastric banding) for morbid obesity. A valve mechanism is used to adjust the inside diameter of the ring for individual requirements. Intrathoracic foreign bodies are discussed more fully in Chapter 9.

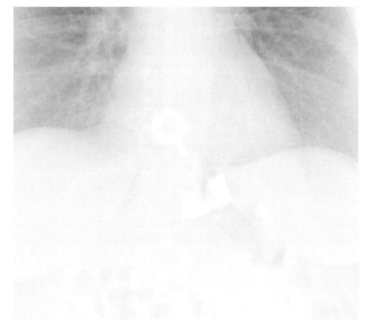

Fig. 47.3

In **Figure 48.1**, a roughly semicircular structure of calcific density (↘ ↗) can be seen just below the left diaphragm leaflet in close proximity to the gastric bubble. This structure is a harmless splenic cyst with a calcified wall. Ménétrier disease is a gastrointestinal disease of unknown cause that is associated with increased mucus production and mucosal hypertrophy with characteristic giant rugal folds. **Figure 48.2** shows a gastric bubble with a highly irregular configuration, which is the conventional radiographic correlate of these giant folds. Because there is a 10% incidence of malignant transformation in Ménétrier disease, the early diagnosis of this condition is of major importance.

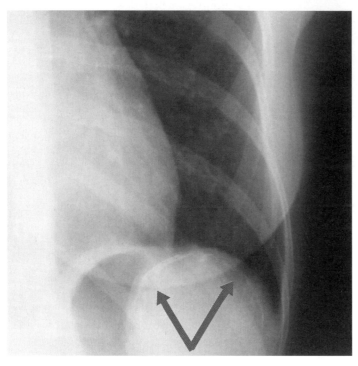

Fig. 48.1

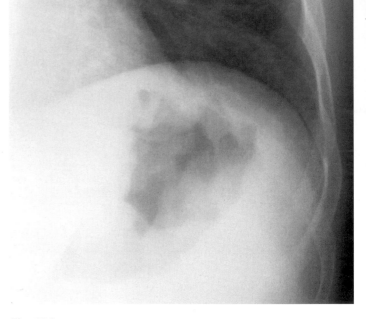

Fig. 48.2

Quiz – Test Yourself!

9   **Figure 49.1** tests your ability to avoid being distracted by conspicuous incidental findings and locate the more significant pathology.

10   The radiograph in **Figure 49.2** is from a 27-year-old woman who had bronchial asthma and recurrent bouts of pneumonia since childhood. She was hospitalized again with clinical suspicion of pneumonic infiltration. What additional finding do you see on her chest radiograph?

11   The radiographs in **Figure 49.3** contain another important finding besides the obvious bilateral pulmonary metastases. What is it? The solutions are at the end of the book.

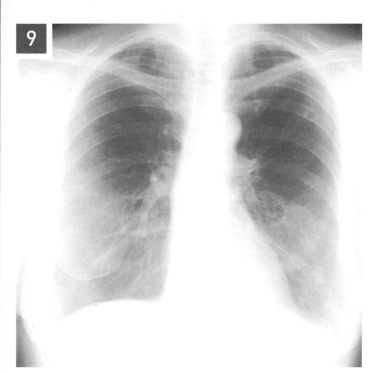

Fig. 49.1

Fig. 49.2

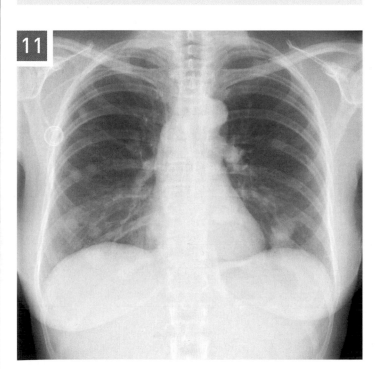

Fig. 49.3 a

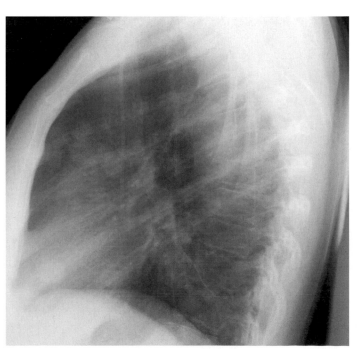

Fig. 49.3 b

Space For Your Notes

Nadine Abanador
Matthias Hofer

Pleura

Chapter Goals:

This chapter deals with the radiographic manifestations and differential diagnosis of pleural thickening. Because the information in this book is arranged according to morphological criteria, pleural effusions are discussed in chapter 6 on patchy lung changes. On completing this chapter, you should be able to:

- distinguish a healthy pleura from pleural abnormalities;

- recognize the various manifestations of pleural thickening;

- recognize grades of severity of pleural thickening and describe their clinical significance;

- differentiate intrapulmonary processes from pleural masses.

4

Normal Findings

The function of the pleura is to allow frictionless movement between the chest wall and lung. The pleura has a normal width of approximately 0.2-0.4 mm. If it is not abnormally thickened, the thin pleural line is visible only at sites where it is struck tangentially by the roentgen ray beam. **Figure 51.1** shows the "para-aortic stripe" (◁), which is formed by the posterior reflection of the pleura at the descending aorta **(8)**. The posterior reflection can also be seen in the apical region. The pleural line (↖ ↗) appears as a medial prolongation of the posterior segment of the second rib on each side.

Both lines unite above the aortic arch **(6)** to form a vertical line. The lateral radiograph **(Fig. 51.2)** shows the retrotracheal stripe (➡) at the posterior border of the trachea **(14)**. Additionally, a retrosternal stripe (▷) can be seen basally in the retrosternal space **(12)**. This stripe is usually formed by epicardial fat and should not be mistaken for pleural thickening. The parietal pleura can be identified at a somewhat higher level, appearing as a wavy line (⬅) that intermittently protrudes into the intercostal spaces.

The pleura normally appears as a thin, smooth, regular line.

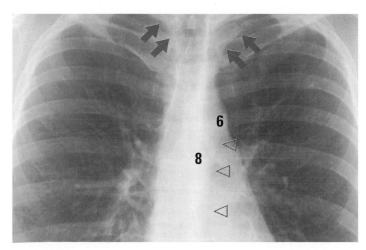

Fig. 51.1

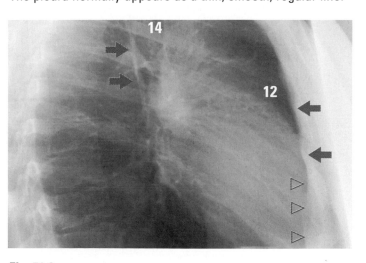

Fig. 51.2

At some sites, however, the pleura may appear widened or irregular, and this should not be mistaken for abnormal pleural thickening. The line of the parietal pleura (▷) is particularly well defined in the posteroanterior (PA) radiograph (**Fig. 52.1**). This line is wavy due to the physiological pleural bulge into the intercostal spaces (compare with **Fig. 51.2**). In **Figure 52.2**, the apical pleura (↑) is tangential to the roentgen ray beam and therefore appears as a companion shadow along the inferior border of the second rib (**22**).

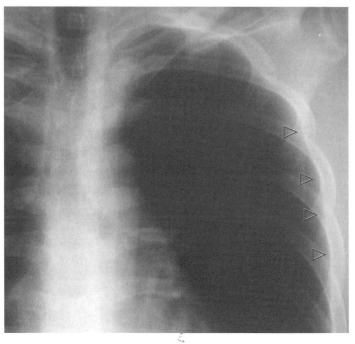

Fig. 52.1

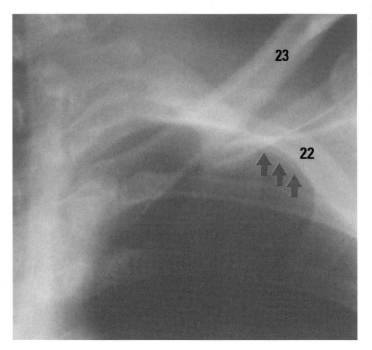

Fig. 52.2

By contrast, the companion shadow of the clavicle (↙) in **Figure 52.3** is formed a layer of skin overlying the clavicle (**23**) that is tangential to the roentgen ray beam; it is not caused by the pleura. The greater the depth of the supraclavicular fossa, the more conspicuous this companion shadow will appear. **Figure 52.4** shows a vertical line (→) at the level of the right pleural dome. This is a normal feature caused by the sternocleidomastoid muscle, whose margin is struck tangentially by the roentgen ray beam. Be careful not to mistake the companion shadow of the clavicle or the vertical shadow of the sternocleidomastoid muscle for a pleural opacity.

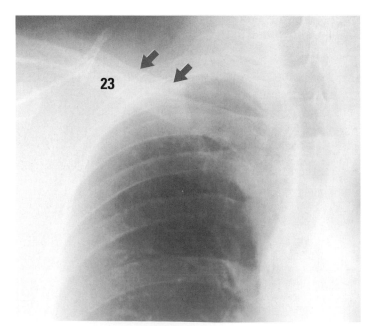

Fig. 52.3

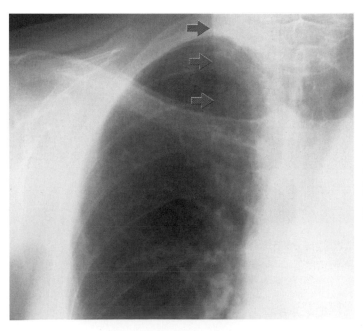

Fig. 52.4

Pleural thickening may be focal or generalized. Its potential causes range from postinflammatory changes (the most common cause) to pleural tumors. It may have various presentations depending on its location and morphology. Sites of pleural thickening on the lateral chest wall may be sharply delineated when they are struck tangentially by the roentgen ray beam in the PA projection. **Figure 53.1** shows a pleural calcification (←) on the right chest wall. The adjacent lower lung zone (↙) and diaphragm **(17)** are slightly distorted by the calcified area. Pleural thickening at an anterior or posterior site is imaged en face in the PA projection and may appear as a diffuse, circumscribed, or patchy opacity.

Figure 53.2 shows bilateral pleural calcifications (↗) that are projected into the lung field because of their anterior and posterior location. They should not be mistaken for intrapulmonary lesions (see Chapter 7). Bilateral pleural thickening (→) is also present.

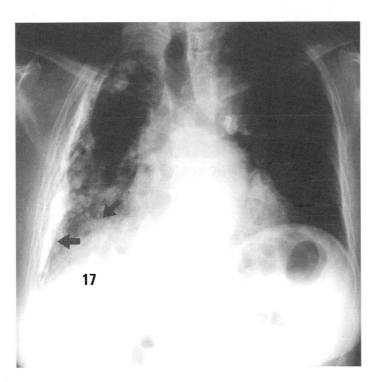

Fig. 53.1

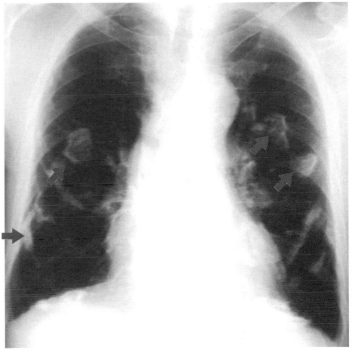

Fig. 53.2

Focal pleural thickening greater than 1 cm should raise suspicion of a tumor [4.1]. Thickening of the visceral and parietal pleura can be differentiated by real-time ultrasound scanning or fluoroscopy: Lesions of the visceral pleura follow the excursions of the lung, whereas lesions of the parietal pleura or extrapleural space move with the ribs and chest wall.

Pleural thickening greater than 3 mm should be investigated further by computed tomography (CT) [4.4]. CT scans are helpful in distinguishing pleural abnormalities from changes in adjacent tissues.

Characteristics of Pleural Thickening

Radiographic appearance	• Anterior or posterior plaques appear diffuse with ill-defined margins • Plaques struck tangentially by the roentgen ray beam are sharply delineated
Frequent causes	• Postinflammatory (postpleuritic) changes; unifocal pleural thickening is most common
Key cutoff values	• Indeterminate pleural thickening > 3 mm: Obtain CT scans • Pleural thickening > 1 cm: Suspicious for tumor

Table 53.3

Pleural fibrosis may develop as a sequel to inflammatory pleural changes or pleural effusions and predominantly affects the visceral pleura [4.1]. It consists of granulation tissue that may undergo secondary calcification. Primary pleural fibrosis has no pathological significance. Various grades of severity are illustrated below. Anterobasal fibrotic lesions (◢) like those shown in **Figure 54.1b** are often visible only in the lateral projection, as they are obscured by the cardiac shadow in the PA projection **(Fig. 54.1a)**. The lesions in this case are postinflammatory changes following a previous coronary artery bypass graft and valvular surgery, although the surgical clips **(52)** are difficult to visualize in this patient.

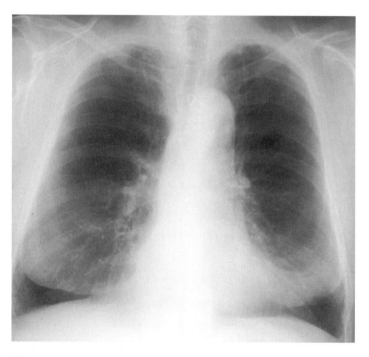

Fig. 54.1 a

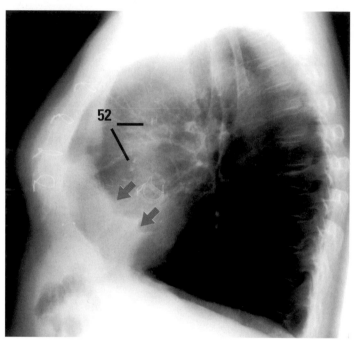

Fig. 54.1 b

Pleural fibrosis may also develop as a sequel to long-term radiotherapy [4.2]. **Figure 54.2a** shows a conspicuous apical pleural cap (⬆) over the left lung. The fibrosis has caused marked upward retraction of the ipsilateral hilum **(10)** (↗). The patient had received radiotherapy years previously for breast cancer and had undergone breast reconstruction with a prosthetic implant (△).

The pleural cap (⬆) is more difficult to identify in the lateral radiograph **(Fig. 54.2b)** than in the PA film due to superimposed structures, and might easily be missed.

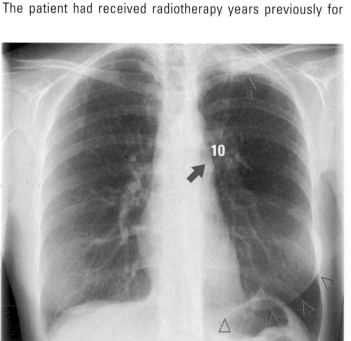

Fig. 54.2 a

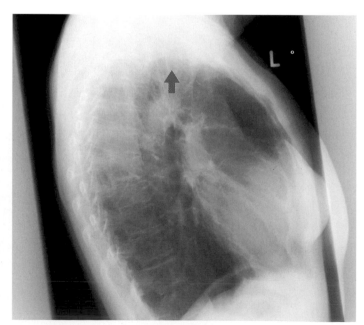

Fig. 54.2 b

Figure 55.1 shows an example of pleural fibrosis in the left basal region (↘). Basal pleural changes can mimic small effusions due to blunting of the costophrenic angle. Interlobar fibrosis (↓) is constrained on both sides by aerated lung and is therefore clearly delineated **(Fig. 55.2)**. This radiograph also shows lateral pleural thickening on the left side (→) with an accompanying pleural effusion **(41)** (see also p. 106-109).

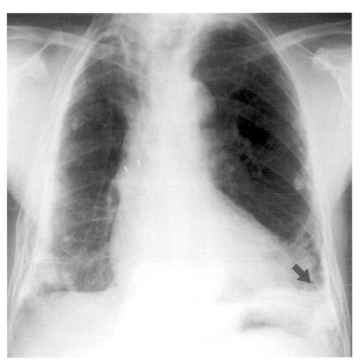

Fig. 55.1

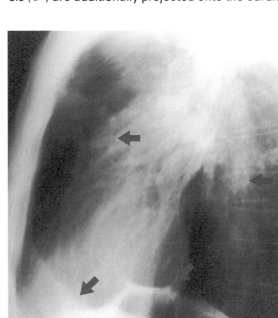

Fig. 55.2

"Apical caps" are a common feature of advancing age but are suggestive of tuberculosis (TB) only if there is concomitant intrapulmonary involvement [4.1]. The findings in these cases are more pronounced. **Figure 55.3a** shows conspicuous, bilateral pleural caps (↖ ↗) in a patient known to have TB.

Traction from the apical fibrotic scar tissue has caused upward retraction of both pulmonary hila (⬆). The lateral radiograph clearly demonstrates the streaklike texture of the dense interstitium (← in **Fig. 55.3b**). Foci of anterobasal fibrosis (↙) are additionally projected onto the cardiac silhouette.

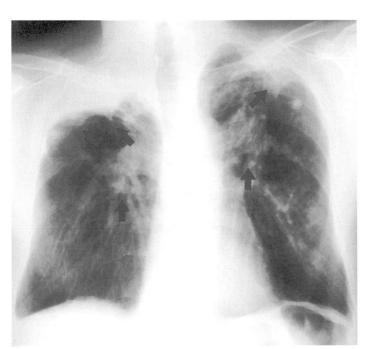

Fig. 55.3a

Fig. 55.3b

Pleural Plaques

Pleural plaques are focal thickenings of the parietal pleura. They consist of aggregations of hyalinized collagen fibers that form almost exclusively as a result of asbestos-related proliferation [4.1, 4.3]. They frequently develop on the lateral chest wall and in the basal region near the diaphragm. Unlike residual postinflammatory changes, asbestos-related pleural changes ("pleural asbestosis") often lead to bilateral thickening of the parietal pleura [4.2]. The patient in **Figure 56.1** had bilateral diaphragmatic (↓) pleural plaques and additional plaques near the pericardium (↙). Possible pleural mani-festations of asbestosis are illustrated in **Figure 56.2**.

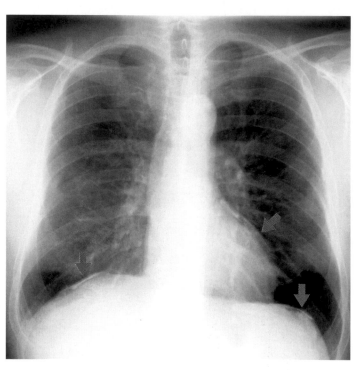

Fig. 56.1

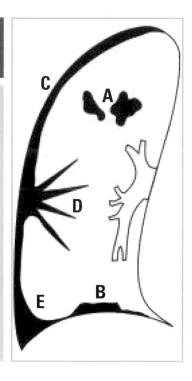

"Pleural Asbestosis"

A   Plaques en face

B   Plaques in profile

C   Pleural peel

D   Fibrotic strands

E   Costophrenic angle fibrosis

Fig. 56.2

Figure 56.3a shows asbestos-related pleural thickening and pleural peels (←, ↗). The corresponding CT scan in **Figure** **56.3b** confirms the lateral fibrotic changes (→) in the left pleura with multiple septal extensions (↗).

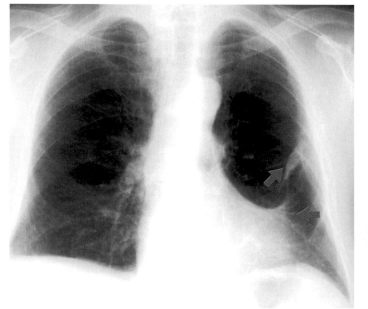

Fig. 56.3 a

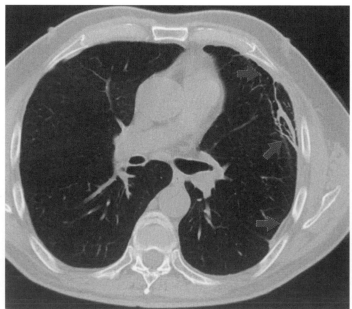

Fig. 56.3 b

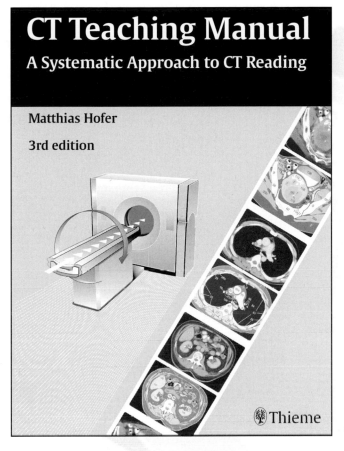
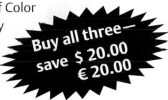
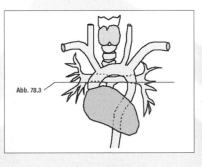
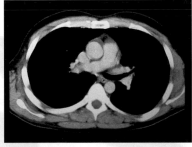

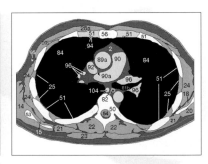
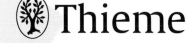

Primary pleural tumors arise from the mesothelium of the pleura, but secondary tumors are far more common [4.4]. These lesions may be metastatic to primary tumors of the lung, breast, pancreas, ovary, and colon, or they may result from invasion of the pleural cavity by malignant tumors. Possible routes of invasion are shown in **Figure 58.1**. Whereas peripheral bronchial carcinomas (BCs) mainly infiltrate the pleural cavity, central BCs are more likely to spread to the hilar lymph nodes (see p. 73). The ultrasound image in **Figure 58.2** shows a pleural metastasis **(21)** accompanied by a malignant pleural effusion **(41)** in a patient with known BC. The metastasis is located on the thoracic side of the diaphragm **(17)** on the parietal pleura, superior to the spleen **(44)**.

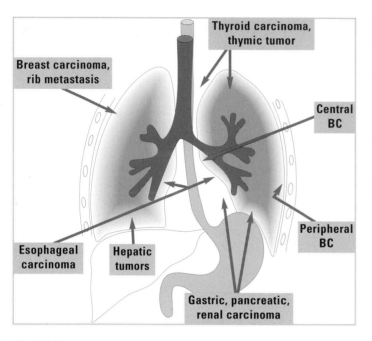

Fig. 58.1

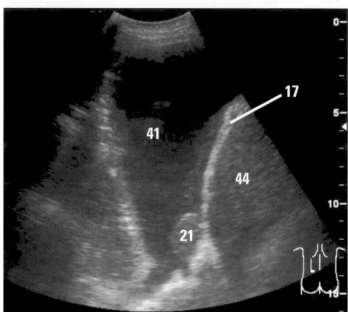

Fig. 58.2

Sectional imaging studies provide more detailed information. **Figure 58.3a** shows a patient with a Pancoast tumor **(21)** of the apical right lung.

The cause of the ipsilateral elevated hemidiaphragm (⬆) was tumor-induced phrenic nerve paralysis on the right side (see p. 117). CT clearly demonstrates the infiltration of the soft-tissue mantle (⬂ in **Fig. 58.3b**). The nonhomogeneous tumor structure **(21)** and the mediastinal shift to the left side (➡) are also evident. The scan with a lung window **(Fig. 58.3c)** still shows no erosion of the upper ribs **(22)**, however.

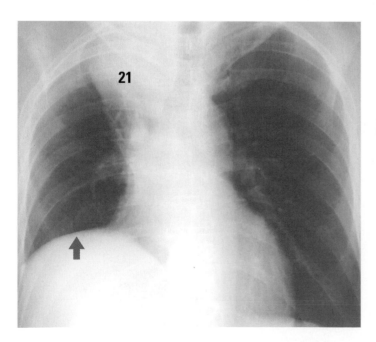

Fig. 58.3a

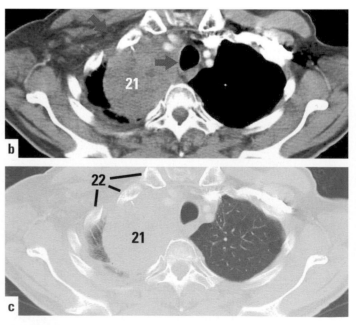

Fig. 58.3b+c

Lenk's rule **(Fig. 59.1)** is helpful in establishing the pleural or pulmonary origin of an intrathoracic mass **(21)**. Pleural masses on the lateral chest wall that are imaged in profile form an obtuse angle (> 90°) with the chest wall **(Fig. 59.2a)**.

This differs from intrapulmonary masses bordering the pleura, which form an acute angle (< 90°) with the lateral chest wall **(Fig. 59.2b)**.

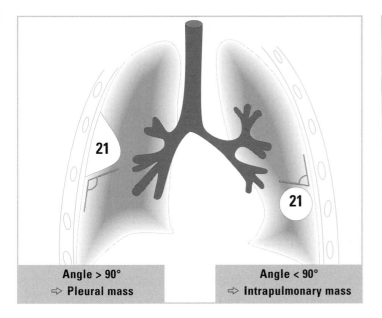

Fig. 59.1

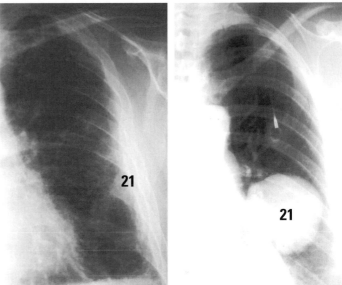

Fig. 59.2a   Fig. 59.2b

Pleural mesotheliomas are predominantly malignant pleural tumors that commonly arise from asbestos-related pleural changes [4.6]. They typically appear as unilateral, diffusely distributed, nodular pleural thickenings that may be located along the border of the lung or mediastinum, may abut the diaphragm, or may occur in the interlobar fissure. Concomitant effusions are often present. Bilateral involvement and infiltration of the lung and pericardium are signs of late-stage disease [4.5]. **Figure 59.3** shows distinct, nodular pleural thickenings ( ) along the border of the right lung and an effusion in the ipsilateral costophrenic angle ( ).

Figure 59.4 shows a large pleural mesothelioma ( ) that has already displaced large portions of the left lung and is not delineated from the left cardiac border. Equivocal findings should be resolved by CT, which may be supplemented if necessary by pleural biopsy.

Densitometry can aid in differentiating simple fibrotic changes from mesotheliomas and secondary tumors **(21)**. Neoplasms typically show a density increase from approximately 40 HU before i.v. contrast administration to approximately 80 HU after contrast administration.

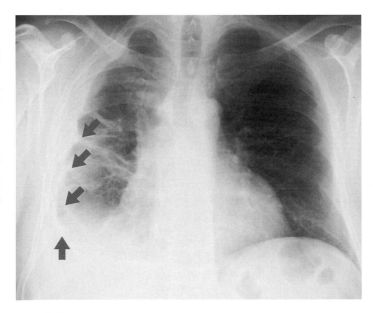

Fig. 59.3

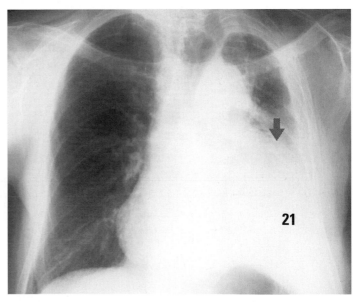

Fig. 59.4

Thoracentesis

The percutaneous aspiration of a pleural effusion (thoracentesis) may be done for diagnostic purposes (is the collection an empyema or does it contain malignant cells indicating a malignant effusion?), or it may be done to decompress the lung in patients with heart failure who have responded poorly to diuretics. Ordinarily the needle is introduced under sonographic guidance in the posterior axillary line (PAL) along an upper rib margin to avoid injury to intercostal nerves and vessels (**Fig. 60.1**).

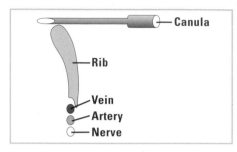

Fig. 60.1

The sterile thoracentesis tray includes a needle and syringe with local anesthetic (**A**), sterile compresses (**B**), a scalpel for making the stab incision (**C**), and an over-the-needle catheter with syringe for aspirating the pleural fluid (**D**). Many thoracentesis sets also include a rigid aspirating needle (**E**), but this poses a greater risk of injury to the visceral pleura when the lung reexpands and approaches the chest wall as the fluid is withdrawn. This is why many colleagues prefer to remove the needle and perform the aspiration with a plastic catheter (see p. 61). The set also includes aspirating tubing (**F**) with a three-way stopcock (**G**), a collection bag (**H**), a sterile fenestrated drape (**I**), and sterile gloves (**Fig. 60.2**). The skin is prepped with antiseptic spray, and the optimum insertion site is located under ultrasound guidance by indenting the skin with pressure from a pen or other object at the upper border of a rib (**Fig. 60.3**). If a skin marker were used, the mark might be obliterated by the second skin prep. The ultrasound image (**Fig. 60.4**) shows the extent of the echo-free (= black) effusion (**41**) above the diaphragm (**17**) and spleen (**44**) and around the lower portions of the lung (**34**).

The following calculation can be used to make a semiquantitative assessment of the effusion volume: Determine the maximum distance from the cranial end of the effusion (↓) to the caudal limit (⬈) of the costodiaphragmatic recess (equal here to 9.5 cm), then determine the minimum distance (⬈) between the lung (**34**) and the diaphragm (**17**, equal here to 1.1 cm). Add both numbers together and multiply the sum by 70 to obtain the approximate effusion volume (in mL). In this example: 9.5 + 1.1 = 10.6 x 70 = approximately 740 mL.

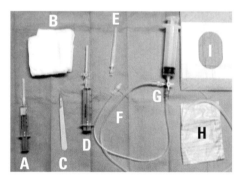

Fig. 60.2

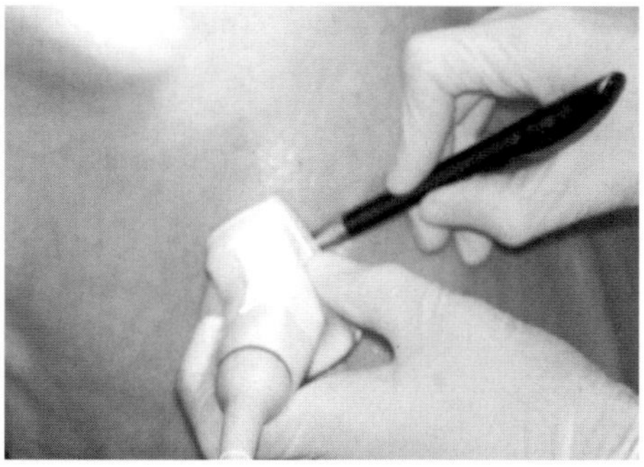

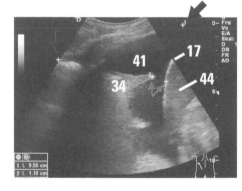

Fig 60.3

Fig. 60.4

After the site has been sterily draped and sprayed again with antiseptic (**Fig. 60.5**), a thin needle is used to raise a skin wheal with local anesthetic (**Fig. 60.6**). The needle track up to and including the parietal pleura is infiltrated (⬈) until the (generally yellowish) pleural fluid can be aspirated (⬈ in **Fig. 60.7**). While doing this, the examiner braces the middle and ring finger of the nondominant hand (↑) against the chest wall so that the needle can be advanced slowly and with maximum control.

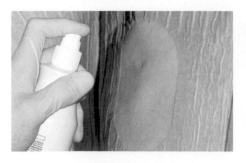

Fig. 60.5

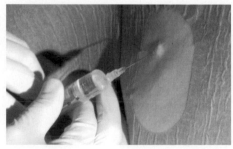

Fig. 60.6

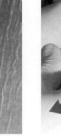

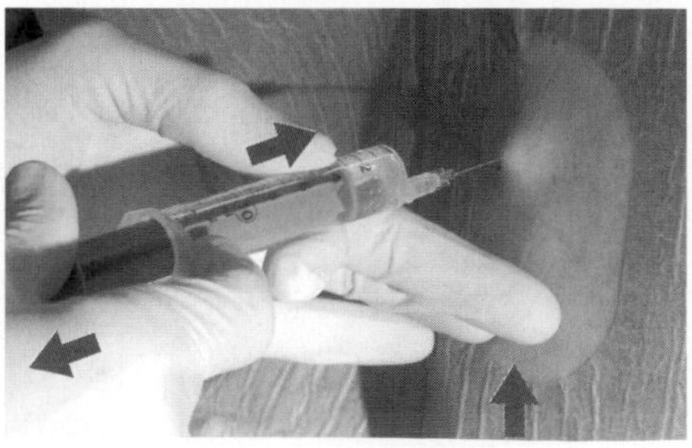

Fig. 60.7

Next a horizontal stab incision is made (**Fig. 61.1**), and the catheter-clad needle is carefully advanced (→) while retracting the plunger (←) until yellowish fluid gushes into the syringe (**Fig. 61.2**). The next step is somewhat critical because immediately after withdrawing the metal needle, the examiner must occlude the catheter port with a finger (**Fig. 61.3**) to avoid causing a significant pneumothorax. Of course, this occlusion should be maintained when the aspiration tubing is connected to the catheter hub. This is the only rationale for the alternative option of using a metal aspirating needle (**E** in **Fig. 60.2**), in which case the tubing could be connected to the needle before it is inserted. We know from experience, however, that the amount of air entering the pleural space is so small that this apparent disadvantage is negligible.

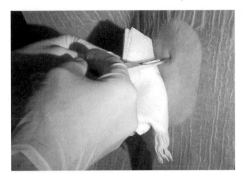

Fig. 61.1

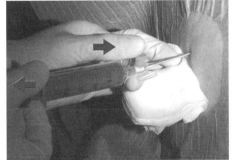

Fig. 61.2

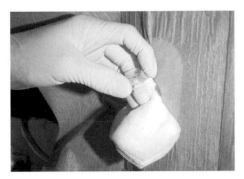

Fig. 61.3

With the catheter and tubing in place, the effusion is drawn slowly and carefully into the syringe (↗ in **Fig. 61.4**). The three-way stopcock is turned 90° (↰), and the fluid is injected into the collection bag (↙ in **Fig. 61.5**). This is done alternately throughout the procedure. You should **not** push the plunger (↓) all the way down when expelling the fluid (**Fig. 61.6**). It is wise to leave a "reserve" in case the plastic catheter tip becomes plugged by visceral pleura. Then you can depress the plunger slightly to free the catheter tip from the pleura and, if necessary, withdraw the catheter a little and redirect it downward as shown in **Figure 61.7**. As the lung reexpands, it will come into contact with the catheter, preventing the further aspiration of fluid. At that point the catheter is removed, the insertion site is covered with a sterile dressing (**Fig. 61.8**), and ultrasound (**Fig. 61.9**) is used to assess the volume of residual pleural fluid (↘). As a safety precaution, no more than 1000 mL of fluid should be drawn in one sitting to prevent reexpansion trauma to the lung (see p. 205). Approximately 730 mL of fluid was collected in the case shown.

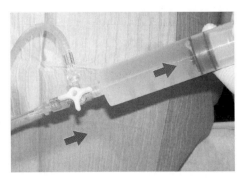

Fig. 61.4

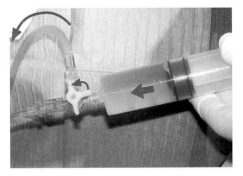

Fig. 61.5

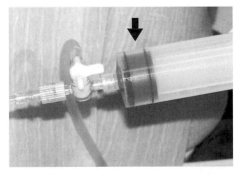

Fig. 61.6

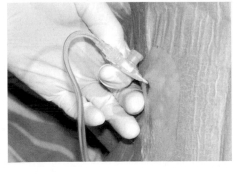

Fig. 61.7

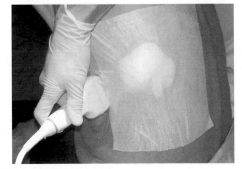

Fig. 61.8

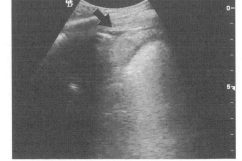

Fig. 61.9

12   What findings can you recognize?

Analyze these PA and lateral radiographs from the same male patient. (The solutions are at the end of the book.)

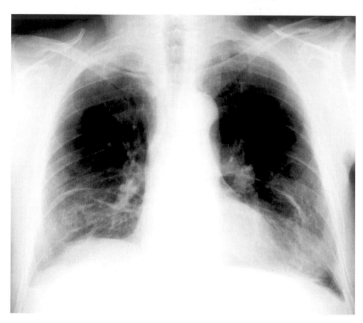

Fig. 62.1 a   **Fig. 62.1 b**

13   Name two important cutoff values for pleural thickening that are used to assess the need for further testing:

14   Name some common primary tumors (at least 10) that metastasize to the pleural cavity:

15   How can you tell whether an intrathoracic mass in the PA radiograph has a pleural or pulmonary origin?

Pleural mass:	Intrapulmonary mass:

Lars Kamper
Matthias Hofer

Mediastinum

Chapter Goals:

This chapter reviews the normal radiographic appearance of the mediastinum, followed by a description of various abnormalities that can lead to mediastinal widening, a mediastinal shift, or mediastinal emphysema. On completing this chapter, you should be able to:

1. recognize the **physiological** appearance of the mediastinal contours on PA radiographs and identify the boundaries of the mediastinal spaces on lateral radiographs;

2. diagnose common mediastinal **abnormalities** on the chest radiograph, e.g.:

   • detect common mediastinal masses,

   • identify the typical locations of mediastinal lymph nodes,

   • distinguish among frequent causes of hilar changes,

   • recognize frequent causes of cardiomegaly,

   • diagnose important abnormalities of the aorta,

   • distinguish among frequent causes of mediastinal shifts.

5

To evaluate the mediastinum, it is necessary to review the anatomy of the normal mediastinal silhouette. The structures that comprise the mediastinal silhouette are numbered in **Figure 64.1a, b**. Please write the names of these structures in the spaces below. First try to label the mediastinal contours from memory, even if it seems tedious at first, for that is the best way to learn them. Refer back to Figure 20.1 only for items that you cannot remember on your own.

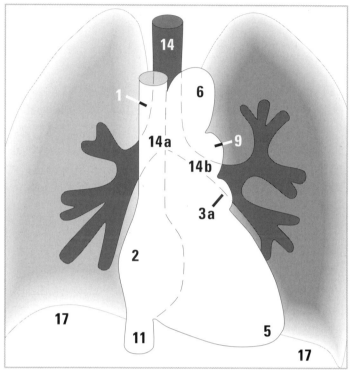

Fig. 64.1 a

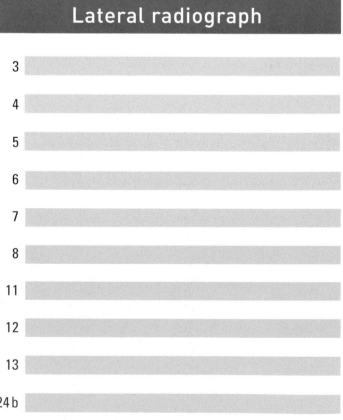

Fig. 64.1 b

PA radiograph
1
2
3a
5
6
9
11
14
14a
17

Lateral radiograph
3
4
5
6
7
8
11
12
13
24b
26

Radiographic evaluation of the mediastinum is aided by dividing it into anterior, middle, and posterior compartments [5.1] (Fig. 65.1a). This makes it considerably easier to identify the possible causes of a mediastinal mass (Fig. 65.1b). The anterior mediastinum (I) extends from the posterior aspect of the sternum to the anterior border of the heart and brachiocephalic vessels. The middle mediastinum (II) contains the heart, ascending aorta, anterior aortic arch, trachea, superior vena cava (SVC), and the brachiocephalic and

pulmonary vessels. The posterior mediastinum (III) consists of the space behind the heart and trachea. It contains the descending aorta, esophagus, azygos vein, autonomic ganglia and nerves, and thoracic duct.

Diseases that occur in all three mediastinal compartments are disregarded in **Figure 65.2**. **Common abnormalities** are shown in **bold** to distinguish them from less frequent conditions.

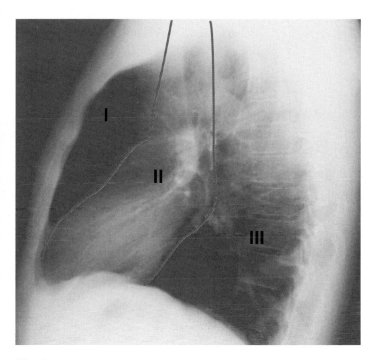

Fig. 65.1 a

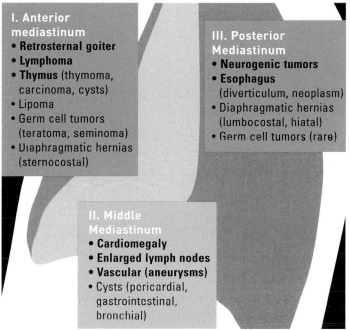

I. Anterior mediastinum
- **Retrosternal goiter**
- **Lymphoma**
- **Thymus** (thymoma, carcinoma, cysts)
- Lipoma
- Germ cell tumors (teratoma, seminoma)
- Diaphragmatic hernias (sternocostal)

III. Posterior Mediastinum
- **Neurogenic tumors**
- **Esophagus** (diverticulum, neoplasm)
- Diaphragmatic hernias (lumbocostal, hiatal)
- Germ cell tumors (rare)

II. Middle Mediastinum
- **Cardiomegaly**
- **Enlarged lymph nodes**
- **Vascular (aneurysms)**
- Cysts (pericardial, gastrointestinal, bronchial)

Fig. 65.1 b

Analysis of the cause is aided further by dividing the mediastinum into superior and inferior compartments (Fig. 65.2). The boundary line between the superior and inferior mediastinum is the tracheal bifurcation. **Figure 65.2b** does not list

diseases that may involve both levels of the mediastinum. As in the previous figure, the more **common abnormalities** are indicated in **bold**.

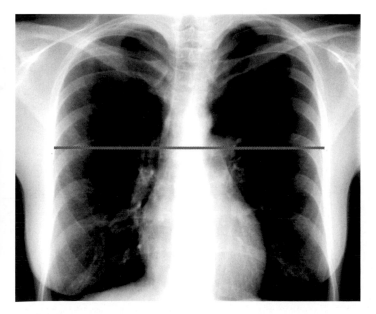

Fig. 65.2 a

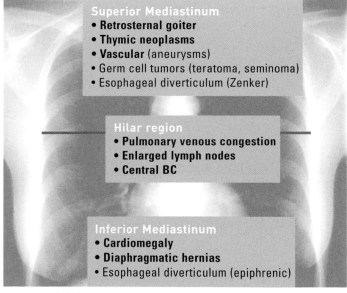

Superior Mediastinum
- **Retrosternal goiter**
- **Thymic neoplasms**
- **Vascular** (aneurysms)
- Germ cell tumors (teratoma, seminoma)
- Esophageal diverticulum (Zenker)

Hilar region
- **Pulmonary venous congestion**
- **Enlarged lymph nodes**
- **Central BC**

Inferior Mediastinum
- **Cardiomegaly**
- **Diaphragmatic hernias**
- Esophageal diverticulum (epiphrenic)

Fig. 65.2 b

The information in **Table 66.1** can help you interpret radiographic widening of the mediastinum. The listing of causes is arranged by compartments to facilitate the differential diagnosis of mediastinal widening and also to help you become oriented within the chapter. Some causes are listed more than once because certain lesions, such as lymphomas, may occur in different compartments.

	Location	Possible Causes	See page
Lateral radiograph	Anterior mediastinum	• Retrosternal goiter	68
		• Lymphoma	69
		• Ascending aortic aneurysm	93
		• Thymus (thymoma, carcinoma, cysts)	70
		• Germ cell tumors (teratoma, seminoma)	71
		• Soft-tissue tumors (e.g., lymphangioma, lipoma)	71
		• Diaphragmatic hernias (sternocostal)	98
	Middle mediastinum	• Cardiomegaly	81
		• Enlarged lymph nodes	72-75
		• Vascular (aneurysms)	83, 93
		• Cysts (pericardial, gastrointestinal, bronchial)	92
	Posterior mediastinum	• Esophagus (diverticulum, neoplasm)	96-97
		• Neurogenic tumors	78
		• Lymphomas	69
		• Diaphragmatic hernias (hiatal, lumbocostal)	98
		• Germ cell tumors (rare)	71
		• Mediastinal abscess	79
PA radiograph	Superior mediastinum	• Retrosternal goiter	68
		• Thymus	70
		• Germ cell tumors	71
		• Esophageal diverticula (Zenker)	96
	Hilar region	• Pulmonary venous congestion	77
		• Pulmonary hypertension	77
		• Enlarged lymph nodes	72-75
		• Central BC	76
		• Bronchiectasis and congenital cysts	92
	Inferior mediastinum	• Cardiomegaly	81
		• Diaphragmatic hernias	98
		• Esophageal diverticula (epiphrenic)	96

Table 66.1

Mediastinal widening caused by a tumor is generally a circumscribed widening that involves one of the mediastinal compartments. Generalized widening of the mediastinum (◀--▶) is more likely to occur after a sternotomy **(Fig. 67.1)** or after trauma to the chest (see Chapter 10). Generalized widening of the mediastinal shadow with ill-defined margins and streaky densities (◥) is also seen after radiotherapy **(Fig. 67.2)** or diffuse mediastinitis **(Fig. 67.3a)**. The mediastinitis in

Figure 67.3a resulted from esophageal perforation, which is confirmed in the lateral radiograph **(Fig. 67.3b)** by the extravasation of orally ingested contrast medium (↙).

Remember to use only water-soluble oral contrast medium (Gastrografin) in patients with a suspected esophageal perforation. Do not use barium sulfate!

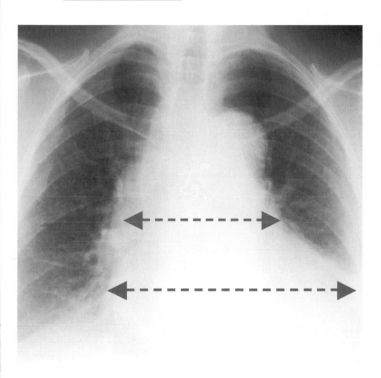

Fig. 67.1

Fig. 67.2

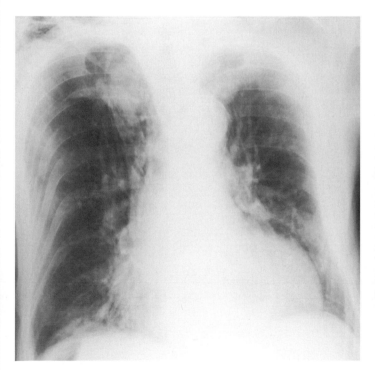

Fig. 67.3 a

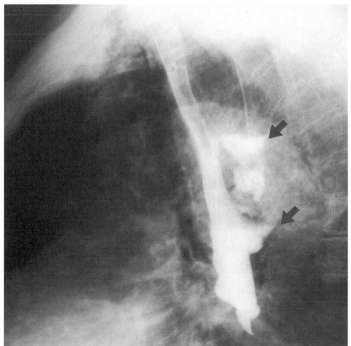

Fig. 67.3 b

5

Retrosternal Goiter

Intrathoracic (retrosternal) goiters (↗) are among the most common masses in the superior mediastinum **(Fig. 68.1)**. The posteroanterior (PA) radiograph shows widening of the mediastinum with displacement of the trachea (→) to the left. The lateral radiograph in a different patient **(Fig. 68.2)** shows the location of the mass in the anterior superior mediastinum (↖). Compression of the trachea may lead to softening of the cartilage rings (tracheomalacia), causing the trachea to narrow or collapse during inspiration. Tracheomalacia can be demonstrated by fluoroscopy **(Fig. 68.3)**: The patient is told to inhale forcefully with the mouth closed and then perform a Valsalva maneuver. During this "sniff test," the luminal diameter of the trachea (↔) should decrease by no more than 50% (→ ←) **(Fig. 68.3)**. Today, spot films of the trachea have been largely superseded by computed tomography (CT; **Fig. 68.4**). CT scans can demonstrate infiltration of the tracheal wall, and the size of the goiter (▽) or tumor can be accurately assessed. CT can also be used to measure the opening area of the trachea **(14)** and its luminal diameter. A 70% inspiratory decrease in the tracheal opening area documented by CT is considered an indicator of tracheomalacia [5.2].

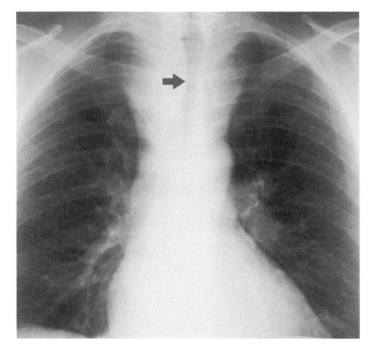

Fig. 68.1

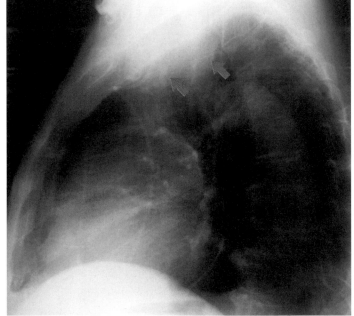

Fig. 68.2

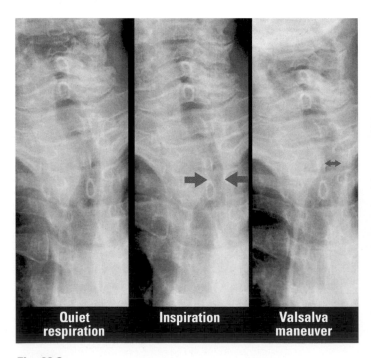

Fig. 68.3

Quiet respiration   Inspiration   Valsalva maneuver

Fig. 68.4

Lymphomas

Mediastinal involvement by malignant lymphoma is particularly common in patients with Hodgkin disease **(Fig. 69.1)** [5.3]. The PA radiograph in these cases typically shows bilateral but asymmetrical widening of the mediastinum (◀--▶, **Fig.**

69.1a). The lateral projection **(Fig. 69.1b)** shows complete opacification of the retrosternal space **(12)**. Lesions may also be manifested in the hilar region (see p. 75) and all other mediastinal compartments (see p. 65) [5.4].

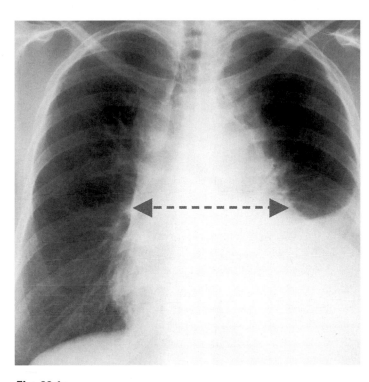

Fig. 69.1a

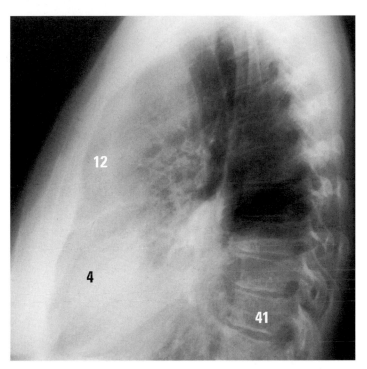

Fig. 69.1b

The enlargement of mediastinal lymph nodes in a setting of acute leukemia **(Fig. 69.2a)** shows a similar distribution pattern in the anterior superior mediastinum (⇨ ⇦) as malignant lymphoma.

Examination by magnetic resonance imaging (MRI; **Fig. 69.2b**) confirms the retrosternal location of the enlarged lymph nodes **(21, 35)** and permits a more accurate determination of tumor extent.

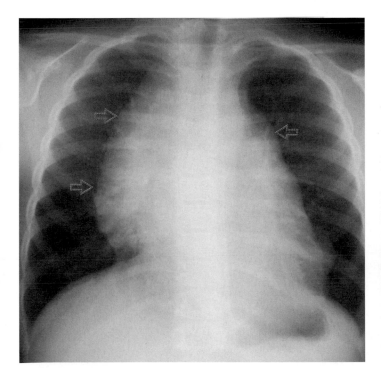

Fig. 69.2a

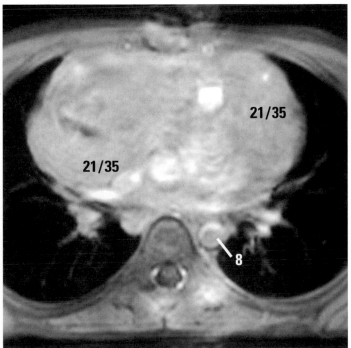

Fig. 69.2b

Thymus

The typical appearance of the normal pediatric thymus on chest radiographs is unfamiliar to most examiners because preschool and school-age children are usually examined by ultrasound or MRI to avoid radiation exposure. In the case shown, the thymus (→) forms the right border of the superior mediastinum instead of the SVC **(Fig. 70.1)**. The shape of the thymus is markedly affected by respiration. On deep inspiration, the expanding lung stretches the thymic tissue and displaces it toward the mediastinum. This may cause the thymus to partially obscure the right cardiac border (↘). The mass in **Figure 70.2** also represents a prominent thymus (↗) rather than a neoplasm.

If uncertainty persists, ultrasound can be used to evaluate the compressibility of the retrosternal tissue. Normal thymic tissue is compressed by the pulsations of the ascending aorta, whereas, say, a tumor-infiltrated pediatric thymus will often show no pulsatile shape changes due to the harder consistency of the infiltrated tissue.

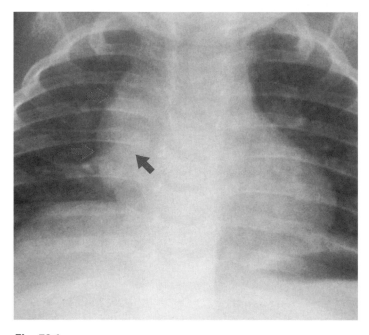

Fig. 70.1

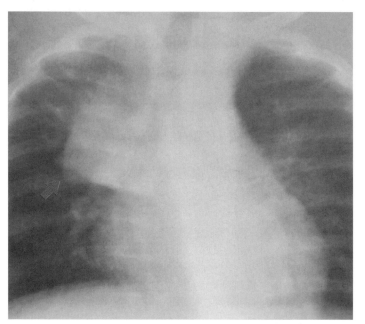

Fig. 70.2

Neoplastic enlargement of the thymus may occur in the setting of a thymoma or a thymic carcinoma, which is less common. Invasion of the thymus by lymphoma has also been described, particularly in the nodular sclerosing form of Hodgkin disease [5.5].

Fatty involution of the thymus is generally complete after puberty. Nevertheless, CT scans will consistently show residual thymic tissue **(42)** in the anterior mediastinum of patients between 20 and 30 years of age **(Fig. 70.3)**.

Reactive thymic hyperplasia in adults may develop after high-dose cortisone therapy or chemotherapy [5.6] or in a setting of myasthenia gravis [5.7]. This hyperplasia appears at CT as a solid mass in the anterior mediastinum (↘ in **Fig. 70.4a**).

As a rule, however, these changes do not become large enough to produce detectable widening of the superior mediastinum on conventional chest radiographs **(Fig. 70.4b)**.

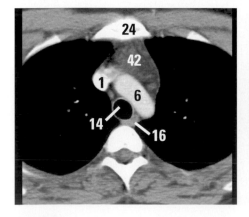

Fig. 70.3

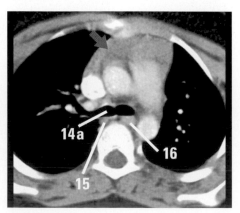

Fig. 70.4a

Fig. 70.4b

Germ Cell Tumors

The upper part of the anterior mediastinum is the most common extragonadal site of occurrence for germ cell tumors. Benign teratomas (▶), while accounting for 60-70% of these tumors [5.8], still constitute a relatively rare diagnosis (**Fig. 71.1a, b**). Since they are composed of tissues from all three germ layers, teratomas may contain bones and teeth, although they consist predominantly of fatty tissue or present a soft-tissue density on radiographs (▽ in **Fig. 71.1b**).

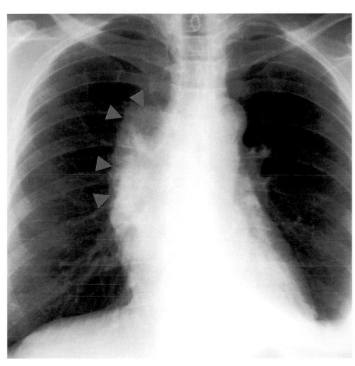

Fig. 71.1a

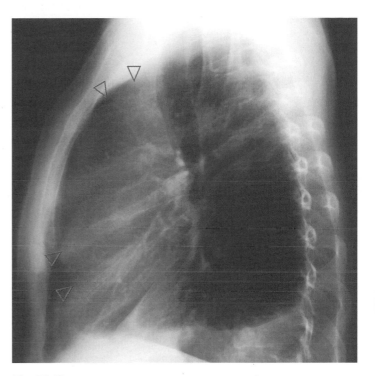

Fig. 71.1b

Lymphangioma

Lymphangioma is a benign soft-tissue tumor of the lymphatic vessels. The lymphangioma in **Figure 71.2** appears in the PA radiograph as a well-circumscribed widening of the entire right mediastinal border (➡). CT (**Fig. 71.2b, c**) reveals the cystic characteristics (◇) of the mass. Lymphangiomas of sufficient size may cause a shift of mediastinal structures such as the SVC (**1**) or ascending aorta (**7**) [5.8].

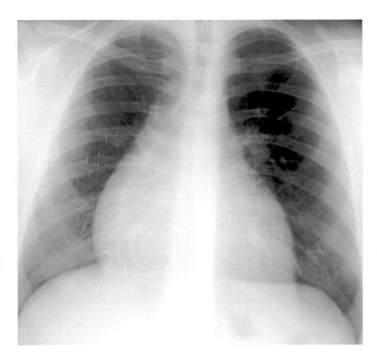

Fig. 71.2a

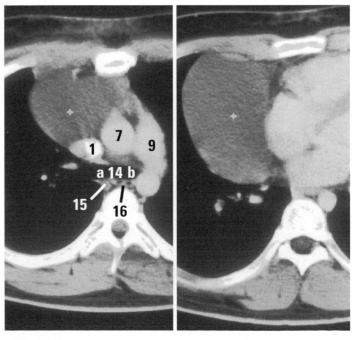

Fig. 71.2b   **Fig. 71.2c**

Lymph Node Enlargement

Lymph node enlargement may occur in all mediastinal compartments. The typical locations of enlarged mediastinal lymph nodes are shown in **Figure 72.1**. The nodes are described by their location as infracarinal **(35a)**, hilar **(35b)**, and right or left paratracheal **(35c)**. Enlarged infracarinal lymph nodes **(35a)** are frequently missed on chest radiographs, as shown in **Figure 72.1b**. In this case the mild lymphadenopathy of indeterminate cause (✎) is detectable only by CT **(Fig. 72.1c)**, which shows slightly enlarged lymph nodes anterior to the tracheal bifurcation **(14c)**.

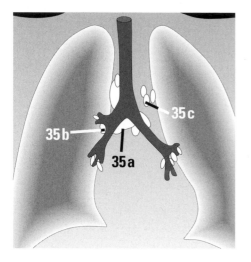

Fig. 72.1 a

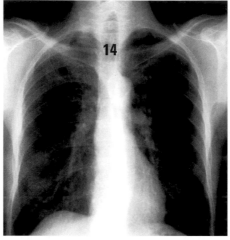

Fig. 72.1 b

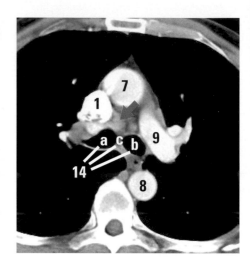

Fig. 72.1 c

When metastatic infracarinal lymph nodes reach sufficient size **(Fig. 72.2)**, they appear on the standard lateral radiograph **(Fig. 72.2c)** as an opacity (▶) in the middle mediastinum. In **Figure 72.2b**, the infracarinal nodal metastases from a left hilar bronchial carcinoma (BC) **(21)** were large enough to cause splaying of the tracheal bifurcation (↖ ↗), which normally forms an angle of 45° to a maximum of 65° in adults [5.9].

The differential diagnosis of splaying of the tracheal bifurcation should also include left atrial dilatation (see p. 82) and a large pericardial effusion (see p. 90). Whenever mediastinal lymphadenopathy is suspected, CT scans should be added to the workup in order to evaluate the mediastinal lymph nodes. The CT scan in **Figure 72.2d** is from a patient with breast cancer and massive infracarinal lymph node metastases **(35a)**.

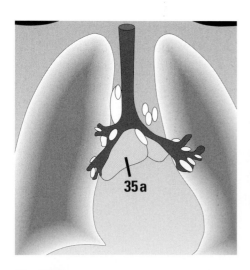

Fig. 72.2 a

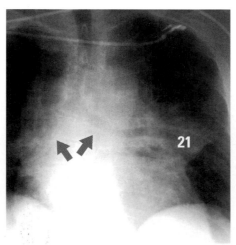

Fig. 72.2 b

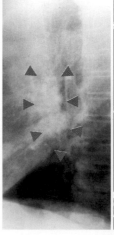

Fig. 72.2 c

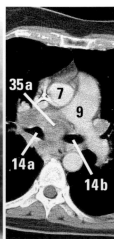

Fig. 72.2 d

Hilar Enlargement

Hilar lymph nodes **(35b)** are easier to identify on PA radiographs **(Fig. 73.1a)** than infracarinal lymph nodes, but they require differentiation from other causes of hilar enlargement (see **Table 66.1**), such as pulmonary venous congestion.

Contrast-enhanced CT scans **(Fig. 73.1c)** can positively distinguish the lymph nodes **(35)** from the pulmonary arteries **(9a, b)** and other vascular segments. Note also the accompanying pleural effusion **(41)** with adjacent dyselectasis **(36)**.

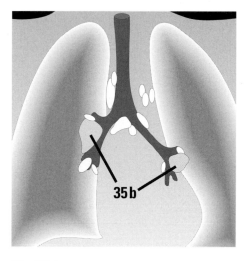

Fig. 73.1 a

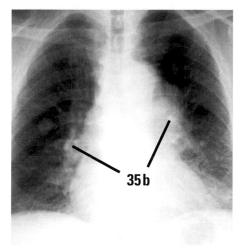

Fig. 73.1 b

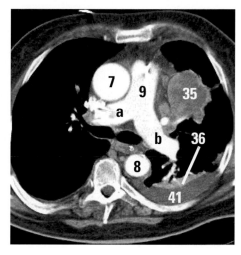

Fig. 73.1 c

Enlarged paratracheal lymph nodes **(35c)** are generally easier to identify on the right side **(Fig. 73.2a)** than on the left side **(Fig. 73.2c)** because enlarged nodes on the left side tend to be obscured by the overlying aortic arch and other mediastinal soft tissues. **Figure 73.2b** shows a right paratracheal lymph node (→) located precisely at the junction of the trachea **(14)**

and right main bronchus **(14a)** in a setting of chronic tuberculosis (TB). In this case the superimposed aortic arch **(6)** and other mediastinal structures make it impossible to evaluate for concomitant left paratracheal lymph node involvement.

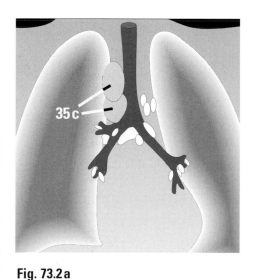

Fig. 73.2 a

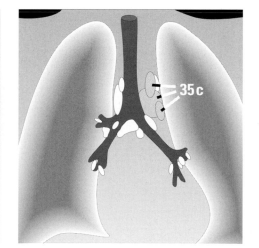

Fig. 73.2 b

Fig. 73.2 c

The differential diagnosis of enlarged mediastinal lymph nodes includes acute and chronic inflammations (sarcoidosis, TB), systemic lymphatic diseases (Hodgkin disease, non-Hodgkin lymphoma), and lymph node metastases. Bilateral enlargement of the hilar lymph nodes **(35b)** is a classic sign of sarcoidosis **(Fig. 74.1)**, particularly in stage I (see p. 131). Strictly unilateral hilar involvement is less commonly observed in sarcoidosis [5.10]. "Bihilar lymphadenopathy" cannot always be definitively diagnosed on chest radiographs, however **(Fig. 74.2)**, and requires differentiation from other conditions such as predominantly central vascular congestion (see **Fig. 77.2**). When lymphadenopathy is present, the differential diagnosis is narrowed by the absence of Kerley B lines, cardiomegaly, and other congestive signs.

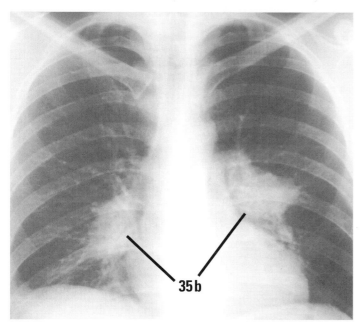

Fig. 74.1

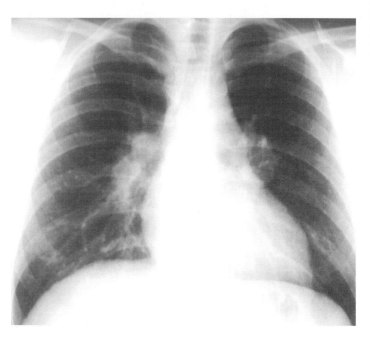

Fig. 74.2

TB of the hilar lymph nodes is marked by an absence of typical signs of pulmonary infection (see p. 116). The only abnormal finding on the chest radiograph is infiltration of the hilar lymph nodes (↘ in **Fig. 74.3**). Later stages of the disease may present with "speckled" calcifications in the hilar lymph nodes (→) (see also **Fig. 73.2b**). In silicosis **(Fig. 74.4)**, the changes in pulmonary markings (see p. 149) are accompanied by hilar lymphadenopathy **(35)**. When the hilar notch of a lymph node becomes calcified, an egg-shell calcification pattern can be seen. The examiner should be particularly alert for silicosis-related lymphadenopathy in patients who work in mining or the ceramic-processing industry.

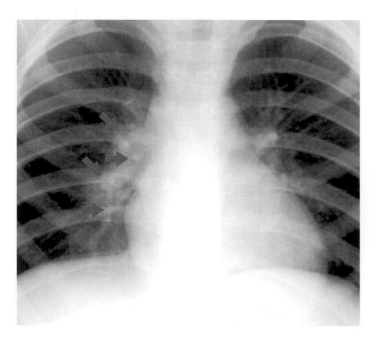

Fig. 74.3

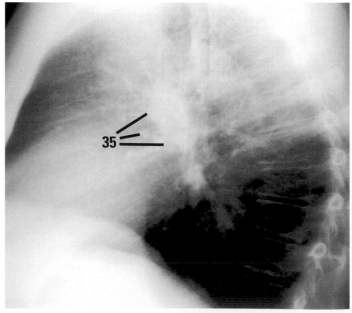

Fig. 74.4

Malignant lymphomas may develop in all mediastinal compartments (see p. 65 and p. 69). With hilar involvement, progressive enlargement of the lymphoma **(Fig. 75.1a, b)** may lead to bronchial obstruction with poststenotic dyselectasis (here in the right basal lung) or infiltration of the phrenic nerve causing elevation of the ipsilateral hemidiaphragm (↟ in **Fig. 75.a b**). Chest radiographs are not useful for excluding the infiltration of surrounding structures or monitoring response to treatment, which require evaluation by CT or MRI [5.11].

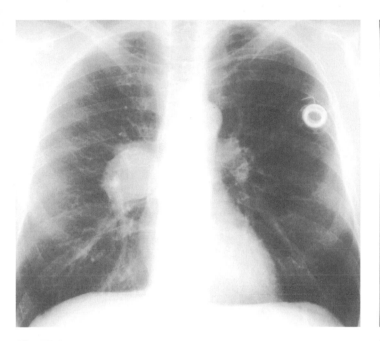

Fig. 75.1 a

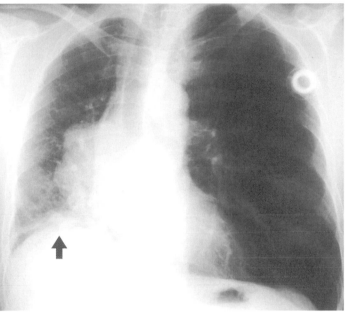

Fig. 75.1 b

Thoracic CT scans in this patient **(Fig. 75.2)** accurately define the mediastinal and intrapulmonary extent of the tumor **(21)** and show partial collapse **(36)** of the right middle lobe, causing the mediastinum (←) to become shifted toward the affected side. Metastatic enlargement of the hilar lymph nodes is consistently seen in association with primary bronchial, breast, and esophageal cancers.

Imaging of patients with bronchial carcinoma (see p. 117) initially shows unilateral involvement of the mediastinal lymph nodes. With small-cell BC, lymph node metastases are often the only change that is detectable on standard radiographs.

Mediastinal lymph node metastases from extrathoracic tumors are less commonly observed [5.12]. They originate from the gastrointestinal or urogenital tract.

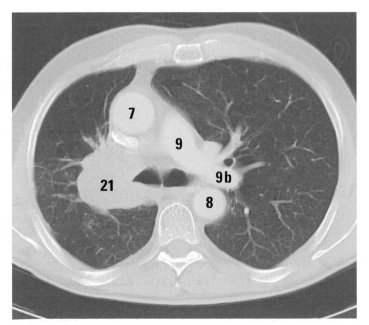

Fig. 75.2 a

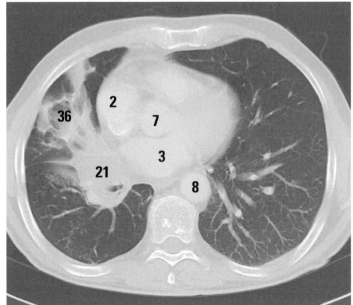

Fig. 75.2 b

Central Bronchial Carcinomas

Central bronchial carcinomas (BCs) located near the hilum (**Fig. 76.1**) lead to hilar enlargement (←). A malignant cause should always be considered, especially in cases with unilateral findings. The radiograph in **Figure 76.1a** shows atelectatic changes in the apicoposterior segment (segments I + II) of the left upper lobe (**36**) due to bronchial stenosis. In a radiograph taken 10 months later (**Fig. 76 1b**), the progression of tumor growth is manifested by complete atelectasis (**36**) of the left upper lobe, a left-sided pleural effusion (↘), metastasis to the contralateral hilar lymph nodes (→), and progressive elevation of the ipsilateral hemidiaphragm (↑).

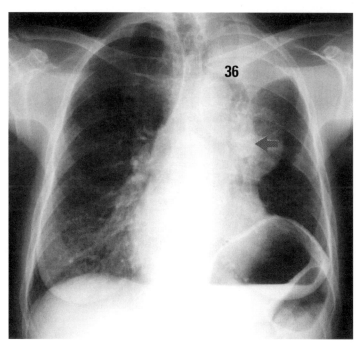

Fig. 76.1 a

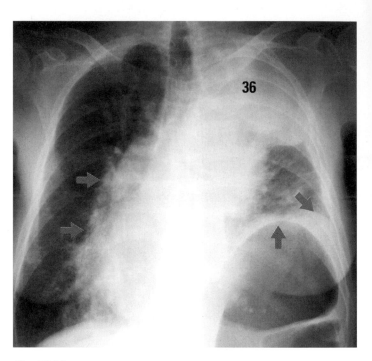

Fig. 76.1 b

Figure 76.2a shows a central BC at the hilum of the right lung (**21**). Treatment consisted of a right lower lobectomy followed by radiotherapy. In a follow-up radiograph taken at seven months (**Fig. 76.2b**), the response to radiotherapy is marked by streaky densities on the right mediastinal border (↖) and a right basal effusion (**41**). Other frequent complications of thoracic irradiation are radiation-induced pneumonitis (see p. 153) and esophagitis.

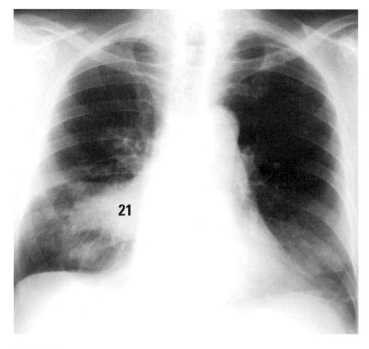

Fig. 76.2 a

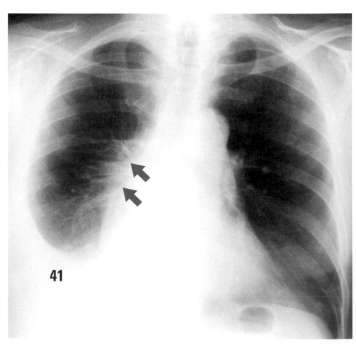

Fig. 76.2 b

Vascular Causes of Hilar Enlargement

Hilar enlargement with a vascular cause may result from pulmonary venous congestion or pulmonary arterial hypertension. The chest radiograph in pulmonary arterial hypertension may show "pruning" of the pulmonary vessels (→ in **Fig. 77.1**), i.e., the enlarged central pulmonary arteries taper rapidly to the constricted peripheral arteries, with an associated decrease in peripheral vascular markings.

Hilar enlargement (**10b**) in the setting of acute pulmonary venous congestion (**Fig. 77.2**) can be distinguished from chronic pulmonary hypertension by the dilatation of the peripheral lung vessels (↘) and associated signs of congestion such as horizontal Kerley B lines (↓) and the development of pleural effusion (**41**) (see p. 21, p. 142).

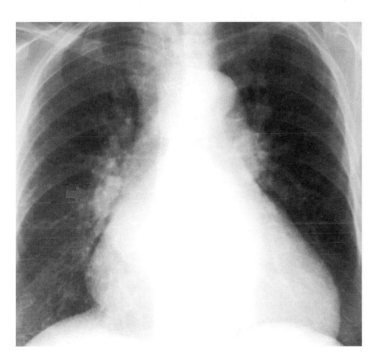

Fig. 77.1

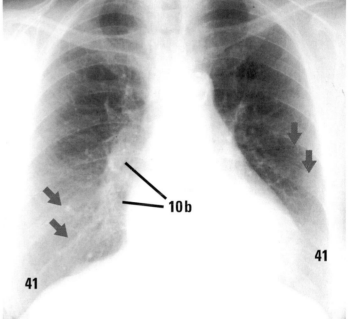

Fig. 77.2

In **Figure 77.3**, aneurysmal dilatation of the left pulmonary artery (**9b**) led to sharply circumscribed, rounded hilar widening in the area of the pulmonary segment. By contrast, the pulmonary segment (↙) may be completely absent in patients with pulmonary atresia (**Fig. 77.4**). In this case the bronchial arteries that supply blood to the lung arise directly

from the aorta and appear as fine lines emanating from the hilum (←) (see also **Fig. 87.1c**). When an MR image in pulmonary atresia (**Fig. 77.5a**) is compared with a normal image (**Fig. 77.5b**), the anomaly is distinguished by absence of the pulmonary trunk (**9**) between the ascending aorta (**7**) and descending aorta (**8**) at the level of the tracheal bifurcation (**14**).

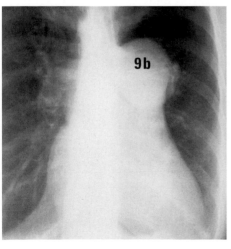

Fig. 77.3

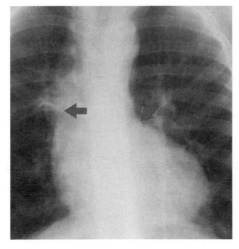

Fig. 77.4

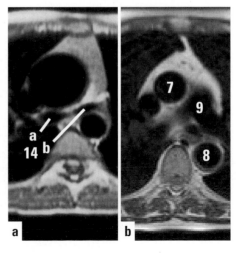

Fig. 77.5

Neurogenic Tumors

Neurogenic tumors are the most common primary neoplasms of the posterior mediastinum [5.4]. Ninety percent of these tumors have a direct paravertebral location. They are somewhat rare in adults and arise from the myelin sheaths of peripheral nerves in the form of schwannomas or neurofibromas. In children, on the other hand, they most commonly arise from neurons of the sympathetic ganglia. This group includes malignant neuroblastomas and benign ganglioneuromas.

Ganglioneuromas appear radiographically as well-circumscribed paraspinal masses **(21)** that form a convex bulge (▶) in the mediastinal silhouette **(Fig. 78.1a)**. The modality of choice for evaluating tumor extent and detecting possible infiltration of adjacent structures is MRI **(Fig. 78.1b)**. In the case shown, MRI confirmed the tumor morphology based on

the classic shape (↗) and paraspinal location of the mass. Many neuroblastomas (↖) also appear as well-circumscribed paraspinal masses in the posterior mediastinum **(Fig. 78.2)**.

With tumors that form a plaquelike growth along the posterior chest wall, the PA radiograph **(Fig. 78.3a)** may show an infiltrating mass with ill-defined margins **(21)**. The lateral projection shows that the tumor is solid (↖) and is located on the posterior rib segments **(Fig. 78.3b)**, but even so the lesion may be easily overlooked, especially if the patient is in a slightly oblique position.

Supplementary CT **(Fig. 78.3c)** defines the extent of the tumor along the posterior chest wall and also shows calcifications **(50)** within the neuroblastoma **(21)**.

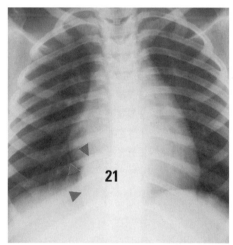
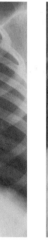

Fig. 78.1 a

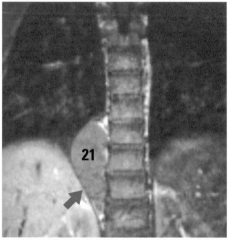

Fig. 78.1 b

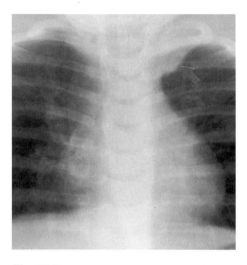

Fig. 78.2

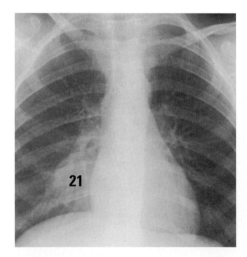

Fig. 78.3 a

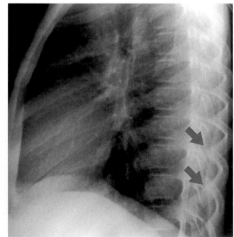

Fig. 78.3 b

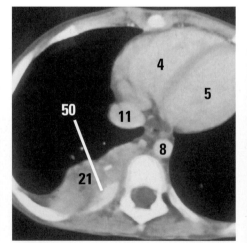

Fig. 78.3 c

Mediastinal Abscess

The focal variant of mediastinitis is a mediastinal abscess **(Fig. 79.1a)**. As in diffuse mediastinitis (see **Fig. 67.3a**), esophageal perforations are a frequent cause. Consequently, these abscesses are often located in the posterior mediastinum and appear as paravertebral opacities (▶) that form a laterally convex bulge. They are easily missed on chest radiographs, depending on the level and width of the cardiac silhouette.

In the case illustrated, the abscess was initially noted during an ultrasound examination of the liver **(Fig. 79.1b)**, appearing as a septated cystic mass (➡) behind the vena cava **(11)**. MRI confirms the cystic nature of the mass (⬆) and the retrocaval location of the abscess **(Fig. 79.1c)**.

Abscesses due to other causes (e.g., surgery or trauma) might occur virtually anywhere in the mediastinum. A disk space infection of sufficient size may also produce a convex paraspinal bulge (⬉ in **Fig. 79.2**).

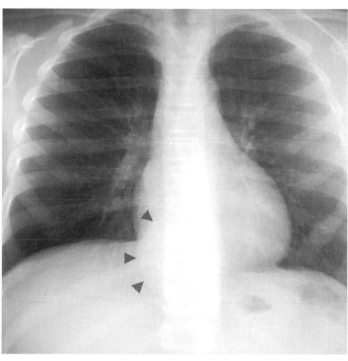

Fig. 79.1 a

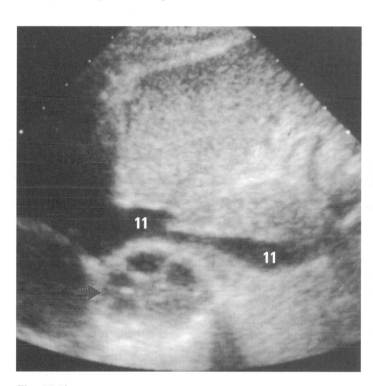

Fig. 79.1 b

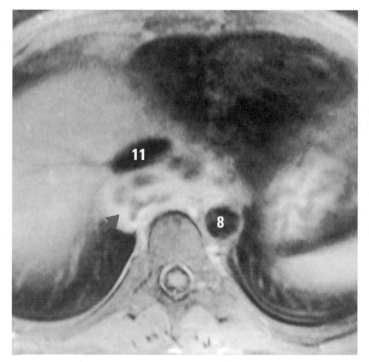

Fig. 79.1 c

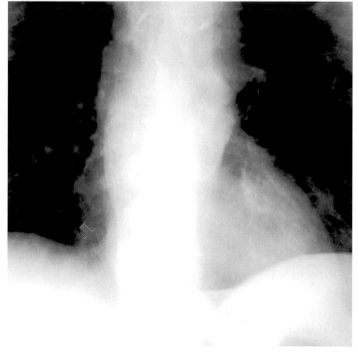

Fig. 79.2

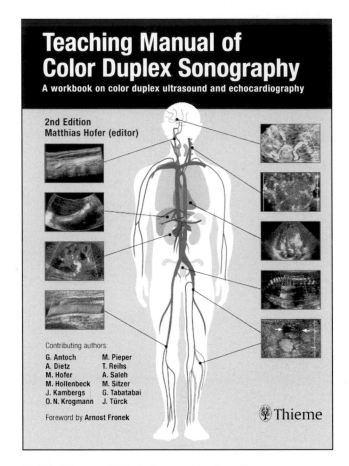
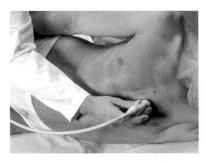
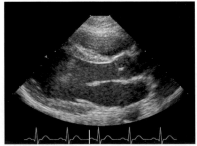
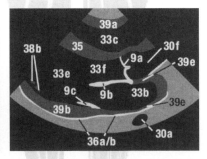
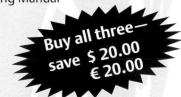

The conventional chest radiograph is a fast, objective, and cost-effective technique for evaluating the heart. It is easily performed by a technologist and does not require the presence of a physician. Of course, echocardiography can provide much more precise information than conventional radiographs with regard to ventricular function and the condition of the pericardium and cardiac valves. The valve opening area, for example, can be accurately determined to assess the need for operative treatment in patients with stenotic valvular disease. But because the chest radiograph can simultaneously evaluate diseases of the lung, mediastinum, and chest wall, it continues to be an indispensable tool in routine examinations of the heart.

Cardiomegaly

The most frequent cause of a broadened cardiac silhouette in the lower mediastinum (cardiomegaly) is dilatation of the cardiac chambers. The size of the cardiac silhouette is described in terms of the cardiothoracic ratio (CTR; see **Fig. 27.1**). Cardiomegaly is present when the CTR is greater than 0.5 (**Fig. 81.1**). In the example shown, the dilated cardiac silhouette has a maximum width of 22.3 cm (**C**), while the total thoracic diameter (**T**) measures 33.5 cm between the inner margins of the lateral ribs (**Fig. 81.1**). The C/T ratio in this case (22.3/33.5) equals 0.66, which confirms the presence of cardiomegaly.

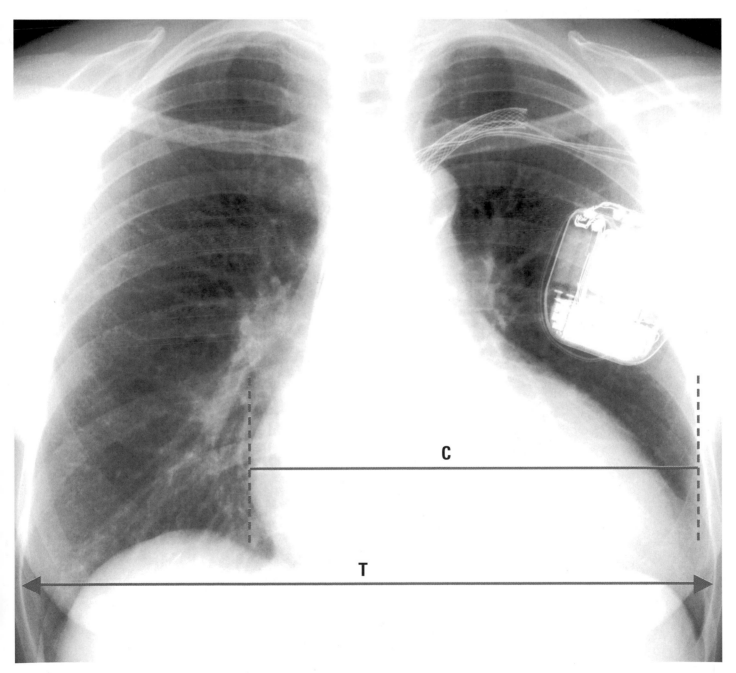

Fig. 81.1

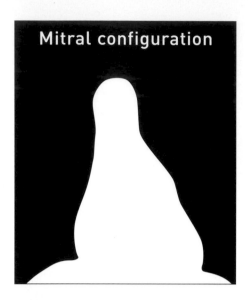

Mitral configuration

Valvular Heart Disease

Stenosis or insufficiency of the mitral valve allows blood to reflux into the left atrium, causing that chamber to become dilated. As a result, mitral valve diseases often produce a mitral configuration of the left cardiac border on the chest radiograph **(Fig. 82.1a)**. The dilated left atrium leads to broadening of the cardiac waist (↗ ↗) and may produce a double contour sign (green area in **Fig. 82.1b**). The atrial dilatation may be so pronounced that the left atrium appears to touch the right mediastinal border (→).

Atrial dilatation may also cause splaying of the tracheal bifurcation (↖ ↗) between the right main bronchus **(14a)** and left main bronchus **(14b) (Fig. 82.2)**, similar to that caused by enlarged infracarinal lymph nodes (see p. 72) or a large pericardial effusion [5.9].

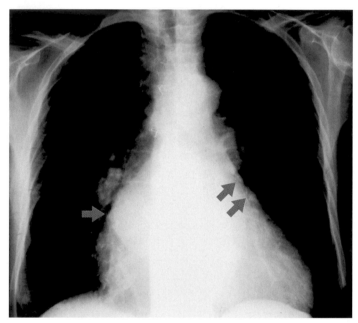

Fig. 82.1 a

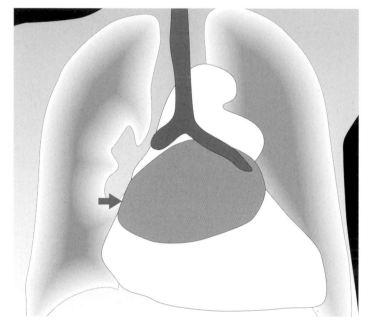

Fig. 82.1 b

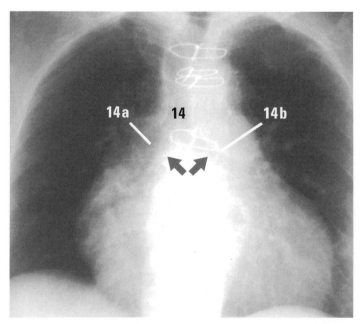

Fig. 82.2 a

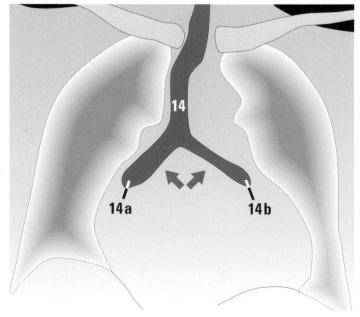

Fig. 82.2 b

Aortic configuration

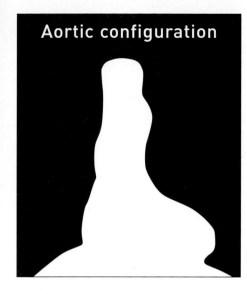

Diseases of the aortic valve often produce an aortic configuration on the chest radiograph **(Fig. 83.1)**. The basic principle is the same as in mitral valve disease, as stenosis or insufficiency of the aortic valve leads to hypertrophy or dilatation of the left ventricle. As a result, the left ventricular border (↗) is shifted toward the left side while the cardiac waist is preserved (↙).

Cor bovinum **(Fig. 83.2)** is the term applied to extreme, bilateral cardiac enlargement with a CTR greater than 0.66. The potential causes include severe aortic insufficiency, cardiomyopathies, and combined valvular disease.

Unlike the harmonious expansion of the cardiac silhouette that results from a dilated heart chamber **(Fig. 83.2)**, a myocardial aneurysm produces a circumscribed bulge (↗) in the cardiac silhouette **(Fig. 83.3)**. In doubtful cases the diagnosis can be established by echocardiography, which will show paradoxical contraction (dyskinesia) of the left ventricular wall at the site of the aneurysm.

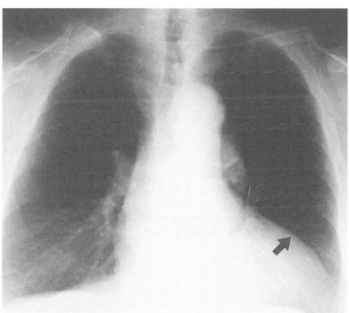

Fig. 83.1 a

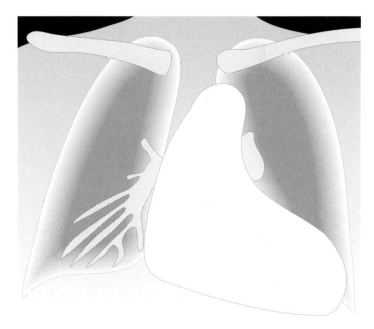

Fig. 83.1 b

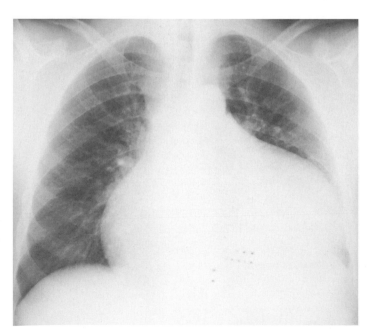

Fig. 83.2

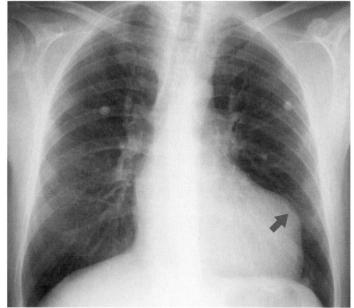

Fig. 83.3

Differentiation Between Stenosis and Insufficiency

Several morphological criteria are available for differentiating the radiographic features of valvular diseases.

In the case of mitral stenosis, the cardiac silhouette will show a typical mitral configuration with a broadened cardiac waist. The reduction of blood flow across the mitral valve leads to dilatation of the left atrium (see p. 82), while the left ventricle remains normal in size. A lateral radiograph after oral contrast administration may define the extent of the left atrial dilatation. The esophagus will deviate markedly from its normal vertical course **(Fig. 84.1)** and will show convex posterior bowing at the level of the left atrium (➔ in **Fig. 84.2**). Radiographs in chronic mitral stenosis will additionally show signs of pulmonary venous congestion due to the damming back of blood into the pulmonary circulation (see p. 77).

Mitral insufficiency leads to left atrial dilatation with an associated mitral configuration of the heart. Additionally, the bidirectional blood flow imposes a volume load on the left ventricle. The resulting left ventricular dilatation (➘) can be appreciated in the lateral radiograph **(Fig. 84.3)** based on narrowing of the retrocardiac space **(13)**. This narrowing occurs at a considerably lower level than that produced by atrial dilatation (➔ in **Fig. 84.2**). As a result, the disappearance of a vena cava triangle **(11)** seen on previous radiographs may provide an early sign of incipient left ventricular dilatation.

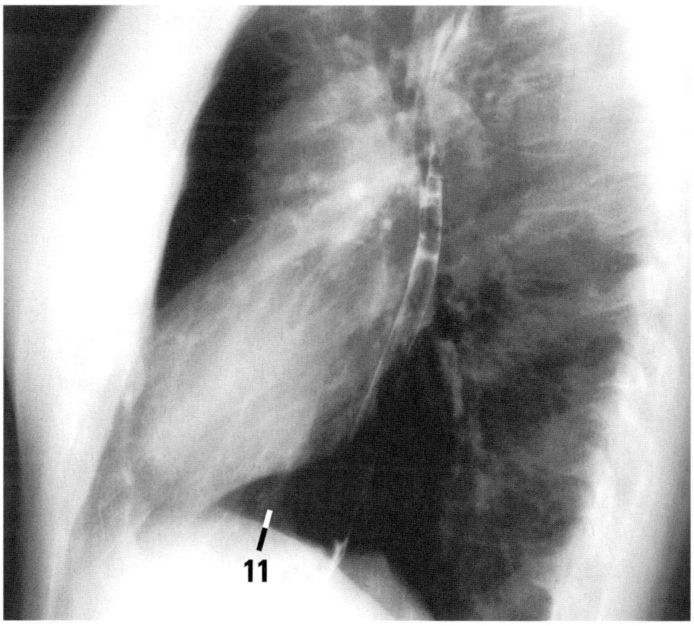

Fig. 84.1 a

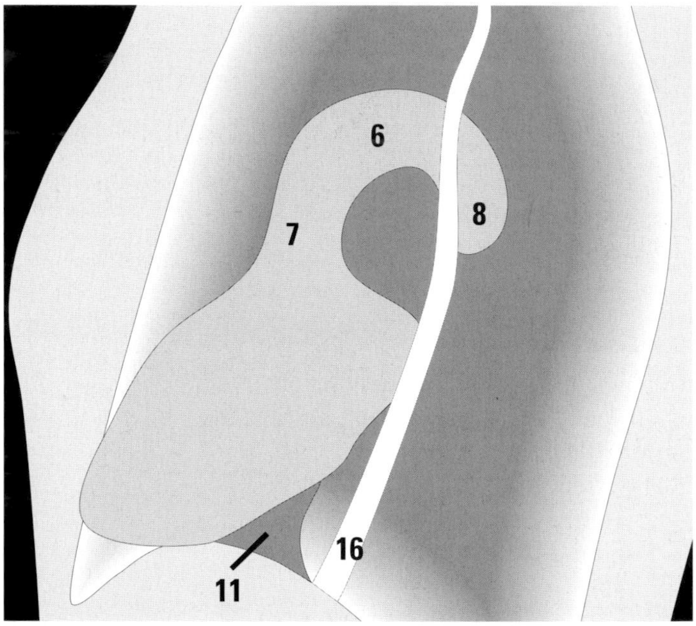

Fig. 84.1 b

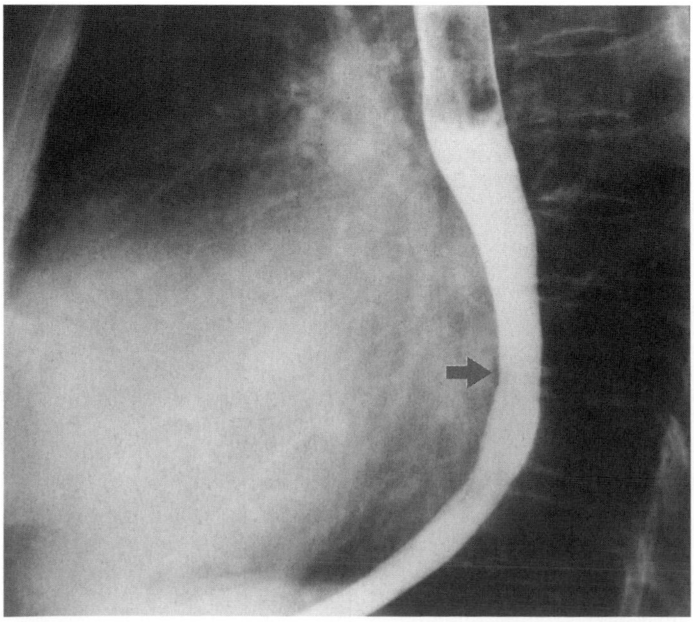

Fig. 84.2

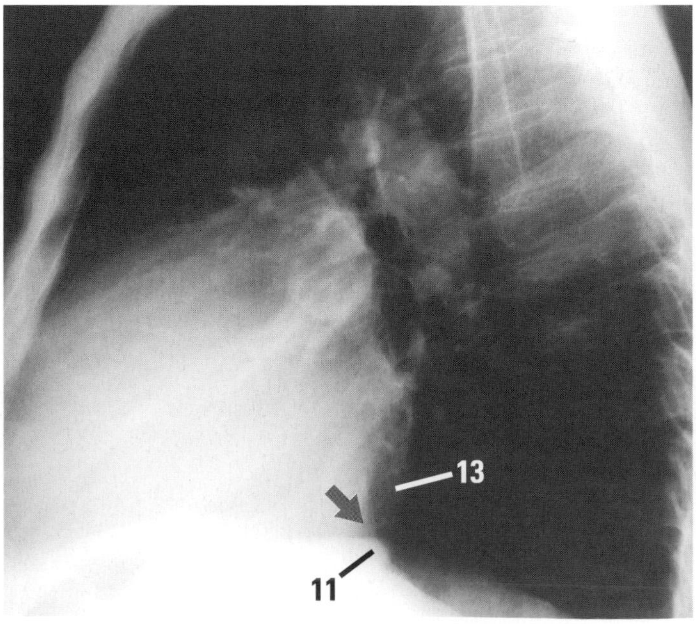

Fig. 84.3

Mitral Stenosis

Cardiac size

- Normal-sized left ventricle
- Dilated left atrium ⇨
  - PA: possible double contour sign
  - Lat: High narrowing of RCS by
    the left atrium **alone**
- Small aortic knob (compared with aortic stenosis)
- With high-grade stenosis: Possible relative
  tricuspid insufficiency

Pulmonary vessels

- Marked signs of pulmonary venous congestion
  (see p. 77)
- Signs of pulmonary hypertension (see p. 77)

Table 85.1

Mitral Insufficiency

Cardiac size

- Left ventricular dilatation plus
- Left atrial dilatation ⇨
  - PA: Possible double contour sign
  - Lat.: Complete narrowing of RCS by
    the left atrium **and** ventricle

Pulmonary vessels

- Relatively mild signs of pulmonary venous
  congestion (periodic pressure load on
  pulmonary circulation)

Table 85.2

In cases of pure aortic stenosis unaccompanied by aortic insufficiency, the cardiac silhouette often maintains a normal size initially, because at first the pressure load causes only a concentric hypertrophy of the left ventricular myocardium. Often there is associated poststenotic dilatation of the ascending aorta, but the extent of the dilatation does not correlate directly with the severity of the stenosis [5.13]. Fluoroscopy will often show calcifications projected over the aortic valve, but these may occur even in the absence of hemodynamically significant stenosis. In patients with aortic insufficiency, on

the other hand, the volume load leads to early, eccentric dilatation of the left ventricle, resulting in an aortic configuration of the left cardiac border (see **Fig. 83.1**). Thus, the PA radiograph will show an earlier increase in the CTR than is observed in patients with aortic stenosis.

In cases of primary valvular insufficiency, the luminal size of the aorta remains unchanged. But when the insufficiency is secondary to an aneurysm of the ascending aorta, the typical signs of aortic dilatation may be found.

Aortic Stenosis

Cardiac size

- CTR is often normal initially, and later is increased ↑
  (pressure load ⇨ concentric hypertrophy)
- RCS: Initially normal; becomes narrowed later

Aorta

- Possible poststenotic ectasia
  (does not correlate with degree of stenosis)
- Fluoroscopy may show aortic valve calcification.

Table 85.3

Aortic Insufficiency

Cardiac size

- CTR increased ↑
  (volume load ⇨ eccentric dilatation)
- RCS: Immediate narrowing

Aorta

- Normal luminal size in primary aortic insufficiency
- Secondary insufficiency (e.g., aneurysm)
  ➡ signs of aortic dilatation (see p. 93)

Table 85.4

Once very rare, primary diseases of the tricuspid valve have become more common in recent years due to the rising incidence of drug abuse. Infectious valvular diseases frequently develop after intravenous injections with non-sterile needles. **Figure 86.1** illustrates a case of tricuspid insufficiency accompanied by a bradycardiac arrhythmia in a female drug user. This case was managed by implanting a prosthetic valve (⬇) and a pacemaker module (see p. 167 and p. 172) **(Fig. 86.1)**.

A much more common condition is relative tricuspid insufficiency, which may occur in a setting of mitral stenosis, for example. The valve becomes incompetent due to myogenic dilatation of the right ventricle and tricuspid valve ring. The resulting dilatation of the right atrium causes massive widening of the cardiac silhouette toward the right side in the PA radiograph (⬅).

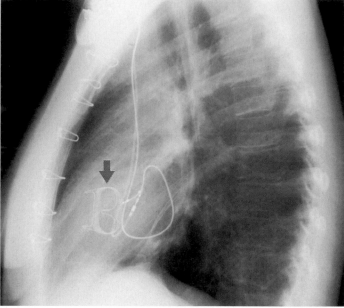

Fig. 86.1

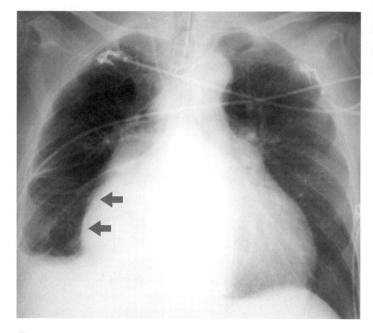

Fig. 86.2

Congenital Heart Diseases

The primary task of conventional imaging studies in congenital heart diseases is to differentiate between conditions that are associated with an increase or decrease in pulmonary blood flow. Nonspecific widening of the cardiac silhouette is a common finding, depending on the degree of severity. The ventricular septal defect (VSD; **Fig. 86.3**) and patent ductus arteriosus (PDA; **Fig. 86.4**) are typical congenital defects characterized by the left-to-right shunt of blood with an increase in pulmonary perfusion. By contrast, diseases such as pulmonary atresia **(Fig. 86.5)** and the tetralogy of Fallot (see p. 87) are characterized by decreased pulmonary blood flow, causing a decrease in pulmonary vascular markings (increased lucency) on the chest radiograph.

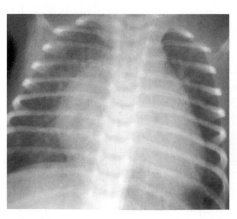

Fig. 86.3

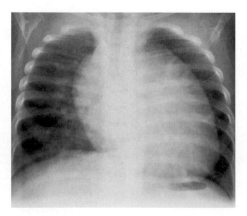

Fig. 86.4

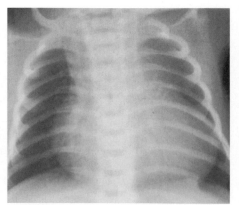

Fig. 86.5

The tetralogy of Fallot (**Fig. 87.1a-c**) is the most common congenital cyanotic heart disease. It is a combination of anomalies consisting of a VSD, a right-sided aorta that "overrides" the VSD, and primary infundibular pulmonary stenosis, which leads to right ventricular hypertrophy.

The radiographic hallmarks are an enlarged right ventricle with an elevated cardiac apex (↖), a small or absent pulmonary segment (↙) and, in approximately 25% of cases, a right-sided aortic arch (↘ in **Fig. 87.1a**). The CTR is 0.66 in the case illustrated but is not necessarily increased in every case. The lateral radiograph also shows the typical right ventricular enlargement (←), which in this case is combined with an enlarged left ventricle (→) (**Fig. 87.1b**).

Pulmonary stenosis leads to attenuation of the pulmonary vessels, which is often associated with a compensatory enlargement of bronchial arteries arising from the aorta. These vessels can be identified as straight intrapulmonary lines (↓ in **Fig. 87.1c**). A common palliative procedure for the tetralogy of Fallot is the Blalock-Taussig operation. In this procedure the subclavian artery is divided proximal to the origin of the internal thoracic artery (ITA) and anastomosed to the pulmonary artery in order to increase blood flow to the lungs. The arm receives retrograde blood flow through the ITA, which in turn is supplied by the intercostal arteries arising from the aorta. The increased blood flow in the intercostal arteries leads to erosive notching the inferior rib margins (↑ in **Fig. 87.1c**). This notching occurs only on the side of the shunt, contrasting with the bilateral rib notches found in coarctation of the aorta (see the Chapter 3 and **Fig. 88.1**).

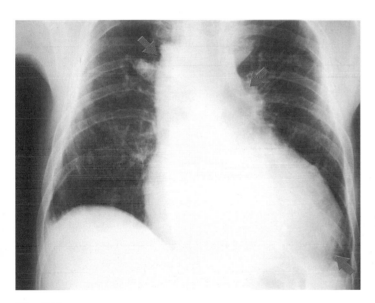

Fig. 87.1 a

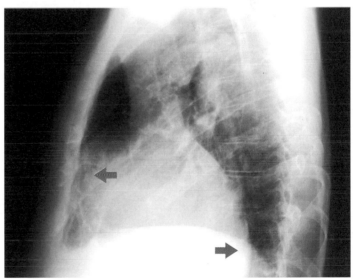

Fig. 87.1 b

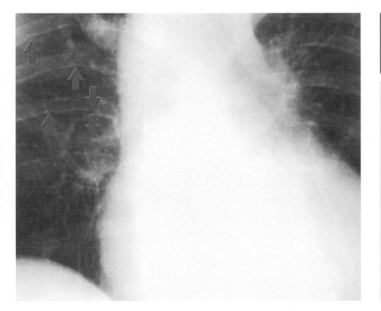

Fig. 87.1 c

Radiographic Checklist for the Tetralogy of Fallot

- Enlarged right ventricle with an elevated apex
- Small or concave pulmonary segment
- Attenuation of pulmonary vessels
- Normal-sized or enlarged aorta with a right-sided aortic arch (in approximately 25% of cases)
- Short, straight intrapulmonary lines (enlarged bronchial arteries from the aorta)
- CTR not necessarily increased
- Ipsilateral rib notches following a Blalock-Taussig operation

Table 87.2

In coarctation of the aorta (COA), the aortic lumen is constricted distal to the left subclavian artery near the insertion of the ductus arteriosus. This raises the blood pressure in the lower half of the body while decreasing blood flow to the upper half of the body. A brisk collateral circulation develops through the intercostal arteries, and the increased blood flow through these vessels causes bilateral notching of the ribs (⬆ in **Fig. 88.1**). The direction of this flow is opposite to that following the Blalock-Taussig operation (p. 87), with blood flowing from the subclavian artery through the ITA into the intercostal arteries. This provides compensatory collateral flow to the descending aorta that circumvents the stenotic segment.

In some cases the prestenotic and poststenotic widening of the descending aorta at the coarctation site may produce a "figure 3" sign (⬅) at the left border of the superior mediastinum **(Fig. 88.3a, b)**.

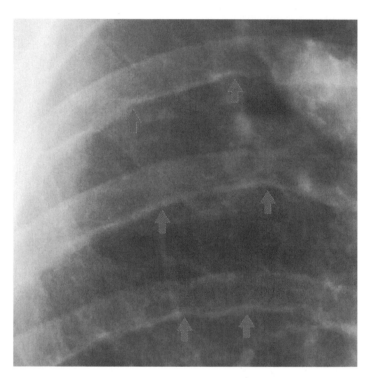

Fig. 88.1

Radiographic Checklist for Coarctation of the Aorta

- Bilateral notching of the third through ninth ribs

- Prominent, dilated ascending aorta

- Prestenotic and poststenotic widening of the descending aorta ("figure 3" sign)

- Possible widening of the superior mediastinum due to dilatation of the subclavian artery

Table 88.2

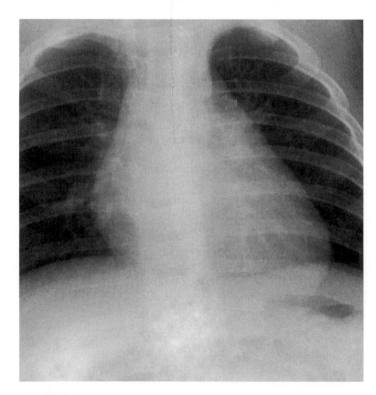

Fig. 88.3 a

"Figure 3" sign

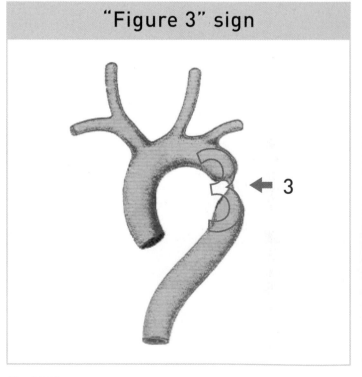

Fig. 88.3 b

Transposition of the great arteries (TGA) is a rotational abnormality in which the pulmonary and systemic circulations are separate and parallel. It is compatible with life only if shunts have been established between the two circulations.

The radiographic changes in the cardiac borders depend on the severity of the associated cardiac anomalies. The case illustrated is marked by a prominent pulmonary segment (✐) and bilateral cardiac enlargement (←→ in **Fig. 89.1**).

When we compare a normal thoracic CT scan (**Fig. 89.2a**) with a scan in TGA (**Fig. 89.2b**), we note that the aortic arch (**6**) in TGA is not oblique but has an almost anteroposterior orientation.

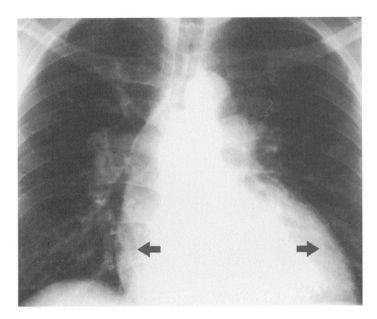

Fig. 89.1

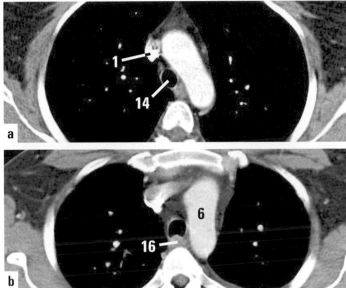

Fig. 89.2

Comparing the normal anatomy at a lower level (**Fig. 89.3a**) with the findings in TGA (**Fig. 89.3b**), we note that the pulmonary trunk (**9**) and ascending aorta (**7**) are transposed. The cyanosis typical of TGA was absent in this case because the patient had a monoventricular heart (**4, 5**), which established an adequate connection between the two circulations (**Fig. 89.4b**). In a monoventricular heart, both arterioventricular (AV) valves open into one large chamber from which the ascending aorta and pulmonary trunk arise. Because the single chamber usually has a left ventricular trabecular structure, the patient is at risk of developing pulmonary hypertension. In the case shown, this is evidenced by dilatation of both pulmonary arteries (**9a, b**) and the pulmonary trunk (**9**) in **Figure 89.3b**.

The normal CT findings in **Figure 89.4a** contrast markedly with the global dilatation of both atria (**2, 3**) and the common ventricle (**4, 5**) seen in **Figure 89.4b**.

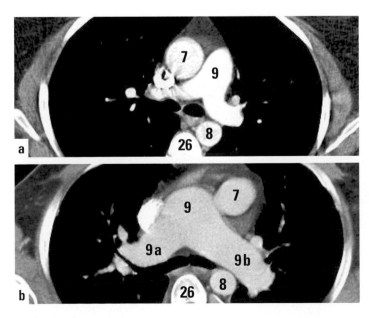

Fig. 89.3

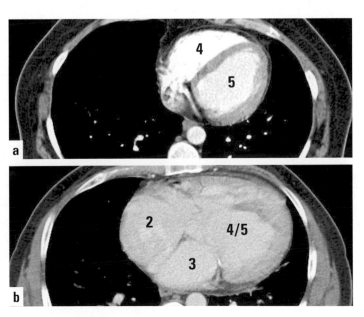

Fig. 89.4

Pericardium

Pericardial effusions may have various causes, including viral and tuberculous infections, rheumatological diseases, uremia, postmyocardial infarction syndrome, and postcardiotomy syndrome. Other possible causes are traumatic hemorrhage (e.g., due to aortic dissection [5.14]) and post-irradiation changes [5.15].

Cardiomegaly in the setting of a pericardial effusion may produce a "tent" appearance with an obscured left cardiac border (✐ in **Fig. 90.1a**). The lateral radiograph **(Fig. 90.1b)** shows global enlargement of the cardiac silhouette with narrowing of the retrosternal space (RSS) **(12)** and retrocar-

diac space (RCS) **(13)**. These contour changes are nonspecific, however [5.16], and the differential diagnosis should always include myogenic dilatation of the left ventricle. CT **(Fig. 90.1c)** or echocardiography **(Fig. 90.1d)** can establish the correct diagnosis. These modalities can detect even very small amounts of pericardial fluid **(40)**.

With a large effusion causing incipient pericardial tamponade (see FAST, p. 194-195), the decreased cardiac output may cause a decrease in pulmonary vascular markings (see p. 25) with prominence of the SVC along the right mediastinal border (see also **Fig. 25.2**).

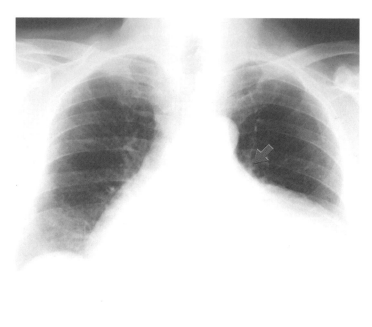

Fig. 90.1 a

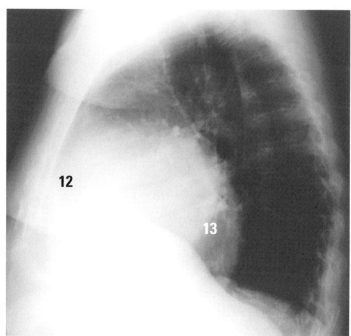

Fig. 90.1 b

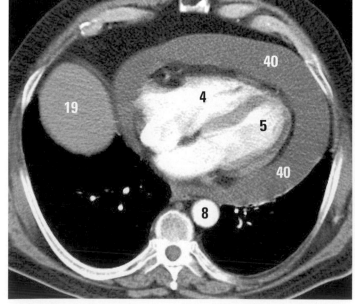

Fig. 90.1 c

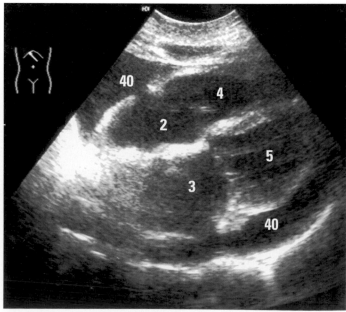

Fig. 90.1 d

Chronic constrictive pericarditis may develop as a sequel to pericarditis or pericardial effusion (**Fig. 91.1**). In typical cases a disproportion exists between the clinical manifestations of right-sided heart failure and the normal-sized heart.
Contraction of the pericardium due to scarring may be associated with the formation of peripheral eggshell calcifications (**50**).

Pneumopericardium (**Fig. 91.2**) may develop postoperatively or following the removal of a pericardial drain (↑ in **Fig. 91.3**). The trapped air forms a double contour along the cardiac borders (↘) and does not extend above the hilar region. This latter feature distinguishes it from pneumomediastinum and from an esophageal reconstruction (see p. 99) by gastric transposition (↙), for example (**Fig. 91.4**).

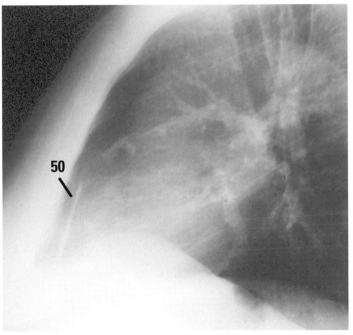

Fig. 91.1

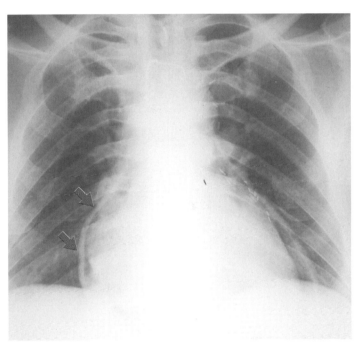

Fig. 91.2

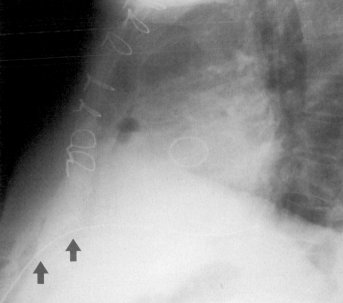

Fig. 91.3

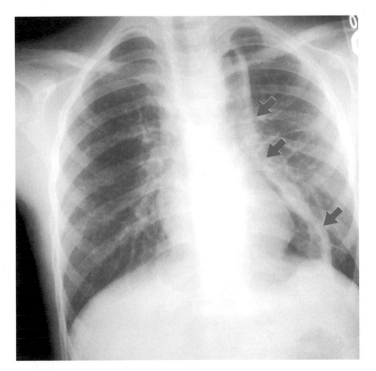

Fig. 91.4

Less commonly, pericardial cysts (49) may be diagnosed as an incidental finding (Fig. 92.1a). Most of these cysts result from a congenital disturbance of pericardial development. Pericardial cysts appear radiographically as a sharply circumscribed round or teardrop-shaped change in the cardiac contour. The radiographic density (attenuation) of the cyst contents can be evaluated by CT. The densitometry image after contrast administration in **Figure 92.1b** shows near–water attenuation values that are consistent with a

benigncyst: A mean value of 8.8 HU (Hounsfield units) with a standard deviation (SD) of 6.7 HU.

Approximately 70% of pericardial cysts are located in the right cardiophrenic angle (Fig. 92.1a) and only about 20% in the left cardiophrenic angle (Fig. 92.2a) [5.17]. CT demonstrates the close relationship of the cyst to the pericardium (Fig. 92.2b), thereby differentiating it from a loculated subpulmonic pleural effusion.

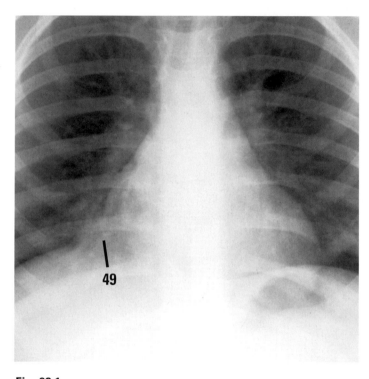

Fig. 92.1 a

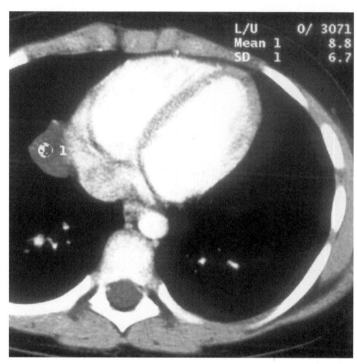

Fig. 92.1 b

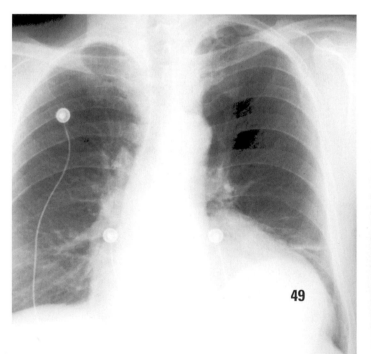

Fig. 92.2 a

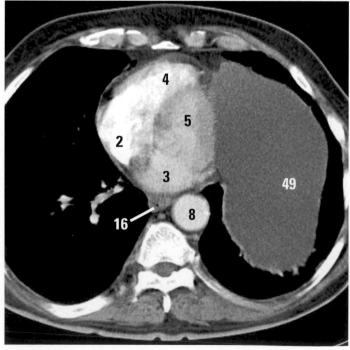

Fig. 92.2 b

Degenerative, inflammatory, or traumatic lesions of the aortic vessel wall may give rise to a thoracic aortic aneurysm (TAA). An aneurysm of the ascending aorta **(Fig. 93.1)** often produces a right-sided bulge (➡) on the PA radiograph, while a TAA of the descending aorta **(Fig. 93.2)** tends to cause a bulge on the left side (⬅).

Several morphological criteria have been established for aneurysm screening on chest radiographs [5.18] **(Table 93.3)**. In the lateral projection, measure the greatest distance between the anterior and posterior walls (D_{AO}) of the descending aorta **(Fig. 93.4)**. This value, if measurable, should be less than 4.5 cm. In the PA projection, measure the greatest distance between the left tracheal border and mediastinal border (D_{TM}) in the horizontal plane **(Fig. 93.5)**. This distance should be less than 5 cm. Additional signs are an ascending aorta that forms the upper right border of the cardiovascular silhouette (➡ in **Fig. 93.1**) and a convex bowing of the trachea toward the right side (⬅ in **Fig. 93.5**). Occasionally, the left main bronchus is also displaced downward by the dilated aorta (⬏ in **Fig. 93.1**).

Taken together, these criteria often permit an accurate evaluation of the aortic diameter. A normal set of values can exclude an aneurysm of the aortic arch and descending aorta with a high degree of confidence. All of the criteria should be analyzed, and no single criterion is diagnostic in itself [5.20].

Other imaging modalities such as CT or transesophageal echocardiography (TEE) are used to make a precise determination of luminal diameter, craniocaudal extent (involvement of supra-aortic branches?), and the shape of the aneurysm (saccular or fusiform?). The axial CT scan in **Figure 93.6** shows peripheral thrombosis **(51)** of the aneurysm involving the aortic arch **(6)** and descending aorta **(8)**.

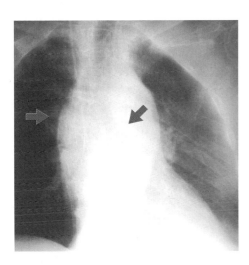

Fig. 93.1

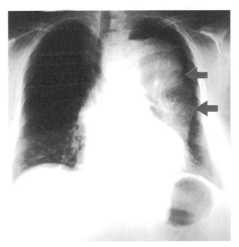

Fig. 93.2

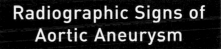

Radiographic Signs of Aortic Aneurysm

Lat.	• D_{AO} > 4,5 cm in lateral projection
PA	• D_{TM} > 5,0 cm • Ascending aorta forms upper right border of cardiovascular silhouette • Trachea displaced to the right side • Left main bronchus displaced upward

Table 93.3

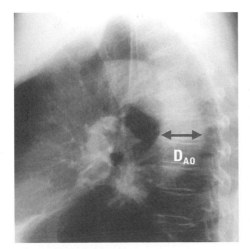

Fig. 93.4

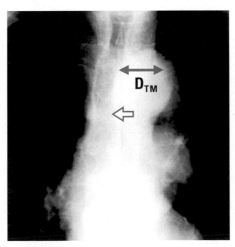
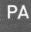
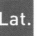

Fig. 93.5

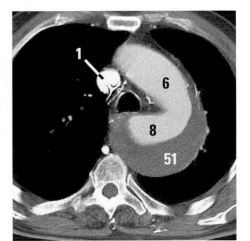

Fig. 93.6

An aortic dissection **(Fig. 94.1)** does not necessarily cause widening of the mediastinal shadow. CT is used to evaluate its extent and make a clinical classification **(Fig. 94.2)**. The intimal flap (✎) is clearly defined in the CT scan **(Fig. 94.3a)**. Multiplanar reconstructions of the CT data can supply valuable information for preoperative planning **(Fig. 94.3b)**. In the case illustrated, the patient had a dissecting aneurysm of the descending aorta **(8)** that did not involve the ascending aorta **(7)**. A pericardial or left-sided pleural effusion may be noted in the chest radiograph of an asymptomatic dissection [5.14].

Endovascular stent insertion is available as a minimally invasive option for the treatment of aneurysms and dissections (see **Fig. 171.4a, b** in Chapter 9).

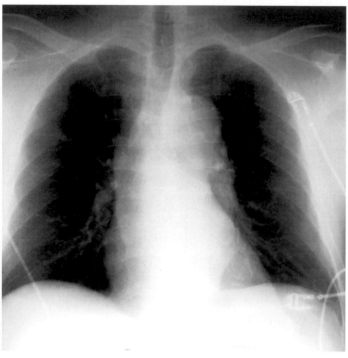

Fig. 94.1

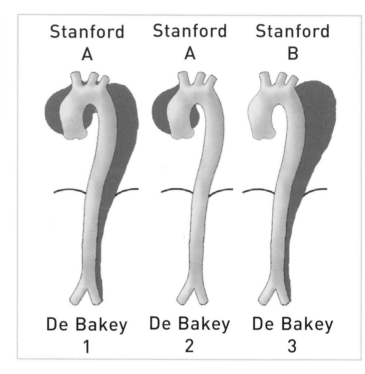

Fig. 94.2

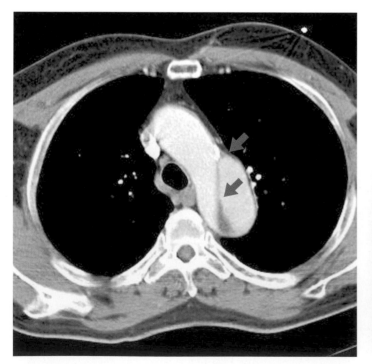

Fig. 94.3a

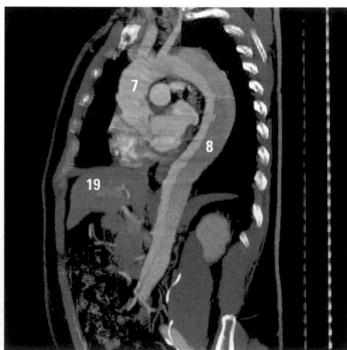

Fig. 94.3b

Calcifications in aortic sclerosis (↖), while a common incidental finding in older patients **(Fig. 95.1)**, are associated with an increased risk of coronary heart disease (CHD) and should therefore be mentioned in the radiology report [5.19].

In the patient in **Figure 95.2**, this association provided an indication for a coronary artery bypass graft. The sternal cerclage wires **(52)** from the operation are visible in the radiograph.

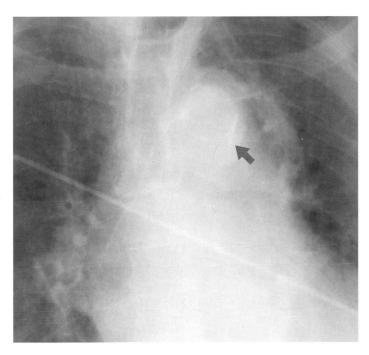

Fig. 95.1

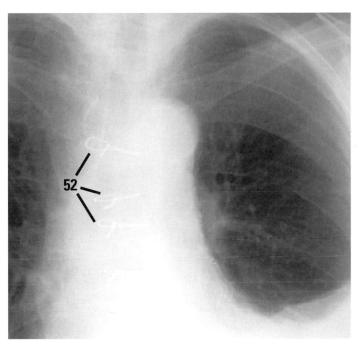

Fig. 95.2

Variants of vascular anatomy can also affect the mediastinal silhouette. The patient in **Figure 95.3** had a right descending aorta, indicated by the absence of the typical aortic knob (↗) above the left main bronchus **(14b)** and the visible segment

of descending aorta along the right mediastinal border (↘). In **Figure 95.4**, the right-sided aortic arch has caused pronounced displacement of the trachea **(14)** toward the left side (→).

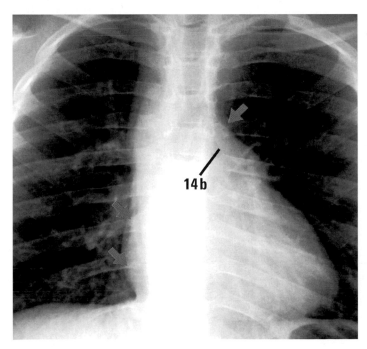

Fig. 95.3

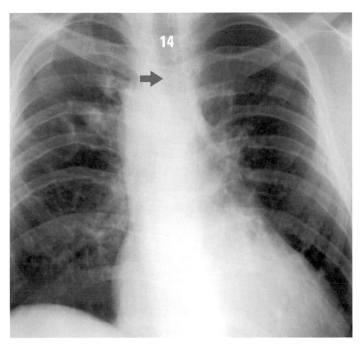

Fig. 95.4

Esophageal diverticula may develop at any level of the esophagus. Cervical Zenker diverticula (**Fig. 96.1a**) are the most common form, accounting for 70% of cases. When large enough, they may cause widening of the superior mediastinum (⇨). Typical, contrast-filled outpouchings can be seen at fluoroscopy (**Fig. 96.1b**).

Esophageal diverticula appear on CT (**Fig. 96.1c**) as sharply circumscribed masses (◄) located between the trachea (**14**) and thoracic spine (**26**). Esophageal atresia can also be demonstrated after the ingestion of a water-soluble contrast medium. This condition can also be diagnosed by passing a bougie down the esophagus under radiographic control. When atresia is present, the bougie will loop back upward (↗) after entering the blind esophageal pouch (**Fig. 96.2**).

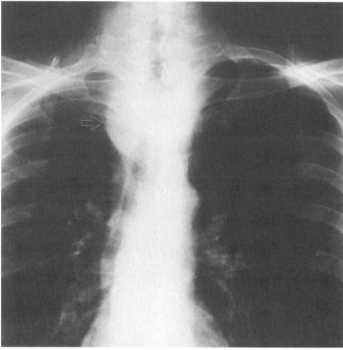

Fig. 96.1 a

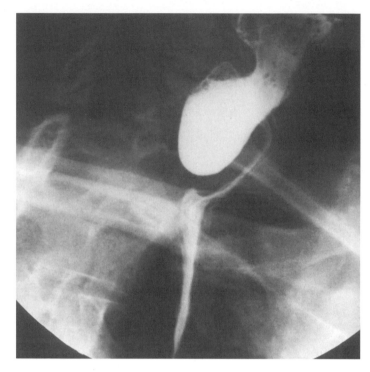

Fig. 96.1 b

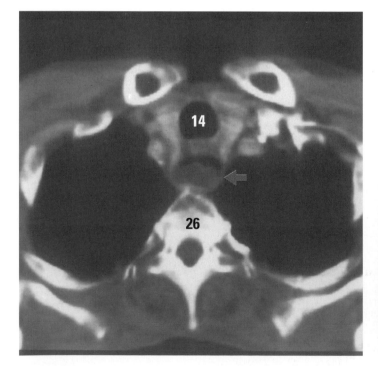

Fig. 96.1 c

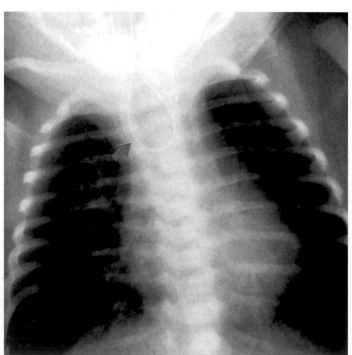

Fig. 96.2

Esophageal carcinomas rarely grow large enough to be visible on chest radiographs, and only a few are detected incidentally by the presence of mediastinal widening (↗ in **Fig. 97.1a**). This tumor should not be mistaken for a retrosternal goiter (see **Fig. 68.1**) or Zenker diverticulum (see **Fig. 96.1a**), especially in the upper part of the esophagus.

Fluoroscopy after oral contrast administration (**Fig. 97.2a**) in this patient shows contrast material coating the tumor surface and outlining its irregular surface structure. This pattern differs markedly from the straight tracks of contrast medium that appear in the normal esophagus (**Fig. 97.2b**). Additionally, the axis of the diseased esophagus (◄) deviates from its normal craniocaudal alignment.

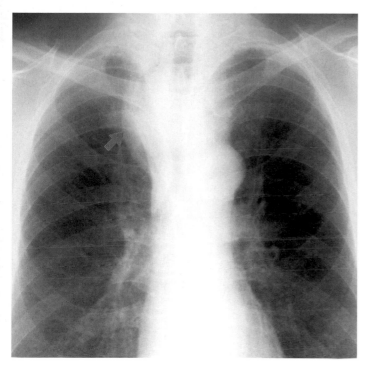

Fig. 97.1

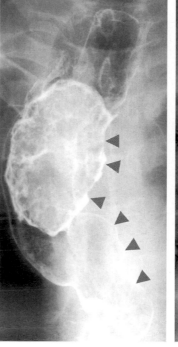

Fig. 97.2a

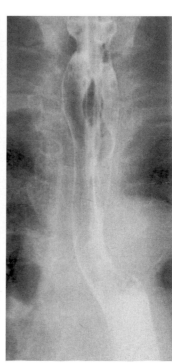

Fig. 97.2b

After the involved segment is resected, alimentary continuity can be restored by a gastric pull-up transposition (➡ ⬅) or similar procedure (**Fig. 97.3**).

If continuity is restored with an interposed colon segment, the air-containing bowel segment (↘) will generally be found directly behind the sternum (**Fig. 97.4**) and not in the normal retrocardiac position occupied by the esophagus.

CT and endosonography can be used to evaluate circumscribed sites of esophageal wall thickening caused by recurrent neoplasia or surrounding lymph nodes.

Alimentary transit can be preserved or restored by stent implantation in patients who have an inoperable esophageal tumor (see **Fig. 171.4a, b** in Chapter 9).

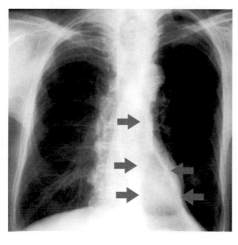

Fig. 97.3a

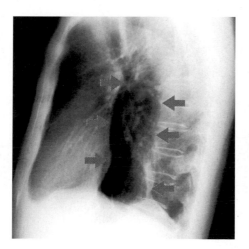

Fig. 97.3b

Fig. 97.4

A hiatal hernia is present when portions of the stomach have herniated into the chest through the esophageal hiatus of the diaphragm. The hernia may cause central widening of the inferior mediastinum. Often this produces a double contour (↙) of the cardiac silhouette (Fig. 98.1) on the PA radiograph, which may be mistaken for free mediastinal or pericardial air (38) (pneumopericardium, Fig. 98.2).

Differentiation is based on the lateral radiograph (Fig. 98.3) or CT scans (Fig. 98.4), which can demonstrate intrathoracic portions of the stomach (18) occupying the RCS anterior to the vertebral column.

Diaphragmatic hernias may also be mistaken for unilateral elevation of the hemidiaphragm on conventional radiographs (see Figs. 58.3a, 75.1b).

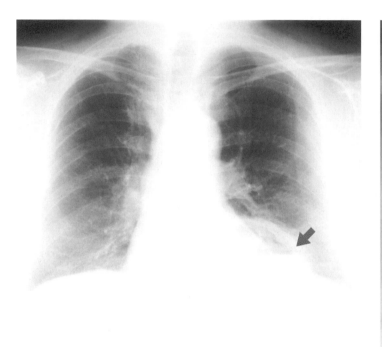

Fig. 98.1

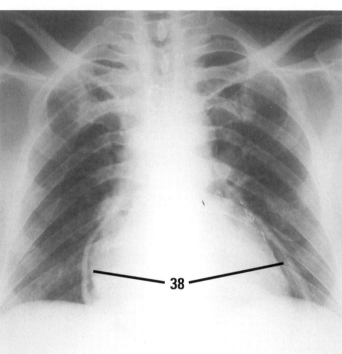

Fig. 98.2

Fig. 98.3

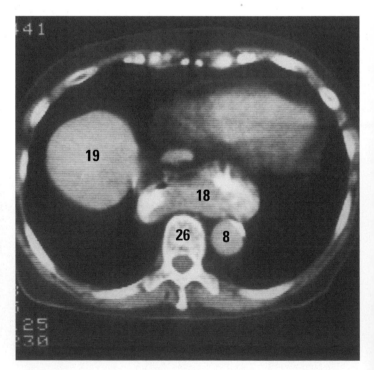

Fig. 98.4

Pneumomediastinum (mediastinal emphysema) is caused by air entering the mediastinal connective tissues, causing enhanced delineation of the mediastinal structures. On PA radiographs, this is often manifested only by a hyperlucent double line along the mediastinal border (↘ ↘ ↘ in **Fig. 99.1**). Air **(38)** may also spread upward through the diaphragmatic crura **(17)** into the mediastinum, usually due to the perforation of a hollow abdominal viscus by a gastric or duodenal ulcer or tumor. This air may accentuate the lateral border of the descending aorta, for example (↙ ↙ ↙ in **Fig. 99.2**). In doubtful cases a lateral radiograph in the supine position may show air separating the heart from the posterior surface of the sternum, or CT scans may help to advance the diagnosis. Examples of posttraumatic pneumomediastinum are shown on p. 193 and p. 202.

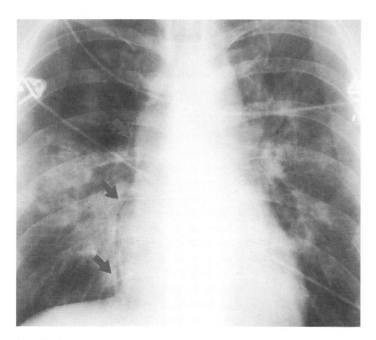

Fig. 99.1

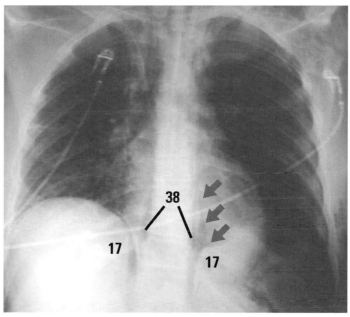

Fig. 99.2

Mediastinal Shift

Three reference points are useful to check for a mediastinal shift on frontal radiographs **(Table 99.4)**. The first is the trachea **(14)**, which should run approximately vertically in the upper part of the mediastinum **(Fig. 99.3)**. The second reference point is the knob of the aortic arch **(6)**, which appears just to the left of the vertebral column. The carina (↑) is normally located slightly to the right of the midline due to the left-sided position of the aortic arch. The third reference point is the border of the right atrium **(2)**, which appears to the right of the vertebral column. Any displacement of these reference points may indicate a mediastinal shift. The mediastinum may be shifted as a result of pressure or traction **(Table 99.5)**.

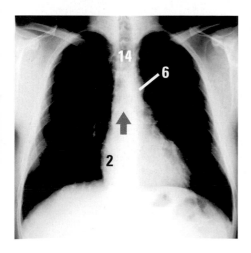

Fig. 99.3

Diagnosis of Mediastinal Shift
Three reference points:
1. Vertical course of the **trachea** (junction with the carina is just to the right of the midline)
2. Left paravertebral **knob of the aortic arch** (approximately at the level of the posterior part of the fifth rib)
3. **Right cardiac border** to the right of the vertebral column

Table 99.4

Causes of Mediastinal Shift
Contralateral pressure:
• Tension pneumothorax
• Diaphragmatic hernia
• Assymetrical emphysema
Ispilateral traction:
• Atelectasis (bronchial obstruction) or previous lobectomy
• Pleural adhesions
• Unilateral pulmonary hypoplasia (rare)

Table 99.5

The mass effect from a pneumothorax or pleural effusion, for example, may exert pressure that shifts the mediastinum toward the contralateral side **(Fig. 100.1a)** compared with the normal mediastinal position **(Fig. 100.1b)**. Meanwhile, the traction exerted by an atelectatic lung area, for example, may shift the mediastinum toward the ipsilateral side **(Fig. 100.1c)**.

These true shifts of the mediastinum require differentiation from "pseudo-shifts." Deformities of the thoracic skeleton (e.g., funnel chest) may lead to rotation and displacement of the heart that can simulate widening or shifting of the media-

stinum. In other cases, however, deformity-related ventilation defects or postinflammatory processes may cause a true mediastinal shift. A rotated position of the chest in the roentgen ray beam can also mimic a mediastinal shift.

Another differentiating criterion is to determine whether the mediastinum moves with respiratory excursions. At fluoroscopy, dynamic position changes associated with a ball-valve stenosis (e.g., caused by an aspirated peanut) can be distinguished from a static mediastinal shift due to atelectasis or pulmonary hypoplasia.

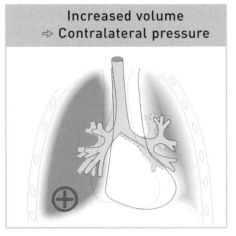

Increased volume
⇨ **Contralateral pressure**

Fig. 100.1 a

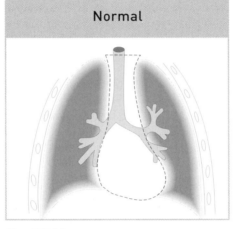

Normal

Fig. 100.1 b

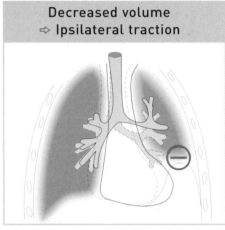

Decreased volume
⇨ **Ipsilateral traction**

Fig. 100.1 c

The involvement of an entire lung leads to a complete mediastinal shift in which all three reference points are displaced in the same direction. **Figure 100.2** shows hypoventilation **(36)** of the right lung with a mediastinal shift to the right side (←). This condition was caused by bronchial obstruction secondary to a perihilar lymphoma **(21)**, resulting in atelectasis of the right middle lobe. There is compensatory hyperinflation of the left lung, which shows increased lucency. When only one upper lobe is affected, the result may be a partial mediastinal

shift like that shown in **Figure 100.3**. In this case only the trachea **(14)** is shifted, while the aortic arch **(6)** and right cardiac border maintain their normal positions. The cause of this partial shift was upper lobe atelectasis **(36)**.

An extreme shift of the mediastinum to one side of the chest gives a clear projection of the thoracic vertebral bodies, similar to the appearance of unilateral pulmonary aplasia (see **Fig. 110.3** in Chapter 6).

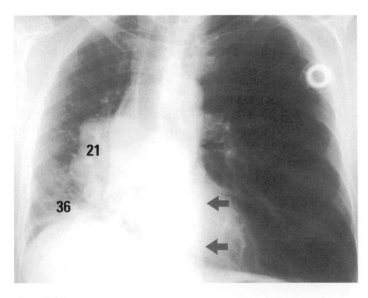

Fig. 100.2

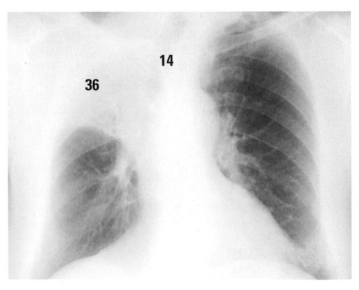

Fig. 100.3

Complete all three quiz pages before checking the answers at the end of the book. This active approach is the best way to learn.

16 What landmarks define the anatomical boundaries of the anterior, middle, and posterior mediastinum in the classification used here?

17 Name several (at least three) frequent causes of a mass in the anterior mediastinum:

18 Name at least two frequent causes of a mass in the middle mediastinum:

19 What findings can you recognize?

Analyze these PA and lateral radiographs from the same patient (**Fig. 101.1**).

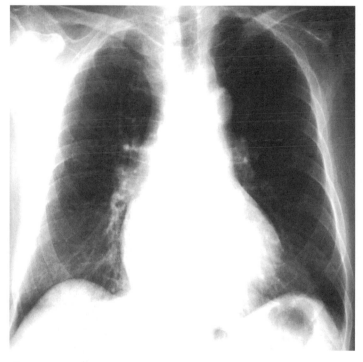

Fig. 101.1 a

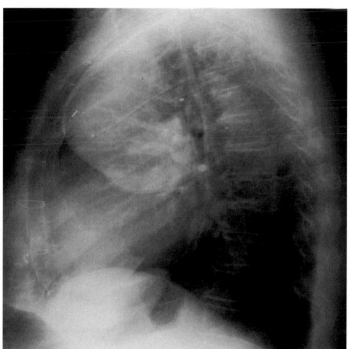

Fig. 101.1 b

What findings can you recognize?

Analyze these radiographs from different patients:

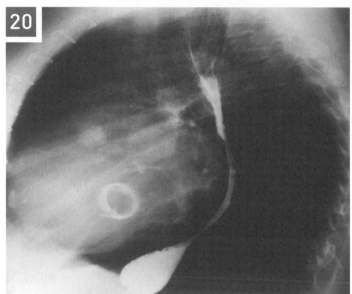

Fig. 102.1

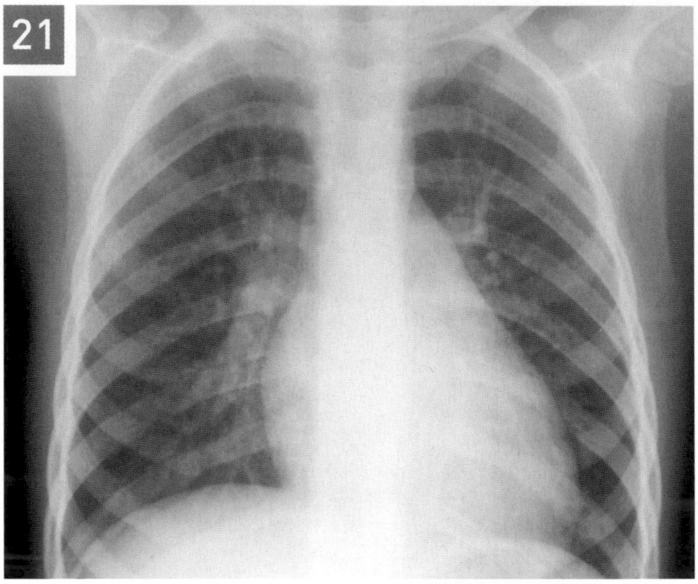

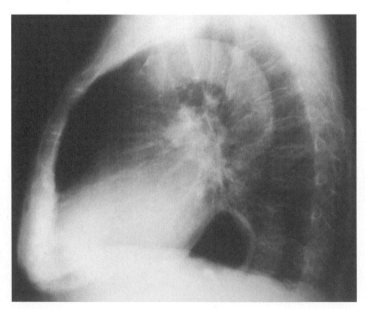

Fig. 102.2

22   What findings can you recognize?

These radiographs are from the same patient **(Fig. 102.3)**:

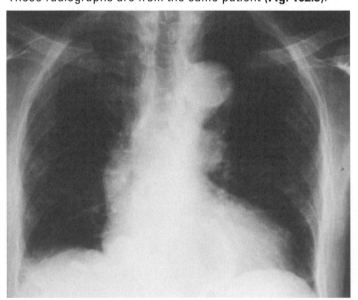

Fig. 102.3a

Fig. 102.3b

23　Can you remember at least two causes of bilateral enlargement of the hilar lymph nodes?

24　How do isolated enlargements of the four cardiac chambers (RA, LA, RV, and LV) appear in the chest radiograph? Write your answers in **Table 103.1**:

25　What type of valvular heart disease leads to narrowing of the RSS? Of the RCS?

RA ↑ =

LA ↑ =

RV ↑ =

LV ↑ =

Table 103.1

RSR ↓ =

RCR ↓ =

26　List the signs of pericardial effusion on the standard chest radiograph and their possible causes. Wait until you complete your list before comparing your answers with page 90 and page 91 or with the answer key at the end of the book.

Causes:		Radiographic signs:	
1.		1.	
2.		2.	
3.		3.	
4.		4.	
5.			

5

27　What are the signs of aortic dilatation on chest radiographs?

Lateral radiograph

PA radiograph

Q

28　Name the criteria for diagnosing coarctation of the aorta on the chest radiograph:

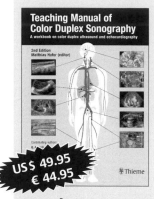
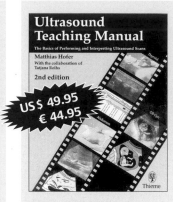
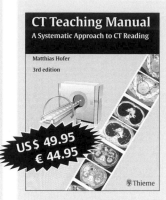
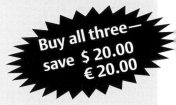
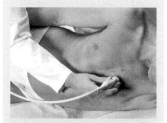
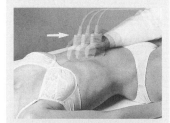
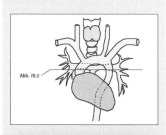
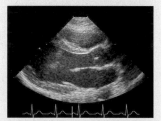
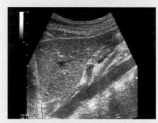
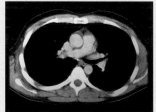
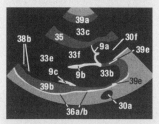
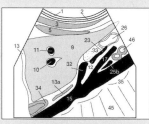
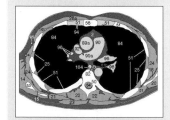
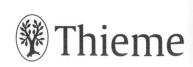

Matthias Hofer

Patchy Lung Changes

Chapter Goals:

When analyzing patchy changes in the radiographic density of the lung, the first step is to differentiate between opacities (areas of increased density, which appear lighter) and hyperlucent areas (areas of increased lucency, which appear darker). After working through this chapter, you should be able to:

- distinguish physiological lung opacities from pathological opacities;

- list the differential diagnoses for a unilateral "white lung";

- distinguish atelectasis (airless lung) from a massive effusion or hemothorax;

- describe adjunctive methods for the investigation of patchy opacities;

- recognize typical forms of atelectasis involving specific lobes and segments;

- explain how radiographic parameters can influence opacities and lucent areas in the lung;

- detect a pneumothorax or impending tension pneumothorax at an early stage;

- correctly classify emphysematous changes.

6

Pleural Effusion

Pleural effusions may occur in the setting of heart failure, renal disease, tumors, and inflammatory processes. Even large pleural effusions usually leave some residual ventilation at the apex (↓ in **Figs. 106.1a, 106.2**) before they become so extensive **(Fig. 106.1b)** that they create a fully established "white lung" **(Fig. 106.1c)**. These films illustrate a malignant effusion in a patient with bronchial carcinoma (BC).

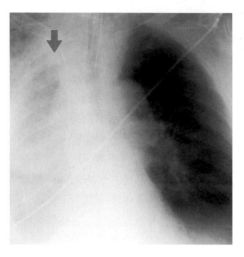

Fig. 106.1 a

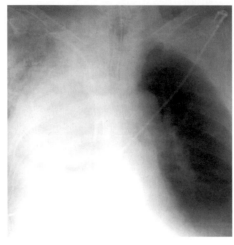

Fig. 106.1 b

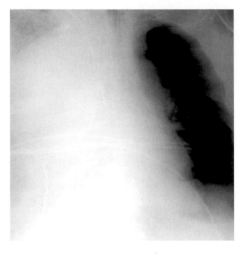

Fig. 106.1 c

Radiographs typically show a slight mediastinal shift toward the contralateral side (←), as in **Figure 106.2**. If the effusion is accompanied by compression atelectasis, however, the volume of the affected lung may remain constant and will not cause a mediastinal shift **(Fig. 106.3)**. In typical cases the opacities caused by the pleural effusion **(41)** will form a raised lateral meniscus in the posteroanterior (PA) radiograph **(Fig. 106.4)**.

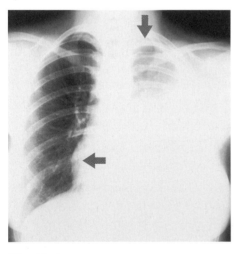

Fig. 106.2

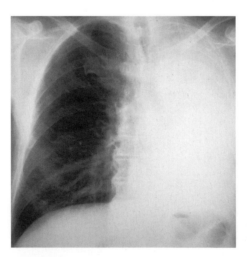

Fig. 106.3

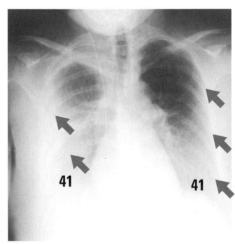

Fig. 106.4

An early sign of a small, incipient effusion is blunting of the costophrenic angle. This refers to the isolated clouding of one or both costophrenic sinuses, which normally taper inferiorly to a sharp, clear angle. This sign may also be a useful differentiating feature from inflammatory infiltrates, which, unlike pleural effusions, tend to spare the cardiophrenic angles in their initial stage. Another, indirect sign of pleural effusion may be broadening of the intercostal spaces, which typically appear normal or narrowed in atelectasis.

Crescent Sign

The "crescent sign" of pleural effusion is a predominantly lateral opacity (◣) that can be attributed to summation effects: The aerated lung parenchyma of the middle lobe (ML) or lower lobe (LL) **(34)** is surrounded by a horseshoe-shaped fluid collection **(41)** that increases the absorption of roentgen rays. Circumferential spread of the effusion is restricted on the medial side by the hilum and pleural reflections. In the PA projection, then, the roentgen rays (⚡) must pass through more fluid in the lateral chest wall than farther medially

(Fig. 107.2). Thus the collection appears to slope upward on the lateral side even though equal amounts of fluid surround the lung anteriorly and posteriorly.

The lateral radiograph often shows definite penetration of the effusion (↗) into the oblique interlobar fissure **(30)** **(Fig. 107.3)**. Extension of the effusion **(41)** into the horizontal fissure **(31)** is often seen in the PA radiograph **(Fig. 107.4)** and may mimic a linear or focal opacity (see also p. 125).

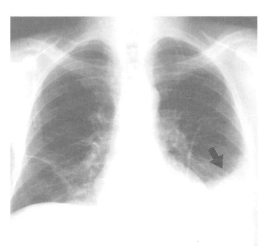

Fig. 107.1

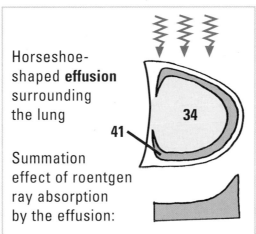

Horseshoe-shaped **effusion** surrounding the lung **34** **41**

Summation effect of roentgen ray absorption by the effusion:

Fig. 107.2

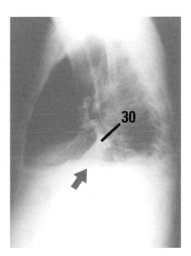

30

Fig. 107.3

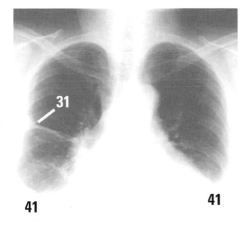

31

41   **41**

Fig. 107.4

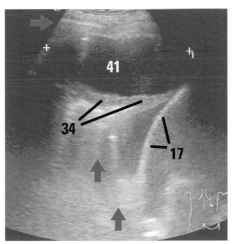

41   **34**   **17**

Fig. 107.5

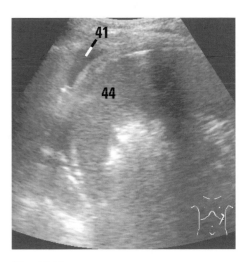

41   **44**

Fig. 107.6

Ultrasound may be used as an adjunctive imaging study or to direct a needle procedure **(Fig. 107.5)**. A scan from the posterior side demonstrates the effusion **(41)** as a dark, hypoechoic mass located between the posterior chest wall (→), the curved echogenic line of the diaphragm **(17)**, and the compressed portion of the LL **(34)**, whose residual air content

casts a faint acoustic shadow (↑). In a scan from the left anterolateral side **(Fig. 107.6)**, the spleen **(44)** can be identified below the diaphragm **(17)**, and a smaller hypoechoic effusion **(41)** can be seen above the spleen. The technique of percutaneous pleural fluid aspiration is described on pages 60–61.

Differential Diagnosis of Pleural Effusion

Regarding the quantification of effusions, it is estimated that a fluid volume of approximately 175-500 mL must be present in order to be detected in the upright PA radiograph. This threshold is only about 150 mL in the lateral radiograph but increases to 500-1000 mL in the supine radiograph **(Fig. 108.1)**. Supine radiographs, however, may give rise to a technical problem that causes decreased lucency in one lung and can mimic the appearance of a layered-out pleural effusion **(Fig. 108.2)**. Do you remember how this effect is produced? If not, please refer back to page 26.

In doubtful cases the differential diagnosis can be further narrowed by obtaining a lateral decubitus radiograph **(Fig. 108.3)**. This position will cause the effusion **(41)** to layer along the lateral chest wall (➔ ←). An ipsilateral decubitus radiograph can detect even a very small fluid collection at a very early stage. It is important to use the correct position, however: LLD for a left-sided opacity and RLD for a right-sided opacity. Occasionally, this is the only way to detect a subpulmonic effusion that was not visible in the PA radiograph.

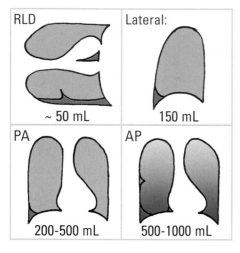

Fig. 108.1

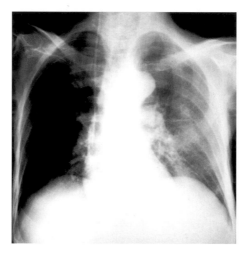

Fig. 108.2

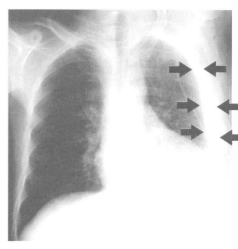

Fig. 108.3

Other diseases may present with patchy, basal opacification that resembles a pleural effusion. Consider the example in **Figure 108.4a** and note the left border of the cardiac silhouette. Would you expect to see this pattern with an effusion, which typically encircles the lung? Of course not. The delineation of the left cardiac border (✎) (see p. 28)

signifies atelectasis **(36)** of the left LL, which appears as a posterior opacity in the lateral radiograph **(Fig. 108.4b)**.

With massive cardiac enlargement in cor bovinum **(Fig. 108.5)**, the heart may extend to the left chest wall and mimic the appearance of a homogeneous pleural effusion.

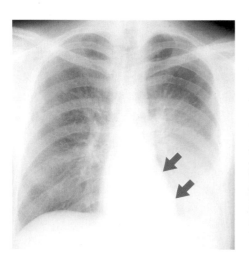

Fig. 108.4a

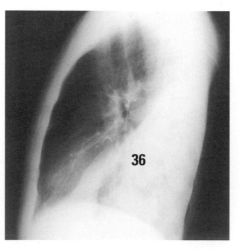

Fig. 108.4b

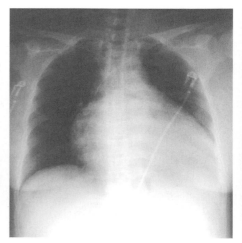

Fig. 108.5

Differential Diagnosis of Pleural Effusion

Other causes of patchy basal opacities include congenital and acquired diaphragmatic hernias involving the displacement of abdominal organs into the thoracic cavity (see also p. 98).

Figure 109.1a shows a plain radiograph of a diaphragmatic hernia. Besides bilateral pleural effusions (⬆ ⬆), the radiograph also shows an indeterminate homogeneous opacity in the left base (⬇). The radiograph after oral contrast administration (⬈) positively identifies the opacity as an abdominal viscus that has herniated into the chest **(Fig. 109.1b)**.

The changes (▷) may be more pronounced in newborns and in patients with large diaphragmatic defects. This case **(Fig. 109.2)** illustrates an enterothorax.

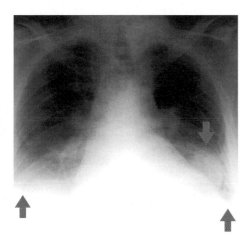

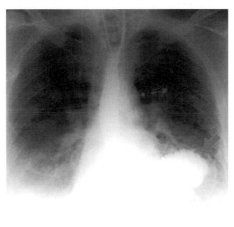

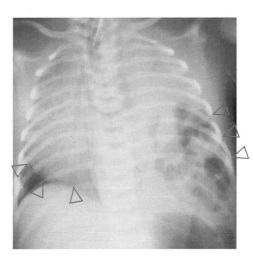

Fig. 109.1 a   Fig. 109.1 b   Fig. 109.2

In rare cases, areas of pneumonic infiltration that no longer contain aerated lung tissue may resemble a homogeneous pleural effusion. This is illustrated by a case of right-sided pneumonia (➡) in **Figure 109.3** (see also p. 116).

In breast cancer patients who have developed very advanced carcinomatous lymphangitis, the normal reticulostriate pattern (see p. 152) sometimes progresses to a more homogeneous opacity like that seen in the right lower zone (LZ) in **Figure 109.4a**. The lateral radiograph of the same patient **(Fig. 109.4b)** shows that the anterior opacity is accompanied by numerous focal pulmonary lesions.

Layered-out effusions also require differentiation from hemothorax, in which a postoperative or posttraumatic hemorrhage collects in the pleural space and may compress the lung. Examples of hemothorax are shown on page 186 and page 207.

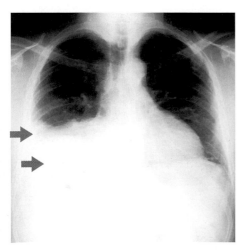

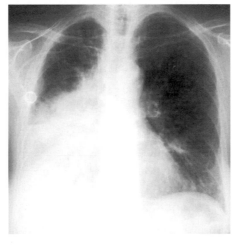

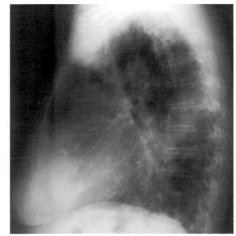

Fig. 109.3   Fig. 109.4 a   Fig. 109.4 b

Differential Diagnosis of "White Lung"

"White lung" refers to the homogeneous, total or subtotal opacification of an entire lung on the chest radiograph. It may be caused by conditions other than pleural effusion. First it is necessary to determine whether the affected side shows an increase in volume, no volume change, or a decrease in volume. **Table 110.1** lists the causes of white lung that are suggested by these findings.

Differential Diagnosis of "White Lung"

Increase in volume	Decrease in volume
• Massive pleural effusion • Large pulmonary tumors • Pleural mesothelioma • Diaphragmatic hernia • Cardiomegaly	• Atelectasis (e.g., in bronchial carcinoma) • Tuberculosis (contraction due to scarring) • Previous pneumonectomy • Aplasia or agenesis of the lung • Pleural plaques or fibrothorax

Table 110.1

Large thoracic tumors like the T-cell non-Hodgkin lymphoma **(21)** in **Figure 110.1a** produce a mass effect that displaces the heart and mediastinum to the contralateral side (◄). While conventional radiographs will not show residual ventilation on the affected side (or at most some apical residual air), the corresponding computed tomography (CT) scan **(Fig. 110.1b)** can demonstrate residual ventilation (↑) as well as chest-wall invasion by the tumor (↗) with much greater clarity. **Figure 110.2a, b** illustrates the same phenomenon in a small child with a thoracic primitive neuroectodermal tumor (PNET). This case shows complete atelectasis **(36)** of the lung, which is compressed from the left side, as well as pronounced displacement of the heart **(4, 5)** toward the right side by the tumor **(21)**, which already contains central hypodense areas of liquefaction.

By contrast, the radiograph of a newborn with right pulmonary agenesis **(Fig. 110.3)** shows an ipsilateral mediastinal shift toward the side of the opacity along with compensatory hyperinflation of the left lung.

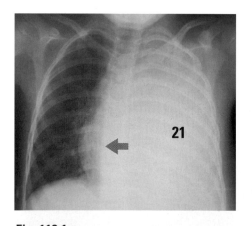

Fig. 110.1a

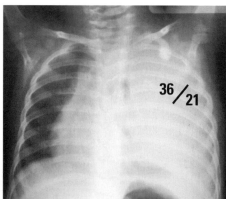

Fig. 110.2a

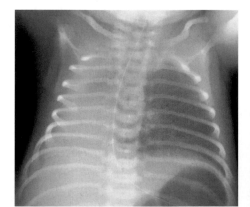

Fig. 110.3a

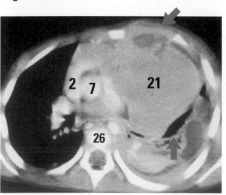

Fig. 110.1b

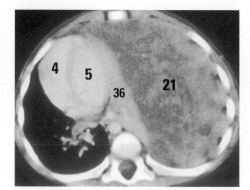

Fig. 110.2b

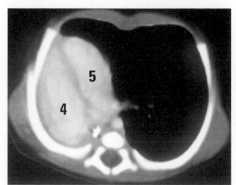

Fig. 110.3b

Upper Lobe Atelectasis

"Atelectasis" is defined as the absence of ventilation (airlessness) in a portion of the lung, while "dyselectasis" refers to a decrease in ventilation (hypoventilation). In the case of the upper lobes (ULs), **Figure 111.1** shows the typical patterns by which the volume of the affected UL **(32)** is reduced to the area shown in dark blue (⌇). Initially, the loss of ventilation may produce a diffusely homogeneous but incomplete haziness like that shown in **Figure 111.2a**. In this case the atelectasis of the left UL is associated with a compensatory upward expansion of the left LL. The decreased lobar volume is manifested in the lateral radiograph by anterior displacement of the oblique fissure (← in **Fig. 111.2 b**). Note the slight shift of the superior mediastinum (→) toward the affected side. The atelectasis may also cause a complete, homogeneous opacification, however **(Fig. 111.3a, b)**, which is again associated with an ipsilateral mediastinal shift and has also caused a slight elevation of the hemidiaphragm (↑). Upward displacement of the horizontal fissure on the right side is a common finding.

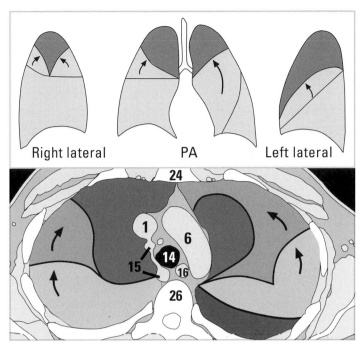

Fig. 111.1

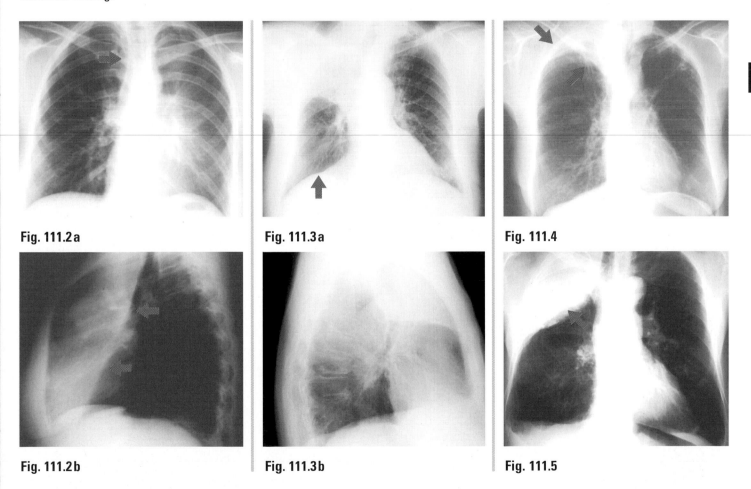

Fig. 111.2 a   **Fig. 111.3 a**   **Fig. 111.4**

Fig. 111.2 b   **Fig. 111.3 b**   **Fig. 111.5**

On the other hand, upward retraction of the hilum or a streaky density (↗) adjacent to the homogeneous opacity in the apical zone (AZ) **(Fig. 111.4)** should raise suspicion of a tumor. In the case shown, the patient also had osteolytic rib lesions (↘) that correlated with malignant chest-wall invasion by a Pancoast tumor.

Homogeneous opacification of the UZs is occasionally found in elderly patients who underwent oil injections into the pleural cavity (↘) for the treatment of tuberculosis (TB) at an earlier age **(Fig. 111.5)**. Typically the opacity has smooth margins and may be mistaken for lobar or segmental atelectasis.

Middle Lobe Atelectasis

Atelectasis of the right ML may have various presentations **(Fig. 112.1)**. In some cases the ML may show homogeneous opacification with no change in size **(Fig. 112.2)**. Sparing of the cardiophrenic angle (↗) is occasionally observed in these cases. In cases with longstanding bronchial obstruc-tion by a mucous plug or a bronchial carcinoma that has penetrated into a bronchus, the atelectatic ML shows a progressive decrease in volume as it contracts toward the right cardiac border and hilum (➡ in **Fig. 112.3**).

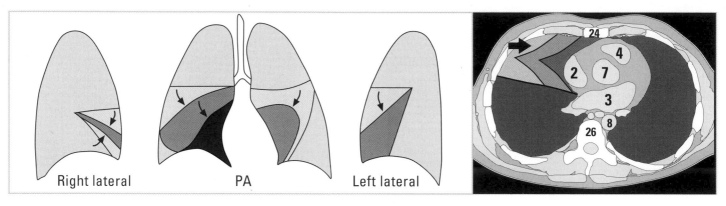

Fig. 112.1

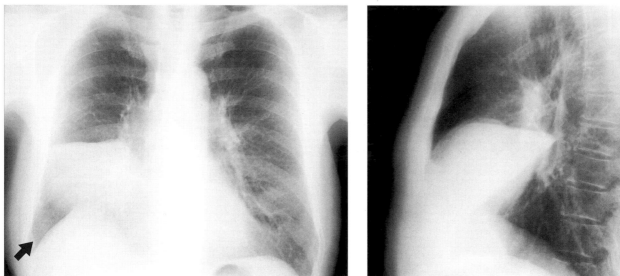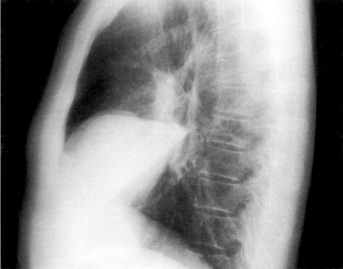

Fig. 112.2a

Fig. 112.2b

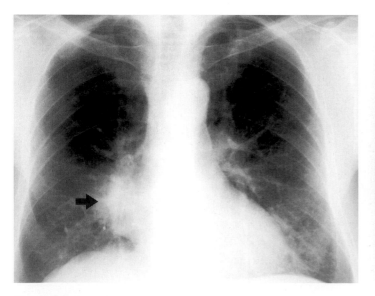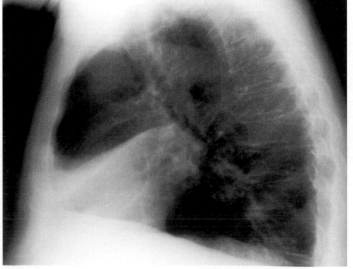

Fig. 112.3a

Fig. 112.3b

Lower Lobe Atelectasis

As the LLs become atelectatic, they also exhibit a fairly typical retraction pattern on radiographs (**Fig. 113.1a**) and axial CT scans (**Fig. 113.1b**). Both LLs contract in the medio- basal direction on PA radiographs and in the posterobasal direction on lateral radiographs.

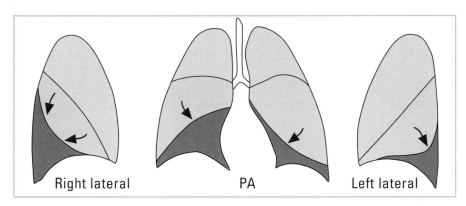

Fig. 113.1a

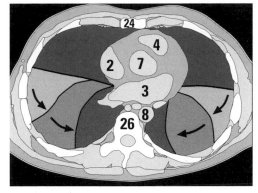

Fig. 113.1b

When LL atelectasis is viewed in the PA radiograph alone, as shown in **Figure. 113.2a**, it may appear as a homogeneous opacity that closely resembles ML atelectasis (see p. 112). In the case shown, the loss of volume in the ML has caused marked elevation of the ipsilateral hemidiaphragm (↟). This patient also shows multiple Central venous catheters (CVCs) and a previous valvular replacement (←). Ask yourself what phenomcnon could be responsible for the streaky horizontal opacity (↙) in the MZ of the right lung (see p. 125 and p. 140). In the CT scan from the same patient (**Fig. 113.2b**), dystelectatic and atelectatic lung tissue (**36**) can be seen posterior to the sections of the diaphragm leaflet and liver (**19**). A fine pleural effusion (**41**) is seen around the posterolateral aspect of this tissue.

Differential Diagnosis of LL Atelectasis

In many cases, however, only CT can determine whether we are dealing with atelectasis alone or with a compression-induced ventilation disturbance that is secondary to a large effusion.

The patient in **Figure 113.3** had a large malignant effusion that resulted in LL atelectasis. The radiograph also shows numerous pulmonary nodules that are metastatic to the malignant underlying disease (here: thyroid carcinoma).

The differential diagnosis of atelectatic opacities also includes bilateral basal opacities caused by neurogenic tumors (see **Fig. 78.1a**), mediastinal abscesses (see **Fig. 79.1a**), pericardial cysts (see **Fig. 92.1a**), and small fat pads along the cardiac border.

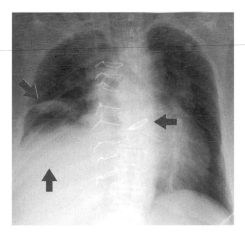

Fig. 113.2a

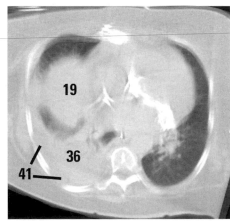

Fig. 113.2b

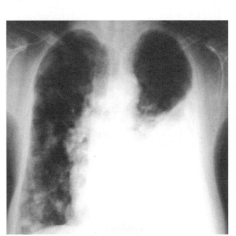

Fig. 113.3a

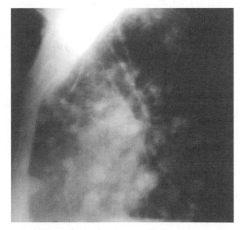

Fig. 113.3b

Segmental Atelectasis

The diagrams below show the typical patterns of opacity that are associated with atelectatic segments in both lungs. One may well encounter variations and deviations from the areas shown here, however. Most segmental atelectases are characterized by relatively narrow intercostal spaces with elevation of the ipsilateral hemidiaphragm and an ipsilateral mediastinal shift **(Table 114.11)**. By contrast, pleural effusions are typically associated with widening of the intercostal spaces, blunting of the cardiophrenic angle, and a contralateral mediastinal shift. For practice, please write the names of the affected segments below the corresponding diagram (remember the mnemonic device!).

Right lateral	PA	Left lateral

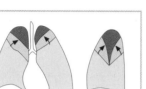
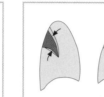
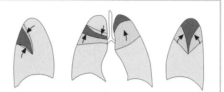
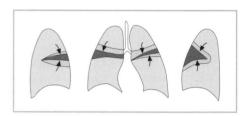

Fig. 114.1

Fig. 114.2

Fig. 114.3

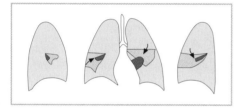
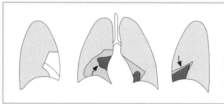
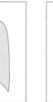
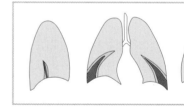

Fig. 114.4

Fig. 114.5

Fig. 114.6

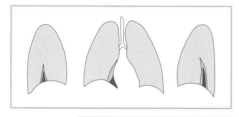
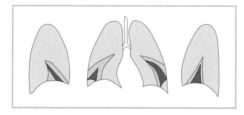

Fig. 114.7

Fig. 114.8

Fig. 114.9

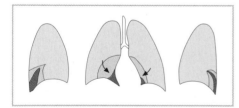

Fig. 114.10

Signs of Atelectasis

- Typical shape and topography of the opacified segments or lobes (see above)
- Displacement of fissures toward the focal change (➜ local decrease in vascularity with increased lucency)
- Hyperinflation of adjacent lung areas

Signs of More Extensive Atelectasis (e.g., affecting an entire lobe)

- Ipsilateral elevation of the hemidiaphragm
- Ipsilateral mediastinal shift
- Narrowed intercostal spaces

Table 114.11

Differential Diagnosis of Segmental Atelectasis

Tumors may also form homogeneous opacities that closely resemble the size and location of a pulmonary segment, as in this example of a plasmacytoma **(Fig. 115.1a)**. This tumor, however, is associated with an anterolateral osteolytic rib lesion (↗) that distinguishes it from atelectasis.

Aided by the diagrams of segmental opacities on the previous page, try to determine what segmental atelectases the tumor would resemble in the lateral or anteroposterior (AP) projections. Write down the number and name of each segment. (The answers are at the bottom of this page.)

PA - view:

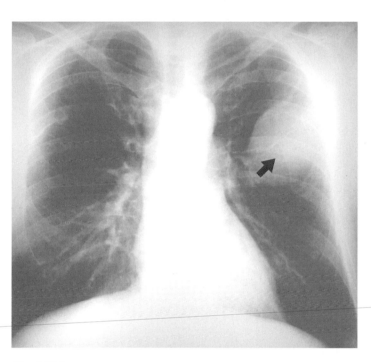

Fig. 115.1a

Lateral view:

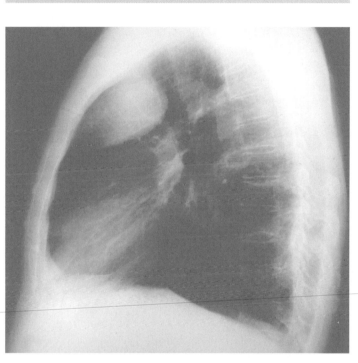

Fig. 115.1b

Interpretation is not always as easy as in the lung cancer case shown in **Figure 115.2**. The patchy opacity in this patient could represent the apical segment (no. 1) of the right UL, and the elevation of the ipsilateral hemidiaphragm (↑) may signify atelectasis. But the shift of the superior mediastinum to the right and especially the upward retraction of the right hilum (↖) suggest that the opacity has a neoplastic cause. When we examine the film closely, we also find postoperative clips **(52)** from previous tumor surgery in the right apical region. The differential diagnosis should also include pericardial cysts (see p. 92) and vertebrogenic or neurogenic masses (see p. 78-79).

Answers to the above question:

The opacity would most likely correspond to the lateral segment (no. 4) in the PA radiograph and to the anterior segment (no. 3) in the lateral radiograph. This makes it unlikely that the opacity in this case is caused by segmental atelectasis.

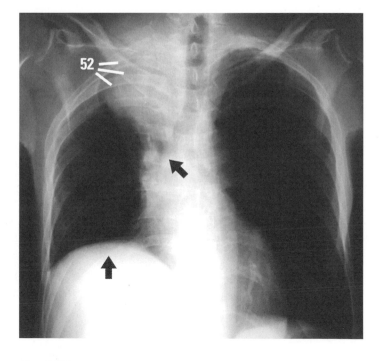

Fig. 115.2

Pneumonia

A classic radiographic sign of pneumonia is the positive air bronchogram. This sign occurs when the density of the peribronchial tissue is increased as a result of inflammatory edema. Normally the bronchial tree (except for the main bronchi) cannot be seen on radiographs, but the sharp contrast between the air-filled bronchi and the surrounding consolidated parenchyma causes the bronchi to become visible. In the slightly rotated view in **Figure 116.1**, radiolucent bronchi (⬋) are outlined in the consolidated lateral UZ of the left lung. Several bronchi in the left LL (↑) are also visible in the retrocardiac area.

Other typical features of pneumonia are a centered mediastinum and symmetrical intercostal spaces. The consolidated area often has a mottled radiographic appearance, depending on the stage of the inflammation. As the infection resolves (e.g., in response to antibiotic therapy), this appearance gives way to a linear or reticular pattern (see Chapter 7). The costophrenic angle often remains clear initially, until an accompanying inflammatory effusion causes it to become opacified. The differential diagnosis of apical lung opacities should include postinflammatory fibrosis (see p. 14-15), tuberculous foci, and retrosternal goiter (see p. 68). The latter can sometimes be identified by the presence of calcifications or by its sonographic features.

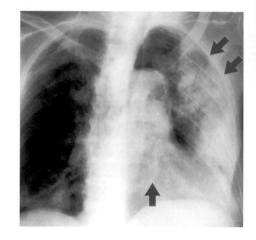

Fig. 116.1

The next two cases illustrate the value of the silhouette sign for assessing lobar involvement by pneumonia (see p. 28). **Figure 116.2** shows a typical case of ML pneumonia (→), in which the cardiac border is obscured, while **Figure 116.3** shows a typical case of LL pneumonia (←), in which the cardiac border remains well defined. The clinical presentation may include a combination of productive cough, fever, leukocytosis, and positive sputum cultures. Abscess formation may develop as a complication. The abscesses may contain fluid levels that appear as lucent cavities (⬊) within the consolidated lung area **(Fig. 116.4)**.

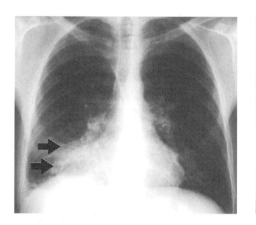

Fig. 116.2a

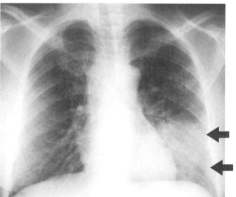

Fig. 116.3a

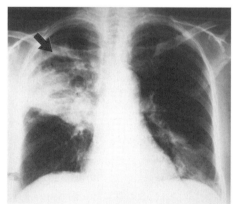

Fig. 116.4a

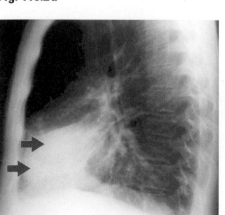

Fig. 116.2b

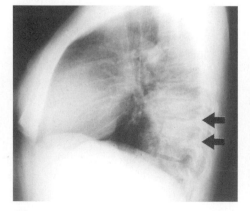

Fig. 116.3b

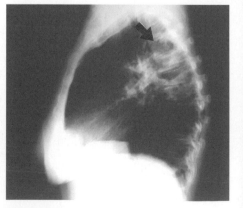

Fig. 116.4b

Misdirected Intubation

Occasionally, an endotracheal tube may be inadvertently inserted into the right main bronchus **(14a)** or even into the intermediate bronchus, or this may result from the dislodgment of a poorly secured tube.

Figure 117.1 shows the case of a preterm infant that required ventilation due to pulmonary immaturity. The endotracheal tube has been placed much too deeply (↖), resulting in atelectasis of the right UL **(32)** and the entire left lung. These areas were quickly reinflated when the tube was withdrawn to the proper level.

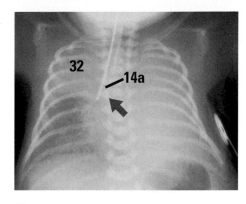

Fig. 117.1

Tumors

A great variety of tumors may produce opaque areas in the lungs. You may recall the "white lung" caused by a pediatric PNET in **Figure 110.2**. Of course, these tumors **(21)** are also detectable at earlier stages when they have infiltrated or displaced only a portion of the lung **(Fig. 117.2a–c)**, resulting in a more circumscribed opacity.

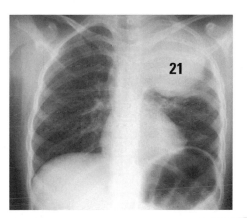

Fig. 117.2a

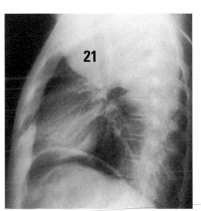

Fig. 117.2b

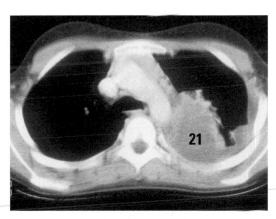

Fig. 117.2c

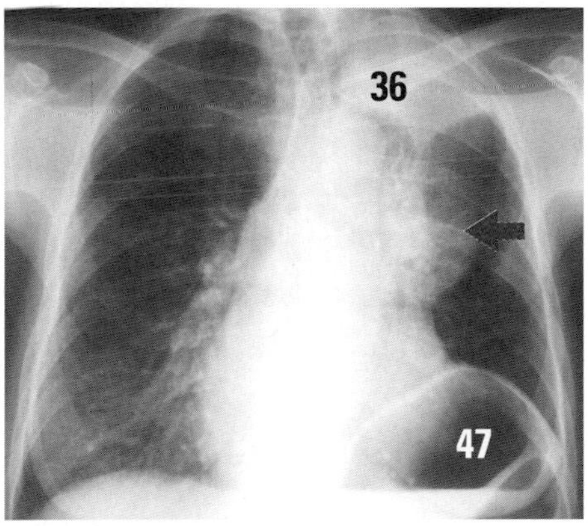

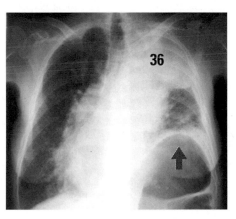

Fig. 117.3a

Fig. 117.3b

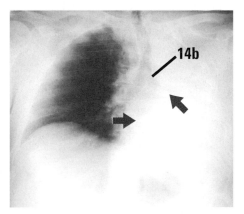

Fig. 117.4

Tumor shadows in adults are most frequently caused by lung cancer (bronchial carcinoma, BC; see p. 18). **Figure 117.3** shows the progression of findings in a woman with left hilar BC (←) and secondary UL atelectasis **(36)** in the left lung. The initial radiograph **(Fig. 117.3a)** already shows marked elevation of the hemidiaphragm and massive gaseous distention of the bowel **(47)**. The findings progressed over time **(Fig. 117.3b)** as the diaphragm leaflet became more elevated (↑) and there was marked clinical progression of dyspnea. By the end stage (shown here in another patient), it is common to find complete atelectasis **(Fig. 117.4)** with a visible cutoff (↖) of the tumor-infiltrated main bronchus **(14b)** and a definite shift of the mediastinum (→) toward the affected side. Pleural mesotheliomas are described on page 59.

General Differential Diagnosis of Hyperlucencies

Recall that hyperlucencies are areas in which roentgen rays are less strongly scattered and absorbed, allowing the radiation to cause greater blackening of the film. Most modern systems use direct feedback from the detector to obtain balanced exposure levels. Even so, overexposure may still occur in children, in thin adults, and especially in supine radiographs. Thus when the entire image appears very dark, it is likely that the film has been overexposed.

When unilateral hyperlucency is noted on a supine radiograph, the most likely cause is an angled scatter-reduction grid (see p. 26 and p. 108). Here is a tip for distinguishing these artifacts from lung pathology: Overexposure and a faulty grid position will also cause excessive blackening of the soft tissues, at least on the affected side. This occurs even in patients who have had a unilateral mastectomy for breast cancer (see p. 36-37). Moreover, some intensive care unit (ICU) patients are in such poor condition that their supine radiograph must be taken in a slightly rotated position, as in patients with severe scoliosis. Sometimes this results in a marked disparity of superimposed cardiac structures between the two sides, causing one side to appear more radiolucent than the opposite side. The depth of inspiration also has a significant effect on pulmonary lucency.

Emphysema

Diffuse hyperlucent areas in a setting of pulmonary emphysema **(Fig. 118.1)** are associated with a decrease in pulmonary vascular markings and interstitial connective tissues. There is associated "pruning" of the pulmonary vessels (↘), in which the enlarged central pulmonary arteries taper rapidly toward the peripheral vessels. Most cases also show a depression of the hemidiaphragm (↓), a barrel chest (◄——►), and a less angled, more transverse orientation of the posterior rib segments. This case additionally showed anterobasal pleural fibrosis (↙), causing less anterior depression of the diaphragm in the lateral projection **(Fig. 118.1b)**. Even the supine radiograph shows an absence of the usual diaphragm elevation, showing instead a flattening of the diaphragm leaflets (↓ in **Fig. 118.2**).

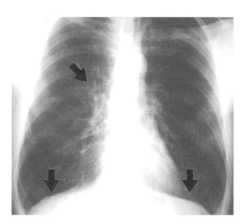

Fig. 118.1a   Fig. 118.1b

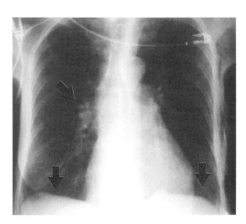

Fig. 118.2

Differential Diagnosis of Frequent Causes of Hyperlucent Areas

Bilateral	Unilateral
Normal lung volume: • Multiple pulmonary emboli • Pulmonary arterial hypertension • Stenosis of pulmonary valve • Congenital heart disease (with decreased lung perfusion) **Increased lung volume:** • Pulmonary emphysema • Bronchial asthma, acute attack • Upper airway stenosis • Acute bronchiolitis	**Due to artifacts or anatomical variants:** • Off-center scatter-reduction grid (in AP only!) • Overexposure (especially in AP) • Rotation (scoliosis, supine, etc.) • Normal variants of the pectoralis muscle **Due to abnormalities:** • Prior unilateral mastectomy • Expiratory check-valve stenosis of a bronchus (e.g., due to foreign body aspiration, see p. 180) • Compensatory hyperinflation due to contralateral atelectasis, effusion • Pneumothorax • Pneumatoceles, large emphysematous bullae • Decreased perfusion, unilateral pulmonary embolism

Table 118.3

CT in emphysema patients shows decreased pulmonary vascularity **(Figs. 119.1, 119.2)**, which usually has a nonhomogeneous distribution, i.e., does not affect all portions of the lung equally. Any infectious foci appear as "ground-glass opacity" in the affected lung areas (⬊) (see also **Fig. 21.2**).

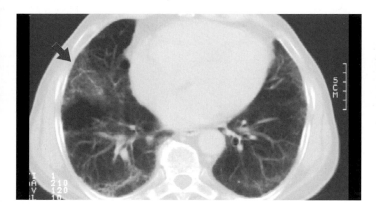

Fig. 119.1

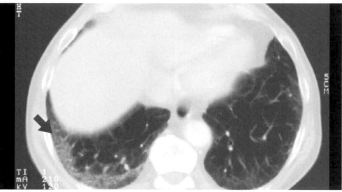

Fig. 119.2

The chronic decrease in pulmonary vascularity leads to an impairment of perfusion and host defense mechanisms in the lung parenchyma. Thus, complications may include bacterial superinfections, and there is an increased incidence of tuberculous infections in emphysema patients. **Figure 119.3** shows an example of a tuberculous primary complex with hilar lymph node enlargement (← →), peripheral lung opacities (⬊ ⬈), and signs of pulmonary arterial hypertension (see p. 118).

Another complication is the formation of emphysematous bullae **(49)**. These lesions may become large enough to cause round atelectasis **(36)** or dyselectasis in adjacent lung areas **(Fig. 119.4)**. It is common to see fine linear opacities bordering the bullae.

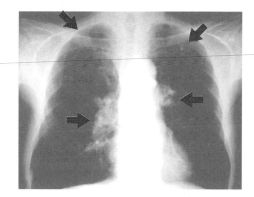

Fig. 119.3a

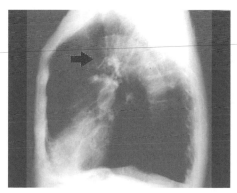

Fig. 119.3b

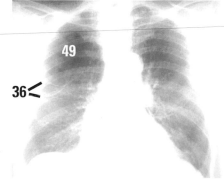

Fig. 119.4

Of course, these bullae may rupture at any time and cause a pneumothorax as air escapes from the lumen of the bulla and enters the interpleural space. Alveolae may rupture in response to sudden and very deep inhalation; this is the mechanism by which a "spontaneous" pneumothorax (not caused by external force or positive-pressure ventilation) may occur in emphysema patients or even in young vocalists. The possible consequences are described in the pages that follow.

A special form is poststenotic emphysema that develops behind sites of bronchial stenosis due to foreign-body aspiration. **Figure 119.5** shows hyperinflation of the left lung caused by a ball-valve mechanism that developed behind an aspirated peanut (nonradiopaque) in a small child. The differential diagnosis of this case would also include atelectasis developing behind a peanut in the right main bronchus.

Similar valve mechanisms may occur in association with bronchial strictures, BC, sarcoidosis, lymphomas, and other lesions. **Note:** Bronchoscopy should be performed whenever bronchial stenosis is believed to be present.

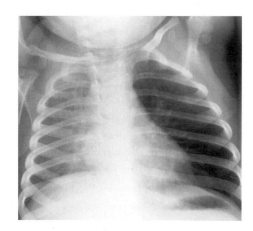

Fig. 119.5

Pneumothorax

Most cases of pneumothorax in Western Europe result from the rupture of small emphysematous bullae that were not previously detected on conventional chest radiographs. Tearing of the visceral pleura permits inspired air to enter the pleural space. This is most likely to occur at the border of the apical UL segments, because this region of the lung is stretched more than other regions during deep inspiration (see p. 29). Traumatic injuries of the pleura due to knife or gunshot wounds are a more common cause in accident victims, crisis regions, and many urban areas. Iatrogenic causes may include inadvertent puncture of the apical lung during the placement of a CVC. The elastic recoil of the punctured lung causes it to retract toward the hilum, and the visceral pleura separates from the parietal chest wall.

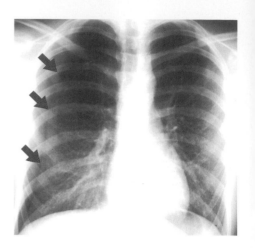

Fig. 120.1

Thus, a typical feature of "mantle pneumothorax" is a fine hairline along the lateral border of the lung (➘) and the absence of pulmonary vascular markings lateral to that line **(Fig. 120.1)**. A small pneumothorax is frequently asymptomatic because small amounts of air can still be reabsorbed.

Tension Pneumothorax

In some cases of pneumothorax, a valvelike mechanism is created that draws air into the pleural space with each breath but does not allow it to escape **(Fig. 120.2)**. As a result, the interpleural air volume **(38)** steadily expands until the lung collapses (➘). This eventually causes a mediastinal shift to the opposite side (←) and ipsilateral depression of the hemidiaphragm (↓) due to the increased intrathoracic pressure on the affected side **(Fig. 120.3)**. Particularly on the right side, this pressure may compromise venous return in the superior vena cava (SVC).

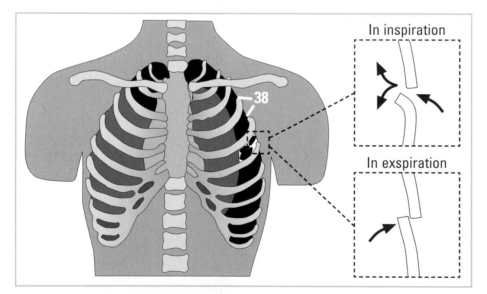

Fig. 120.2

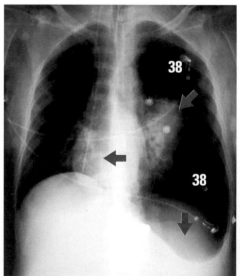

Fig. 120.3

Auscultation reveals diminished breath sounds and hyper-resonance to percussion on the affected side. Because of the decreased cross-sectional area of the pulmonary vascular tree, the heart is subjected to an acute right-sided overload. The surface area available for gas exchange is substantially decreased, producing clinical manifestations of apprehension and severe dyspnea. Most patients experience a sudden onset of chest pain with respiratory distress and progression. Treatment consists of thoracentesis, the details of which are described in Chapter 11 (Intensive Care Unit, see p. 204-206).

In the green boxes below each of the figures, first write some key words to describe the radiographic findings. Then make your differential diagnosis (DD), and finally write down your presumptive diagnosis (PrD). By consistently following this routine, you will be less likely to make a hasty or erroneous diagnosis. To make sure that the quiz is challenging, we have included several case reports with a higher degree of difficulty than before. Approach these problems with a sporting attitude. We hope that you do well!

29   A 72-year-old man with approximately 50 "pack years" of smoking presents with progressive dyspnea and has had a fever of 39° C since the previous day.

30   A 35-year-old man presents with chronic sinusitis, acute lethargy, high fever, and purulent sputum.

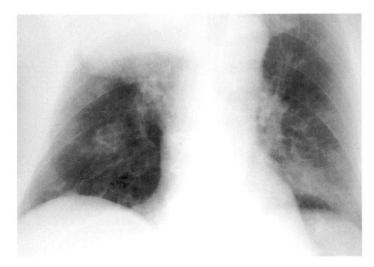

Fig. 121.1

Description:

DD:

PrD:

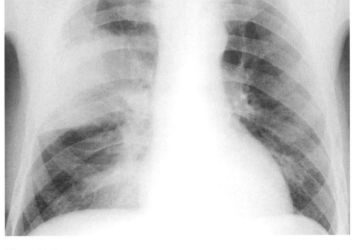

Fig. 121.2

Description:

DD:

PrD:

31   A 55-year-old man with known gastric carcinoma presents with swallowing difficulties of recent onset.

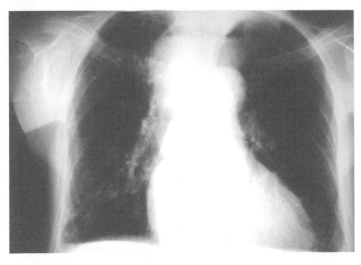

Fig. 121.3a

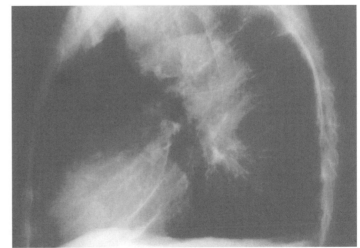

Fig. 121.3b

Description:

DD:

PrD:

32 An 80-year-old woman is referred from a nursing home in a debilitated state with mild respiratory distress and back pain. She also has arterial hypertension.

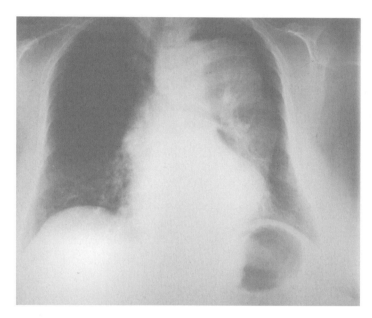

Fig. 122.1

Description:

DD:

PrD:

33 A man presents with high fever and gives a prior history of a severe pedestrian injury in a traffic accident. Where is the abnormality?

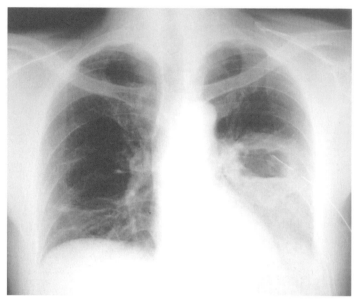

Fig. 122.2

Description:

DD:

PrD:

34 A young man presents with fever and a productive cough. (This is the only information available.)

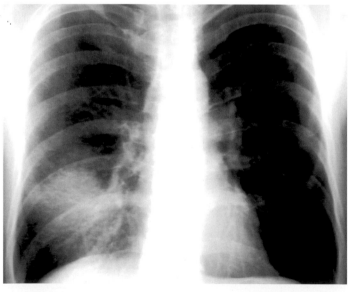

Fig. 122.3

Description:

DD:

PrD:

35 In this case the request form contains no information!

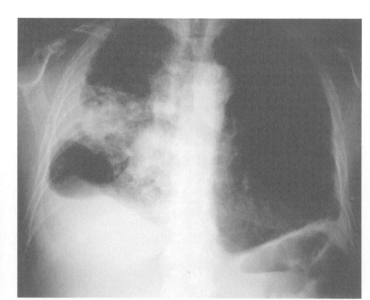

Fig. 122.4

Description:

DD:

PrD:

Matthias Hofer

Focal Opacities

Chapter Goals:

In the differential diagnosis of focal lung opacities, we first make a distinction between solitary and multiple opacities or nodules. It is also helpful to differentiate calcified densities from ring shadows with central lucency. Ring shadows are more often caused by tumor necrosis, cavities, or cysts. After completing this chapter, you should be able to:

- state the benignancy criteria for focal opacities,

- describe the possible appearances and complications of bronchial carcinoma,

- name at least five criteria for establishing the identity of pulmonary nodules,

- describe the radiographic features of the different stages of sarcoidosis,

- recognize the typical characteristics of pulmonary tuberculosis, and

- make an accurate differential diagnosis of pulmonary ring shadows.

7

General Differential Diagnosis of Focal Opacities

While there are many potential causes of nodular opacities in the chest, by far the most common are tuberculomas, bronchial carcinomas, and benign hamartomas. Together, these lesions account for more than two thirds of all pulmonary nodules found on radiographs **(Table 124.1)**. Generally speaking, the likelihood of malignancy rises sharply after 40 years of age [7.1].

Causes of Pulmonary Nodules	
Very common:	**Less common:**
• Tuberculoma • Bronchial carcinoma • Hamartoma • Metastases	• Pneumonia and abscesses • Bronchial cysts • Bronchial adenoma • Neurofibroma

Table 124.1

Criteria for Benignancy
• Size unchanged for 2 years or more • Fat attenuation on CT scans • Clumped or popcorn-like calcifications

Table 124.2

Criteria for Benignancy

Lesions that contain clumped or popcornlike calcifications are interpreted as benign. This feature is considered pathognomonic for benign hamartomas, which are composed of cartilage, muscle, and fatty tissue. This rule has its limitations, however, because many hamartomas contain no calcifications and, unfortunately, certain rare metastases from chondrosarcoma or osteosarcoma (approximately 1% of all metastases) may also contain calcifications. Otherwise, however, it is a good rule of thumb that calcified pulmonary nodules are generally benign **(Table 124.2)**.

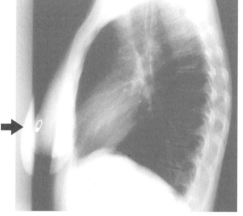
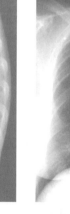

Fig. 124.3

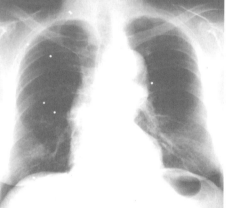

Fig. 124.4

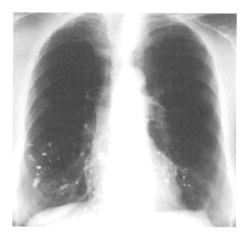

Fig. 124.5

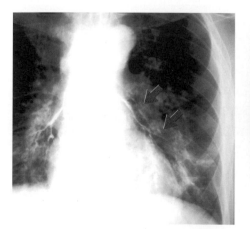

Fig. 124.6a

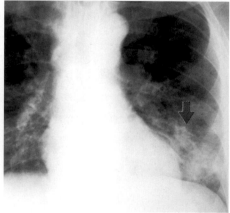

Fig. 124.6b

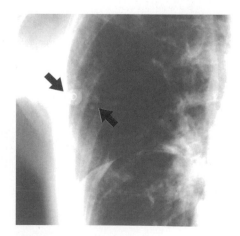

Fig. 124.7

Focal opacities of calcific density may also be caused by metallic nipple piercings (➡ in **Fig. 124.3**) and shotgun pellets **(Fig. 124.4)**. A similar pattern is sometimes seen after contrast administration **(Fig. 124.5)**. Aspirated radiographic contrast medium does not always form focal opacities, however; it may also coat the inner walls of bronchi (➘), making it much easier to identify the cause of the opacity **(Fig. 124.6a)**. In the case shown, the aspirated contrast medium has become so widely distributed that it could easily be mistaken for left basal pneumonia (⬇) if the prior history were not known **(Fig. 124.6b)**. Some findings are more difficult to interpret in the absence of calcifications: The densities next to the electrocardiogram (ECG) electrode (➘) in **Figure 124.7** are several benign granulomas (➘) that resemble metastatic nodules (see p. 126, p. 134).

Differential Diagnosis of Solitary Focal Opacities

The term "pulmonary nodule" generally refers to a rounded opacity less than 1 cm in diameter. Benign-malignant differentiation is not always an easy task. For example, the benign hamartoma (➘) in **Figure 125.1** is virtually indistinguishable from the malignant tumor in **Figure 126.1**. Benign arteriovenous malformations (AVM, ➘) often appear as multiple rounded densities spaced closely together **(Fig. 125.2)**.

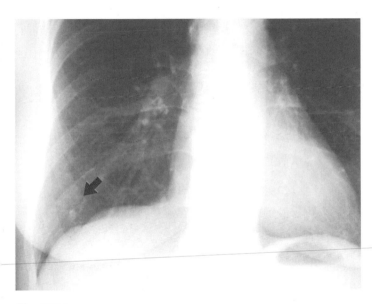

Fig. 125.1

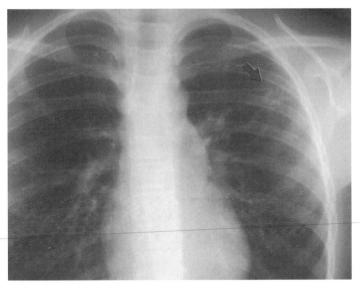

Fig. 125.2

It is somewhat more common to find loculated effusions in the horizontal fissure of the right lung. This type of effusion typically presents a lemon shape (⬇) that is projected onto the horizontal fissure in both the anteroposterior (AP) and lateral views **(Fig. 125.3)**. Were it not for the typical location, it could easily be mistaken for a tumor mass.

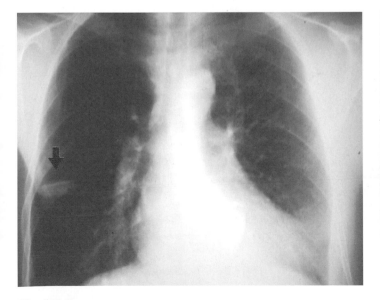

Fig. 125.3a

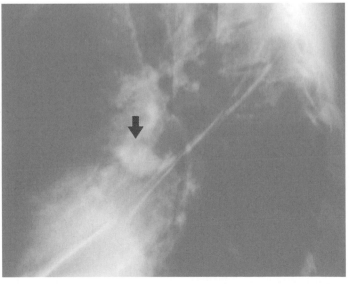

Fig. 125.3b

The principal goal of diagnostic imaging is the detection of small, early-stage tumors that have not yet metastasized or have spread only to their immediate surroundings. The large nodule in the right upper zone (UZ) in **Figure 126.1** was suspicious for malignancy and was surgically removed.

Postoperative follow-up **(Fig. 126.1c)** shows elevation of the right hemidiaphragm (↑) and signs of postoperative soft-tissue emphysema (→). Postoperative clips can be seen along the mediastinal border. The tumor proved to be malignant.

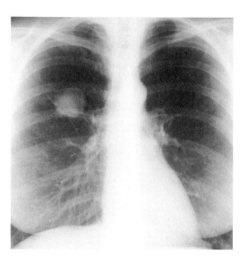

Fig. 126.1a

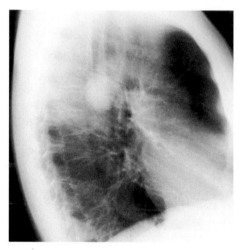

Fig. 126.1b

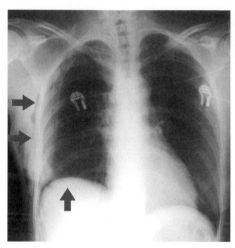

Fig. 126.1c

Pulmonary Metastases

There is always a danger of overlooking other metastatic lesions, particularly small ones, on conventional radiographs in patients who have been selected for a partial lung resection. Of course, the detection of such lesions would have a major bearing on the planning of treatment. Thus, when indeterminate pulmonary nodules are found, the chest radiographs are generally supplemented by thoracic and abdominal computed tomography (CT) scans to look for associated lesions or a primary tumor. The images in **Figure 126.2a-c** show metastatic lesions in a patient with rectal carcinoma. The largest metastasis (↗) is easy to recognize on the chest radiographs **(Fig. 126.2a, b)**, but a second contralateral metastasis (↖) is poorly defined. The CT scans reveal several additional metastases in all pulmonary lobes **(Fig. 126.2c)**, proving that a lobectomy could not be performed for curative intent. The primary tumors that most frequently metastasize to the lung are listed on the next page.

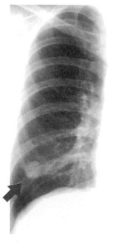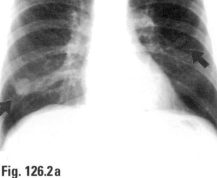

Fig. 126.2a

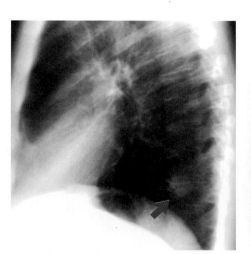

Fig. 126.2b

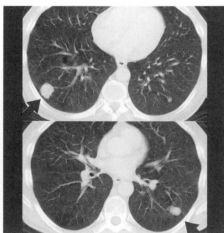

Fig. 126.2c

The primary tumors that are most likely to seed pulmonary metastases are carcinomas of the breast and kidney, colorectal cancers, and cancers of the head and neck **(Table 127.1)**. **Figure 127.2** shows a metastasis that has already reached considerable size (↓). In patients with breast cancer, it is common to find associated carcinomatous lymphangitis (see p. 152) with an accompanying malignant effusion in the pleural space. Thoracentesis (see p. 60-61) can be performed in these cases to collect a fluid sample for cytological testing. Calcified metastases are rare and occur mainly in association with chondrosarcomas and osteosarcomas, thyroid carcinoma, and adenocarcinoma of the gastrointestinal tract.

Common Primary Tumors that Metastasize to the Lung
• Breast carcinoma
• Renal carcinoma
• Head and neck malignancies
• Colorectal carcinoma
• Uterine and ovarian carcinoma
• Pancreatic carcinoma
• Prostatic carcinoma
• Gastric carcinoma

Table 127.1

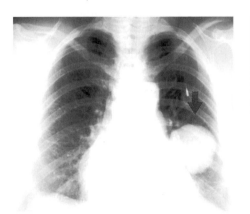

Fig. 127.2a

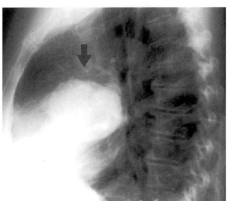

Fig. 127.2b

Azygos Lobe

Whenever you find a solitary focal opacity in the UZ of the right lung (↑), always check to see whether there is a fine line (→) extending upward from the mass **(Fig. 127.3)**. If so, it represents a double fold of visceral pleura caused by the curved, convex course of the azygos vein. This is a normal variant in which the azygos vein does not run along the medial pleural boundary next to the lung **(Fig. 127.4a)** but dips into the visceral pleura to form a small, separate bit of lung tissue called the azygos lobe **(Fig. 127.4b)**. The corresponding CT scans **(Fig. 127.5)** demonstrate the course of the azygos vein **(15)** from the posterior thoracic spine **(26)** to the anteriorly located superior vena cava (SVC) **(1)**.

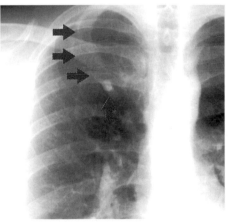

Fig. 127.3

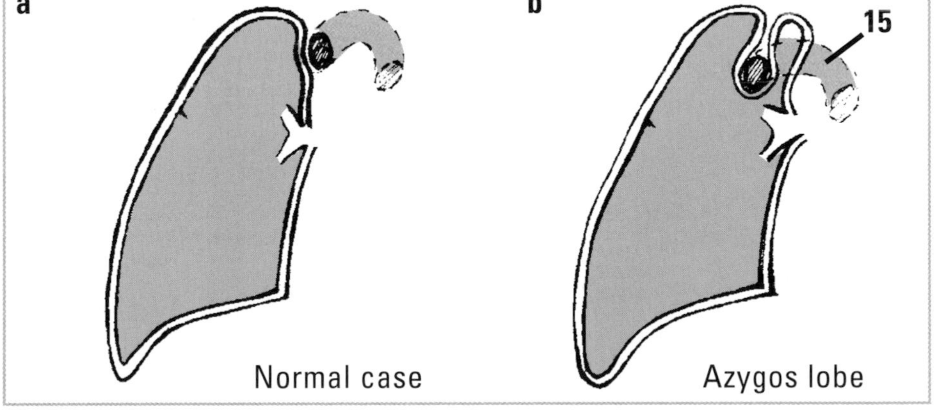

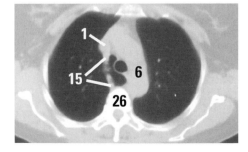

Normal case

Azygos lobe

Fig. 127.4

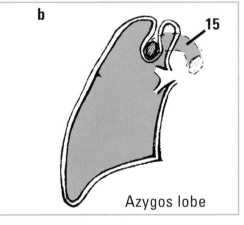

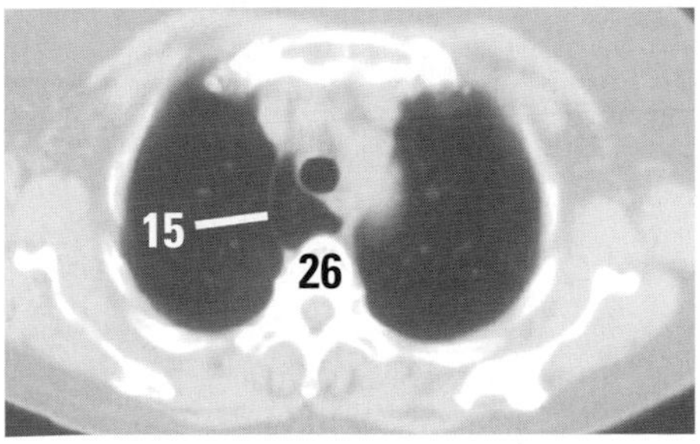

Fig. 127.5a

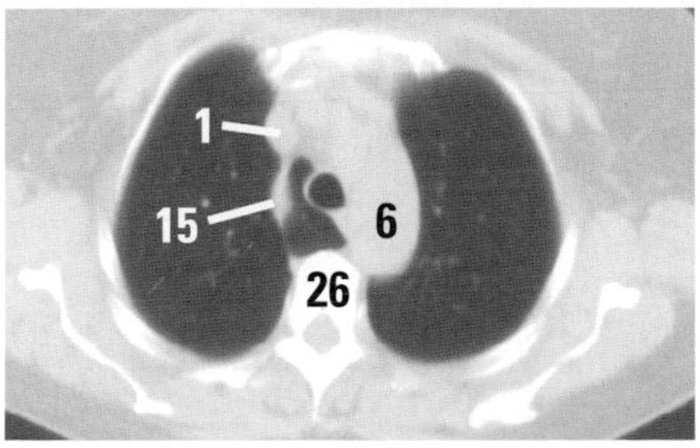

Fig. 127.5b

Fig. 127.5c

TNM Classification of Non-Small-Cell Lung Cancer Published by the UICC [7.2]

A tumor is assigned to a particular TNM category if at least one of the following criteria is met:

T X	Malignant cells are detected in sputum or bronchial washings, but a tumor cannot be seen during imaging or bronchoscopy
T 0	No evidence of a primary tumor
T is	Carcinoma in situ
T 1	Tumor 3 cm or less in its greatest dimension No contact with the visceral pleura No bronchoscopic evidence of invasion of the main bronchus
T 2	Tumor > 3 cm in its greatest dimension Invades the visceral pleura Involves the main bronchus, but 2 cm or more distal to the carina Associated segmental or lobar atelectasis that does not involve the entire lung
T 3	Tumor invades the chest wall, mediastinal pleura, pericardium, or diaphragm Involves the main bronchus < 2 cm distal to the carina Associated atelectasis or pneumonia involving the entire lung
T 4	Tumor invades the heart, great vessels, trachea, esophagus, or vertebral column Malignant pleural effusion (aspiration cytology positive for tumor cells) Satellite lesions detected in the same lobe (separate from the primary tumor)

N X	Regional lymph nodes cannot be assessed
N 0	No regional lymph node metastasis
N 1	Metastasis to ipsilateral peribronchial or hilar lymph nodes (see p. 12)
N 2	Metastasis to ipsilateral mediastinal or subcarinal lymph nodes
N 3	Metastasis to contralateral mediastinal, contralateral hilar, ipsilateral or contralateral scalene lymph nodes

M X	Distant metastasis cannot be assessed
M 0	No distant metastases are found
M 1	Distant metastases are present, including tumor nodule(s) in a different lobe!

Lung cancers are staged as follows based on their TNM classification:

Stage Groupings for Non-Small-Cell Lung Cancer in the TNM System [7.2]

Stage	T	N	M	5-year survival rate
0	is	0	0	
I A	1	0	0	~ 60 %
I B	2	0	0	~ 40 %
II A	1	1	0	~ 35 %
II B	2	1	0	~ 25 %
	3	0	0	~ 35 %
III A	3	1	0	~ 10 %
	1-3	2	0	~ 15 %
III B	4	0-2	0	~ 7 %
	1-4	3	0	~ 3 %
IV	1-4	0-3	1	~ 1 %

For small-cell lung cancer, UICC stages I and II are classified as "very limited disease" and have similar 5-year survival rates. Beyond stage II, the 5-year survival rate falls off sharply to approximately 10% or less. The "extensive disease" stage is characterized by malignant effusion, chest-wall invasion, and metastasis to the opposite lung (stage I), or by carcinomatous lymphangitis or distant metastases (stage II).

Bronchial Carcinoma

Peripheral bronchial carcinoma (BC) may resemble a pulmonary metastasis in its early stage. But the presence of strands or spicules radiating from the nodule into the perifocal lung ("corona radiata," **Fig. 129.1**) is suggestive of BC. These spicules (⤹) are the radiographic correlate of tumor cells invading the surrounding tissue. In the case shown, there is a second contralateral lesion with central necrosis (⤹ ; see also p. 136), which might also represent the peribronchial extension of a BC near the hilum. Aided by the TNM classification on the opposite page, try to stage the tumor in **Figure 129.1**, to the extent that this can be done without seeing the CT scans.

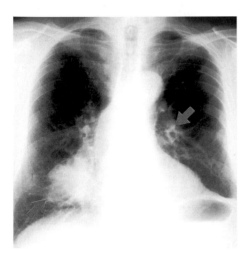

Fig. 129.1 a

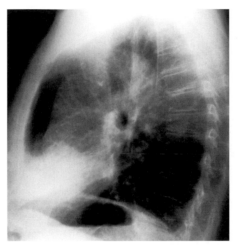

Fig. 129.1 b

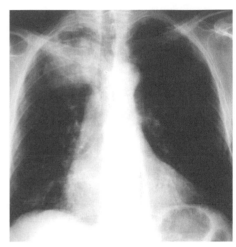

Fig. 129.2

Classification

BC can be classified by its location as central (~ 75%) or peripheral (~ 15%). Histologically, the highest percentage of lung cancers are squamous-cell carcinomas (30-40%) that arise in the mucosa of the (sub)segmental bronchi, or occasionally in the peripheral lung, and spread initially by nodular endobronchial extension. The second most common type is small-cell carcinoma, which usually arises in the central lung, metastasizes very early, and spreads along preexisting tissue spaces. Adenocarcinoma and large-cell carcinoma are the third most common type and most commonly arise in the peripheral part of the lung. Bronchoalveolar carcinoma ("pulmonary adenomatosis") is a rare type (~ 2.5%) characterized by intra-alveolar tumor growth.

BC undergoes early lymphogenous metastasis to hilar, mediastinal and supraclavicular lymph nodes (see p. 22). Hematogenous spread is most commonly to the brain, adrenal glands, and skeleton. Reference was made earlier to possible complications such as poststenotic atelectasis (see pp. 112, 117) and phrenic nerve palsy (see p. 115) with elevation of the ipsilateral hemidiaphragm. Lung cancer tends to have a poor prognosis because it is often detected too late. The 5-year survival rate depends on the tumor stage and may be less than 10%, especially in patients with small-cell cancers. Additional cases of bronchial carcinoma are illustrated on p. 76.

Clinical Manifestations

Unfortunately, suggestive signs and symptoms often appear only after the tumor has reached an advanced stage. General symptoms (weight loss, lethargy, anorexia) may be predominant in the initial stage, before a chronic productive cough and dyspnea supervene. Any member of a high-risk group (especially smokers with more than 20 pack years) who develops pneumonia that is recurrent or refractory to treatment should be investigated for lung cancer.

Hoarseness (recurrent laryngeal nerve palsy), dysphagia (invasion of the esophagus), brachialgia, and Horner syndrome (miosis, ptosis, and enophthalmos due to sympathetic trunk invasion) are strong indicators that a tumor initially confined to the apical part of the lung has spread to involve the mediastinum and adjacent soft tissues ("Pancoast tumor") (**Fig. 129.2**).

Intrapulmonary Hemorrhage

A solitary focal opacity may also represent an intrapulmonary hemorrhage, which may result from trauma or an invasive procedure such as pulmonary catheterization. **Figure 130.1a** shows a focal opacity in the right lower zone (LZ) that has a dense center and a less dense perifocal region (↘ ↙). The patient had undergone pulmonary catheterization, and the corresponding CT scan **(Fig. 130.1b)** showed a focal hemorrhage (↑) in the right middle lobe (ML). The hemorrhagic area is sharply demarcated by the lobar fissure **(30)**, which it does not transcend. Apparently the catheter had been positioned too deeply, causing the hemorrhage.

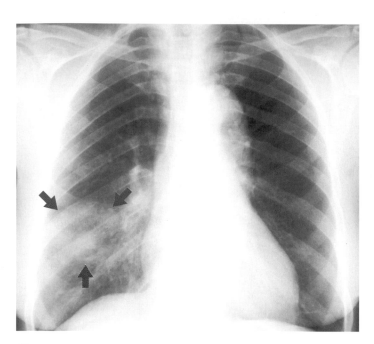

Fig. 130.1a

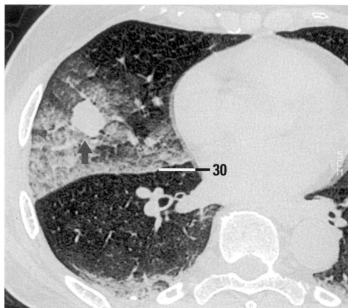

Fig. 130.1b

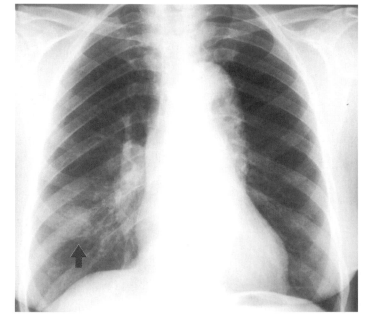

Fig. 130.1c

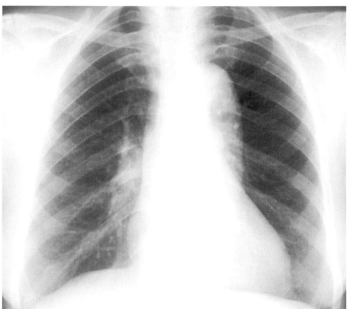

Fig. 130.1d

An initial follow-up radiograph taken two days later **(Fig. 130.1c)** showed partial resolution of the hemorrhage, and a radiograph taken at one week **(Fig. 130.1d)** showed complete resolution. Pulmonary contusions in trauma patients may have a similar appearance. Radiographs typically show confluent focal opacities that are usually located on the injured side (see p. 189) and resolve within a few days. Contralateral hemorrhages resulting from a "contrecoup" mechanism are uncommon.

Sarcoidosis

Sarcoidosis (Boeck disease) is a generalized, epitheloid-cell granulomatosis that predominantly affects the thoracic lymph nodes and lung but may also involve other organs such as the eye (iridocyclitis), liver, spleen, salivary glands, and skin (erythema nodosum).

The classic radiographic feature of stage I sarcoidosis is bilateral enlargement of the hilar lymph nodes (↘ ↙ in **Fig. 131.2**). Unilateral adenopathy may also occur **(Fig. 131.1)** but is rare (~ 5%). In this case enlargement of the left hilar lymph

nodes (↙) is less obvious than enlargement of the right-sided nodes. This is particularly likely to occur on films taken in a slightly rotated position. The disease may regress over a period ranging from a few months to two years, or it may progress to miliary stage II, which predominantly affects the central lung and the MZs near the hila (see p. 133). In most cases the disease eventually progresses to stage III, which is the end-stage marked by pulmonary fibrosis (see p. 150). Radiographs at this stage may demonstrate irregular strands of scar tissue or even a "honeycomb" pattern (see **Fig. 135.2**).

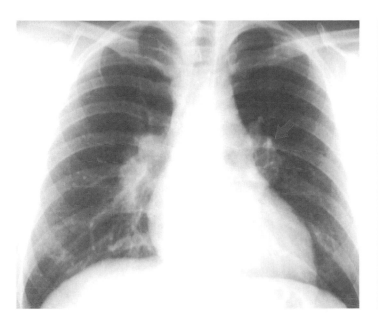

Fig. 131.1a

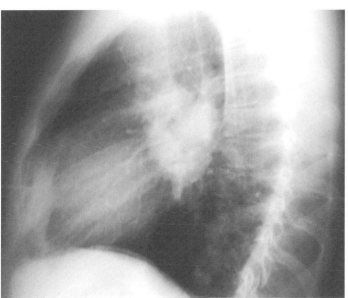

Fig. 131.1b

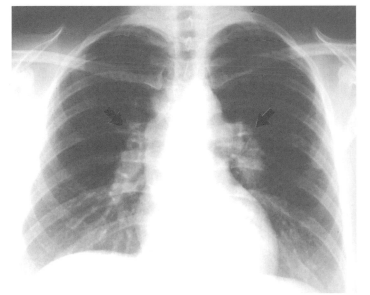

Fig. 131.2a

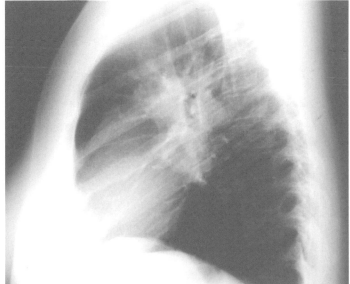

Fig. 131.2b

A special form is Löfgren syndrome **(Fig. 131.2)**, which predominantly affects young women 20-30 years of age. It is characterized by bilateral arthritis (often involving the ankle joint) combined with acute fever, erythema nodosum, and bilateral enlargement of the hilar lymph nodes (↘ ↙).

Tuberculosis

Tuberculosis (TB) is an infectious disease caused by myco-bacteria. It occurs predominantly in individuals who are immunocompromised due to old age, diabetes, HIV infection, cortisone therapy, etc. Its incidence has been rising due in part to more resistant bacterial strains and immigration from Eastern to Western Europe. In stage I of the primary infection, an area of nonspecific alveolitis develops over about a 10-day period into a specific "Ghon focus" (←) with central colliquative necrosis ("caseation") surrounded by a ring of granulation tissue (Fig. 132.1b). These foci are not always easy to detect on standard chest radiographs (Fig. 132.1a).

Most cases undergo lymphogenous spread to the hilar region, inciting a specific lymphadenitis and forming a "primary complex" (↙ ↓), which resolves in most cases and frequently calcifies (Fig. 132.2). In patients with a very poor immune status, the focus may erode into a bronchus and infect the rest of the lung (as well as persons in close contact). This bronchogenic spread leads to cavitating tuber-culosis (see p. 135).

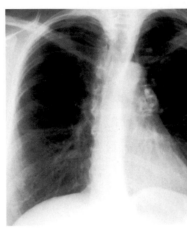

Fig. 132.1a

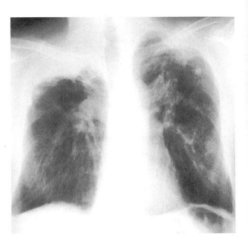

Fig. 132.2a

Fig. 132.3a

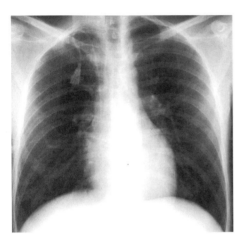

Fig. 132.1b

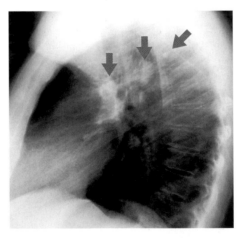

Fig. 132.2b

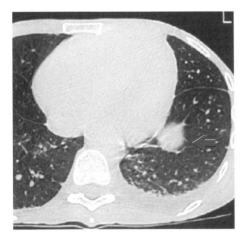

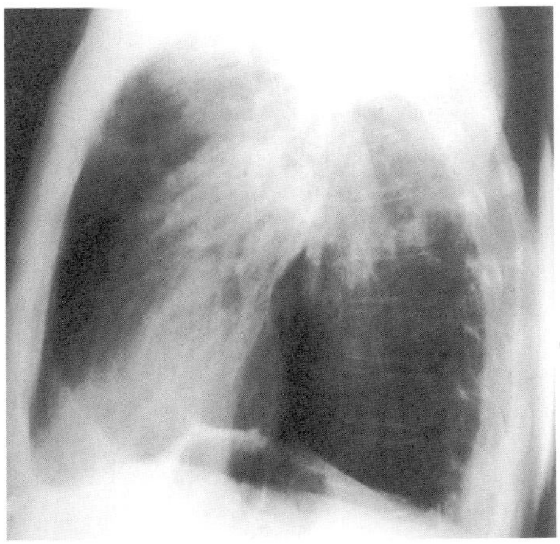

Fig. 132.3b

Organ tuberculosis is a stage of the disease characterized by ill-defined, confluent focal opacities accompanied by cavitation and fibrocirrhotic changes, especially in segments 1 (apical), 2 (posterior), and 6 (superior) (Fig. 132.3). Two tips on differential diagnosis: The changes in TB tend to occur slowly, generally over a period of several weeks, contrasting with the more rapid progression seen in nonspecific forms of pneumonia. The diagnosis can be confirmed by the tuberculin skin test or by identifying acid-fast rods in sputum, gastric juice, or bronchial secretions (bronchoscopy).

If blood eosinophilia is also present in patients with small patchy infiltrates, the differential diagnosis should include parasitic infection by toxoplasmosis, amebae, or helminths (ascarids, echinococci, or schistosomes). This type of infection may lead to an eosinophilic Löffler infiltrate (Fig. 132.4).

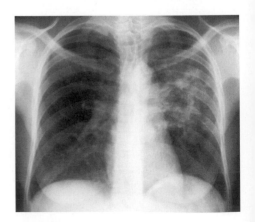

Fig. 132.4

Differential Diagnosis of Multiple Focal Opacities

In the generalized stage of TB, the mycobacteria enter the bloodstream and are disseminated to other lung regions and other organs. The pulmonary manifestation is miliary TB, in which the numerous, small nodular densities are actually a summation effect produced by myriad smaller lesions **(Fig. 133.1)**. Stage II sarcoidosis also forms numerous small foci in the lung parenchyma **(Fig. 133.2)**, which may closely resemble miliary TB.

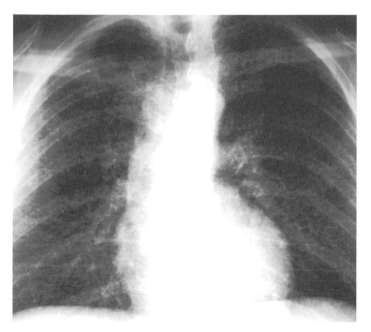

Fig. 133.1

Fig. 133.2

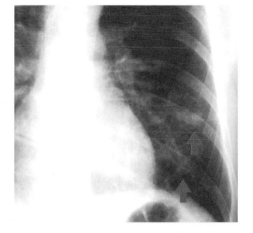

Fig. 133.3 a

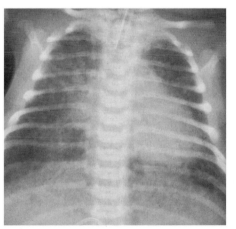

Fig. 133.4

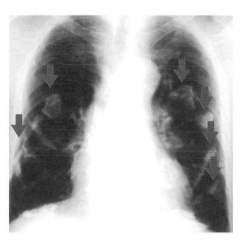

Fig. 133.5

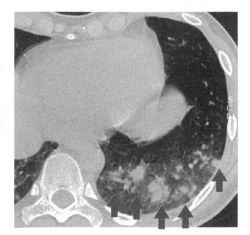

Fig. 133.3 b

A miliary pattern may also result from fungal pneumonia **(Fig. 133.3)** and from meconium aspiration in newborns **(Fig. 133.4)**. Calcific pleuritis **(Fig. 133.5)** is another possibility, although the individual foci are generally calcified and are larger in size (↓) than in the other conditions.

The size and number of lesions in fungal pneumonia (↑) can often be evaluated much more accurately with CT **(Fig. 133.3b)** than on a standard chest radiograph **(Fig. 133.3a)**. The detection of these lesions is particularly important in patients on immunosuppressant therapy or chemotherapy, as it would warrant an immediate change in therapy. The detection of perifocal ground-glass opacity on CT scans **(Fig. 133.3b)** is conclusive for distinguishing fresh infiltrates from older scars [7.3].

Wegener Granulomatosis

Wegener granulomatosis is based on a vasculitis that predominantly affects the small vessels in the kidneys and lungs but additionally involves the upper respiratory tract (sinusitis, ulcerating rhinitis, otitis media, rarely subglottic tracheal stenosis). The radiographic pattern in the lung is that of multiple nodular infiltrates **(Fig. 134.1)** with ground-glass opacities (↘ ↙) on CT **(Fig. 134.2)**. Cavitating foci (↓) with air-fluid levels (→) may be seen in more advanced stages **(Fig. 135.1)**.

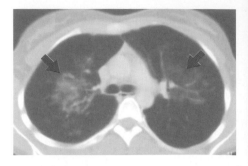

Fig. 134.2

Common Primary Tumors that Give Rise to Pulmonary Metastases [7.4]	
Breast carcinoma	~20%
Renal carcinoma Head and neck tumors Colorectal carcinoma	~10% each
Uterus, ovary, prostate, pancreas, stomach	~5% each

Fig. 134.1a   Fig. 134.1b   Table 134.3

Multiple Metastases

Miliary metastases usually result from the hematogenous seeding of multiple small metastases, particularly from primary tumors of the breast, thyroid gland, and lung. The general frequency distribution of primary tumors is shown in **Table 134.3**. The individual lesions may be too small to be seen on conventional radiographs **(Fig. 134.4a)**, whereas CT will reliably detect even small metastases **(63) (Fig. 134.4b)**. Metastatic lesions of different sizes may reflect a metachronous pattern of spread, as illustrated by **Figure 134.5** in a patient with rectal carcinoma.

Coarse nodular metastases are more characteristic of renocellular carcinoma **(Fig. 134.6)**, seminoma, and sarcoma. Generally, however, the imaging features of pulmonary metastases are very diverse and require differentiation from stage II sarcoidosis (see **Fig. 133.2**), miliary TB (see **Fig. 133.1**), silicosis, and Langerhans cell histiocytosis.

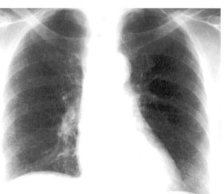

Fig. 134.4a

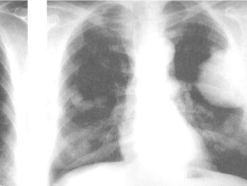

Fig. 134.5a

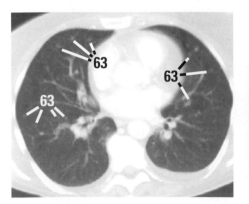

Fig. 134.4b

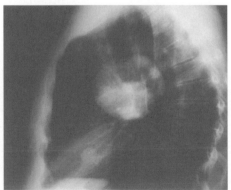

Fig. 134.5b

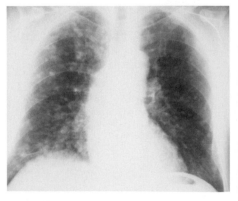

Fig. 134.6

Differential Diagnosis of Ring Shadows and Cavities

Bronchiectasis (➘) may also have a cystic appearance, and multiple affected areas may resemble a "honeycomb lung" **(Fig. 135.2)**. Abscess cavities typically have a shaggy outer wall caused by inflammatory infiltration of the surrounding tissues, accompanied by a sharp inner margin formed by the abscess membrane. **Figure 135.3** is from an HIV patient who had multiple abscess cavities in the right lung (➚) with scattered air-fluid levels (➙).

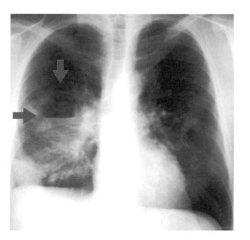
Fig. 135.1

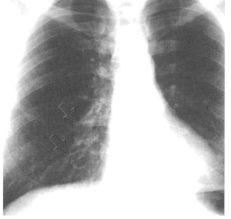
Fig. 135.2a

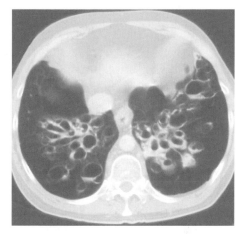
Fig. 135.2b

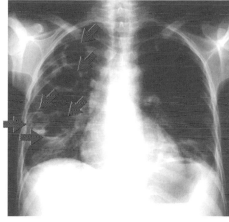
Fig. 135.3

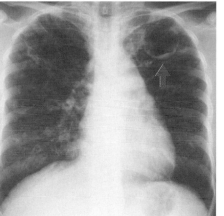
Fig. 135.4

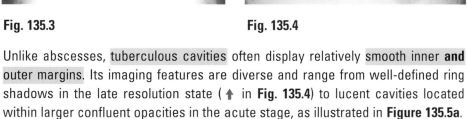
Fig. 135.5a

Unlike abscesses, tuberculous cavities often display relatively smooth inner **and outer margins**. Its imaging features are diverse and range from well-defined ring shadows in the late resolution state (⬆ in **Fig. 135.4**) to lucent cavities located within larger confluent opacities in the acute stage, as illustrated in **Figure 135.5a**.

The correlative CT scan **(Fig. 135.5b)** clearly demonstrates the solid, hyperdense tissue infiltration in the acute stage, causing markedly increased attenuation values. Tuberculous cavities in the lung **(64)** are typically located in the UZs, and TB should always be considered when this UZ predominance is noted.

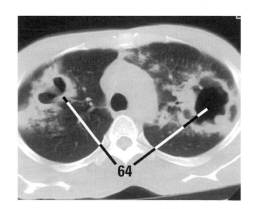
Fig. 135.5b

7

The differential diagnosis should also include echinococcal (hydatid) cysts and amebic abscesses, especially in patients from Mediterranean regions. Amebic abscesses are associated with blood eosinophilia. Suspicious cases should be investigated by ultrasound or CT scanning of the liver and spleen to check for coexisting lesions in those organs. If abscesses continue to progress in an immunocompromised patient despite broad-spectrum i.v. antibiotic therapy, a mycotic abscess should be suspected (see p. 133).

Aspergillosis

Fungi of the genus Aspergillus are opportunistic pathogens that most commonly infect patients with weakened host defenses. A primary infection is acquired only by inhaling massive amounts of fungal spores during the harvesting of grains or hay. Infection with Aspergillus fumigatus is usually marked by the formation of a fungus ball (aspergilloma) in a preexisting cavity or focus of bronchiectasis. Generally the ball (➡) is surrounded by a crescent of air (↙ ↖ in **Fig. 136.1**) and changes its position when the patient is moved. Immunocompromised patients may develop an invasive pulmonary aspergillosis **(Fig. 136.2)** leading to acute pneumonia with abscesses (⬇) and air–fluid levels (⬅).

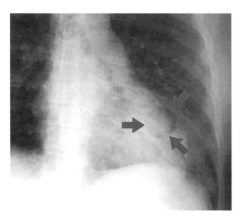
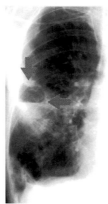
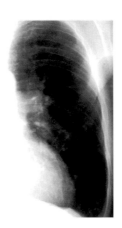
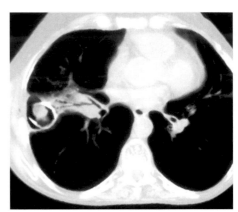

Fig. 136.1   **Fig. 136.2a**   **Fig. 136.2b**

Tumor Necrosis in BC

Advanced, fast-growing BCs may cavitate as a result of central ischemic necrosis. When the tumor erodes through a bronchial wall, not only does it spread to the rest of the lung by the bronchogenic route but the patient may cough up portions of the necrotic tumor center (⬆ in **Fig. 136.3a**). The result is a necrotic cavity **(64)** that is easily mistaken for an abscess cavity. A radiograph taken after bronchoscopic aspiration **(Fig. 136.3b)** shows a decreased depth of the fluid level within the central necrotic cavity.

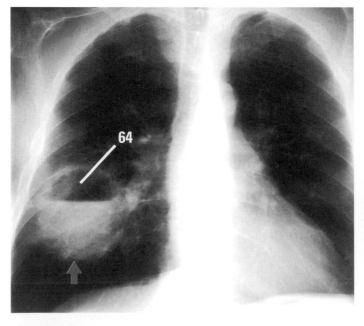
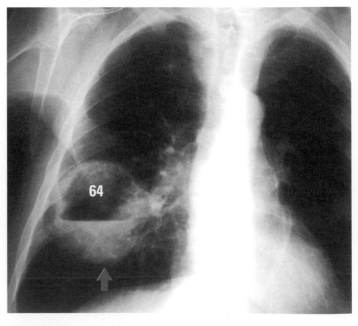

Fig. 136.3a   **Fig. 136.3b**

36 An elderly man presents with pain and limited movement in the upper chest and shoulder region. What do you notice in **Figure 137.1**? What is your presumptive diagnosis?

37 An emaciated small child from a war zone is evaluated for respiratory distress **(Fig. 137.2)**. What does the radiograph suggest?

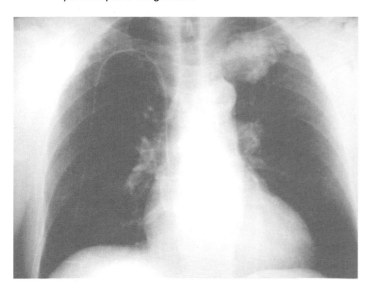

Fig. 137.1

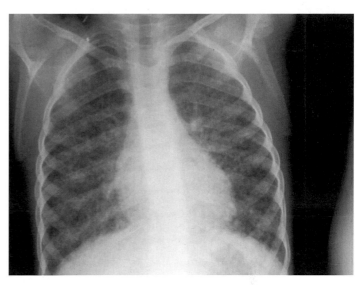

Fig. 137.2

Description:

DD:

PrD:

Description:

DD:

PrD:

38 A man in his mid-60s experiences respiratory distress while in a cardiology unit **(Fig. 137.3)**. Write down **all** of your observations and offer a presumptive diagnosis.

39 A diabetic woman in her late 50s with chronic bronchitis and dysuria is complaining of fever and malaise. In what lung segment is the opacity located **(Fig. 137.4)**? How would you interpret it?

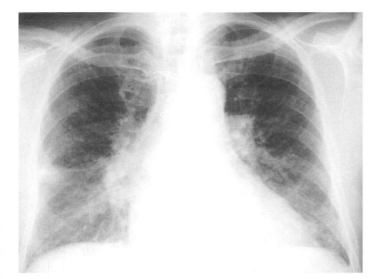

Fig. 137.3

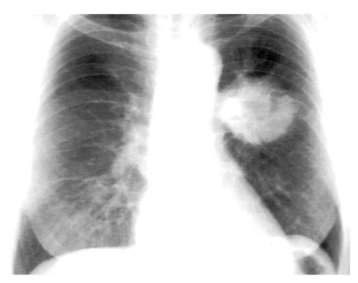

Fig. 137.4

Description:

DD:

PrD:

Description:

DD:

PrD:

40 Guards have brought a coughing prisoner to you for evaluation, and you must determine if he is well enough to be incarcerated with other inmates. Do you have any concerns **(Fig. 138.1)**? Take a close look!

41 A woman approximately 40 years of age presents with respiratory complaints and erythema nodosum **(Fig. 138.2)**. What are your impressions?

42 A homosexual male presents in an almost cachectic state. Describe the abnormalities that you see in **Figure 138.3**:

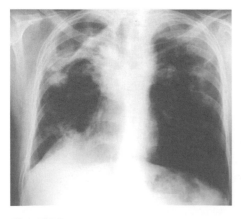

Fig. 138.1

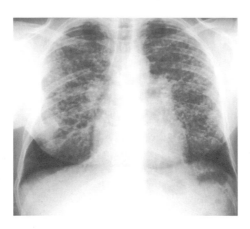

Fig. 138.2

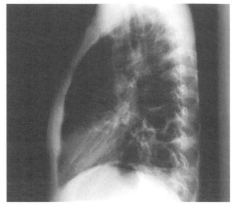

Fig. 138.3

43 This radiograph of an elderly man from Ukraine shows numerous changes **(Fig. 138.4)**. Note the location of the changes when you interpret the film!

44 An elderly woman presents with a recent history of undesired weight loss and lethargy **(Fig. 138.5)**. Signs of Horner syndrome are noted on physical examination. What are your findings?

45 You are given a "follow-up" case in which no history or previous radiographs are available **(Fig. 138.6)**. This time you're on your own.

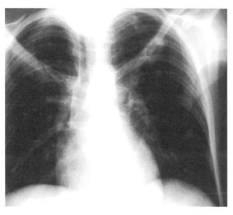

Fig. 138.4

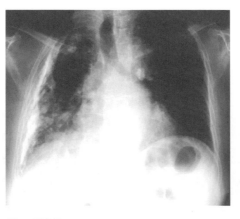

Fig. 138.5

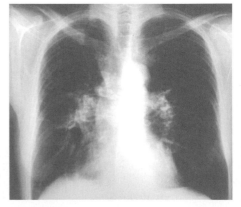

Fig. 138.6

Matthias Hofer

Linear and Reticular Opacities

Chapter Goals:

This chapter will return to several of the diseases in previous chapters that may cause not only large and small opacities but also linear or reticular (weblike) changes in the radiolucency of the lung. After completing this chapter, you should be able to:

- correctly identify normal variants that produce linear or streaky changes in the lung interstitium;

- differentiate normal linear or streaky opacities from true pathological changes;

- distinguish signs of pulmonary venous congestion from inflammatory changes;

- distinguish early pulmonary venous congestion from alveolar pulmonary edema;

- describe the typical features of the various forms of pneumonia;

- recognize an interstitial pattern of lung infiltration;

- describe the typical features of carcinomatous lymphangitis and list the most likely primary tumors.

8

Variants

The most common linear variant that you may encounter in the right apical region of posteroanterior (PA) radiographs is the fine line of a double pleural fold (➡) formed by an atypical course of the azygos vein terminating in the superior vena cava (SVC; see p. 127) (Fig. 140.1). The pleural fold ends at the arch (➚) of the azygos vein (15), which is viewed end-on in the radiograph. Less common findings are partial anomalous terminations of specific pulmonary veins in the azygos vein, inferior vena cava (IVC), hepatic veins, or even the portal vein. Figure 140.2a shows an anomalous termination of the right lower lobe vein (↘ ↖) in the IVC. Figure 140.2a shows a variant in which the lobar vein (↟) terminates in the hepatic venous system, causing unsharpness of the right hemidiaphragm.

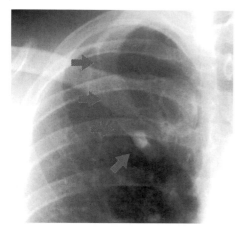

Fig. 140.1a

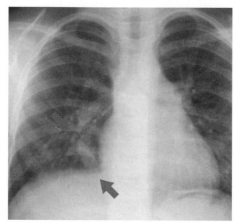

Fig. 140.2a

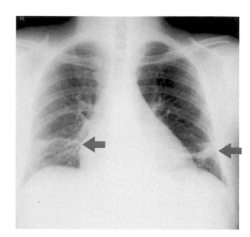

Fig. 140.3

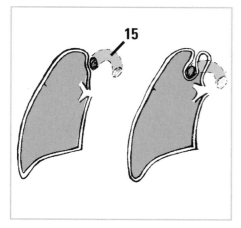

Fig. 140.1b

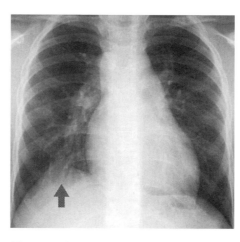

Fig. 140.2b

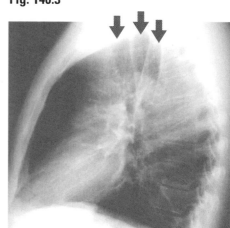

Fig. 140.4

Horizontal linear opacities (⬅) are a relatively common finding on postoperative radiographs and in intensive care unit (ICU) patients. They represent sites of round atelectasis in the lower lung zones, which often result from decreased respiratory excursions due to pain (Fig. 140.3). This type of atelectasis responds well to respiratory exercises or positive end-expiratory pressure (PEEP) ventilation.

Quiz – Test Yourself!

46 In the lateral radiograph in **Figure 140.4**, you will see three vertical, lucent bands (↓) in place of the normal tracheal air column. What could cause these bands? (The answer is at the end of the book.)

47 Do you remember how to distinguish the craniocaudal boundary line of a mantle pneumothorax from the medial border of the scapula?

48 Why does the clavicle occasionally have a horizontal companion shadow? If you have trouble with this question or with question 47, refer back to page 52 and page 120 or check the answers at the end of the book.

Pulmonary Congestion and Edema

When pulmonary venous drainage is impaired, as in a patient with congestive heart failure or mitral valve disease, there is a damming back of blood into the pulmonary veins, causing a rise in pressure. At the capillary level, this causes increased amounts of fluid transudation first into the interstitium and later into the alveoli.

The interstitial component of the congestion is often more pronounced in the basal portions of the lung **(Fig. 141.1)**. This leads to linear and reticular interstitial opacities in the lower lung zones with associated unsharpness of the vessels, cardiac borders, and diaphragm leaflets. We may conclude that the opacities have a cardiac pathogenesis by noting the associated cardiomegaly (⟷), the dilatation of the left atrium (→) in the lateral radiograph **(Fig. 141.2b)**, and the presence of pleural effusions (↑) as shown in **Figures 141.2a, 141.3**.

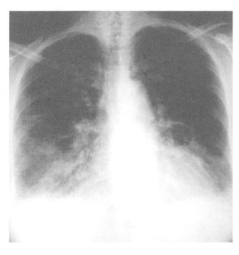

Fig. 141.1

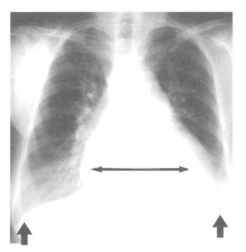

Fig. 141.2a

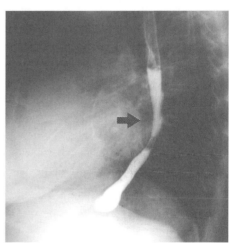

Fig. 141.2b

The interstitial edema compromises gas exchange, especially in the basal lung zones. Sometimes this evokes an Euler-Liljestrand reflex (see p. 29), causing increased calibers of the upper and apical pulmonary vessels **(Fig. 141.3)** due to a basal-to-apical redistribution or upper lobe (UL) diversion of pulmonary blood flow even in the standing position (see p. 25). The typical computed tomography (CT) appearance of interstitial edema **(Fig. 141.3b)** is a ground-glass opacity of the lung parenchyma that spares a narrow peripheral zone (see p. 21). Note again the presence of pleural effusions (↑).

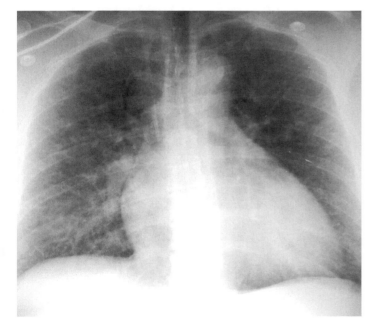

Fig. 141.3a

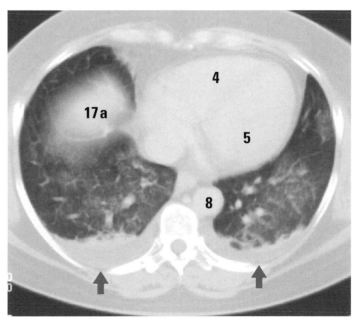

Fig. 141.3b

8

Interstitial edema due to pulmonary congestion does not always affect the basal lung regions more than the upper zones, however. When a "butterfly" pattern of linear and reticular opacities is noted in the central lung region (see p. 10) and is combined with cardiomegaly and pleural effusions **(Fig. 142.1a)**, it is unlikely that the opacities are caused by inflammatory infiltration. **Figure 142.1b** shows a complete

regression of the changes following diuretic therapy and cardiac recompensation.

Occasionally, the accompanying effusion may be so pronounced that the typical butterfly pattern is obscured and is not appreciated when the radiograph is first seen **(Fig. 142.2)**.

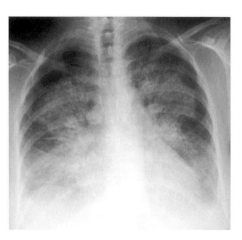

Fig. 142.1 a

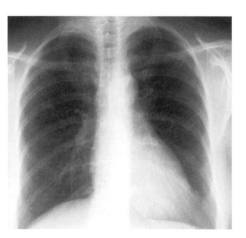

Fig. 142.1 b

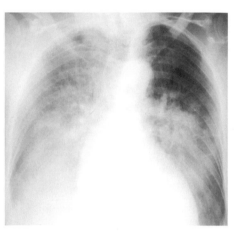

Fig. 142.2

Congestion Due to Pulmonary Emphysema

It is particularly challenging to recognize pulmonary congestion in cases where the pulmonary interstitium is rarefied due to emphysema, for example (see p. 118). In **Figure 142.3a**, you must look very closely in order to recognize the accentuated pulmonary vascular calibers (↖) and the faint Kerley B lines

(➡). The initial lung congestion becomes obvious only when you look at the follow-up film taken several days later **(Fig. 142.3b)**, which also shows resolution of the subtle pleural effusions (⬆). **Table 143.3** should aid you in the interpretation of doubtful cases.

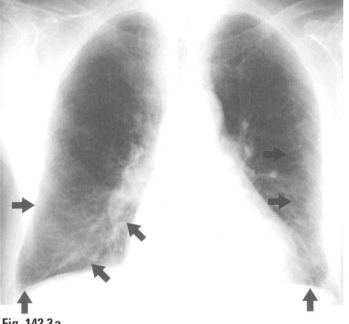

Fig. 142.3 a

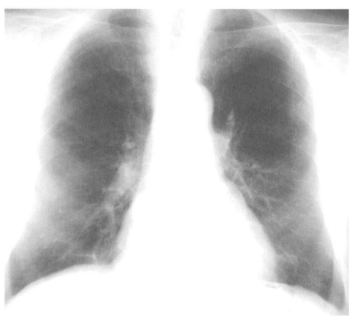

Fig. 142.3 b

Signs of Congestion

When linear and reticular lung opacities are due to congestion, it is typical to find not only a combination of pleural effusions and cardiomegaly (Table 143.3) but also a rapid progression of findings within a period of days or even hours. Figure 143.1 shows a patient who underwent aortocoronary bypass surgery. The initial radiograph shows cardiomegaly in the absence of significant pulmonary congestion (Fig. 143.1a). The radiograph taken the next day shows initial fluid retention in the lung (Fig. 143.1b) in a setting of left-sided heart failure, accompanied by numerous Kerley B lines (→). The Kerley lines cleared within a short time (Fig. 143.1c).

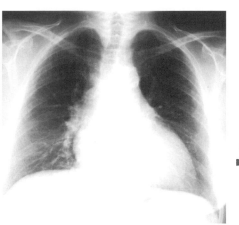
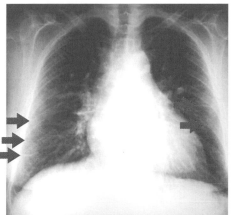
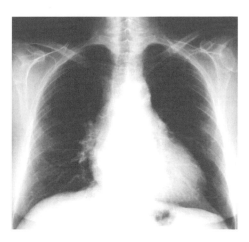

Fig. 143.1 a   Fig. 143.1 b   Fig. 143.1 c

Alveolar Pulmonary Edema

In advanced stages the edema begins to enter the alveoli from the interstitium. The fluid-filled acini and lobules appear as focal opacities 3-5 mm in diameter. These confluent airspace shadows (Fig. 143.2) are difficult to distinguish from inflammatory infiltrates, due in part to the possible appearance of a positive air bronchogram (↖) (see p. 144). If the congestion becomes chronic, it may culminate in pulmonary fibrosis (see p. 150).

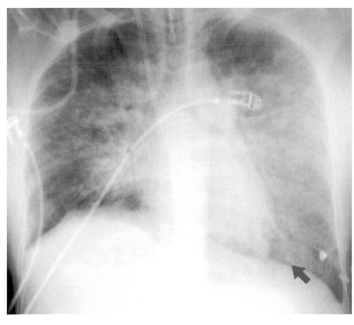

Fig. 143.2

Checklist for Detecting Signs of Pulmonary Congestion

a) Direct signs (generally symmetrical)

- Increased pulmonary vascular markings
- Right LL artery   > 18 mm in diameter (♂)
- Right LL artery   > 16 mm in diameter (♀) (see p. 18)
- Detection of Kerley lines (see p. 21)
- Ill-defined vascular outlines and cardiac borders
- Ill-defined diaphragm leaflets
- Accentuated and hazy hila
- Thickened interlobar fissures
- Possible upper-lobe blood diversion
- Later, confluent focal opacities (alveolar edema)

b) Additional signs

- Cardiomegaly (particularly, left atrial enlargement in lateral radiograph)
- Rapid progression of signs
- Pleural effusions: Often right > left

Table 143.3

Forms of Pneumonia

Classic lobar pneumonia, which is caused by organisms such as Staphylococcus, Klebsiella, and Legionella and infiltrates entire lobes, has become very rare in the modern antibiotic era. The forms most commonly seen today are focal pneumonias, bronchopneumonias, and interstitial forms of pneumonia caused by a variety of bacteria, viruses, and parasites that may infect the lungs by inhalation or the hematogenous route. **Figure 144.1a** is from a patient with a Hickman catheter (←) who was immunosuppressed by chemotherapy. The radiograph shows a reticulolinear infiltration pattern (↘) with associated confluent airspace shadows (↑) in the right middle zone (MZ) and lower zone (LZ). Notice that these

changes, unlike pulmonary venous congestion (see p. 141-143), are focal and unilateral and are not accompanied by cardiomegaly. An associated inflammatory effusion would be consistent with a diagnosis of pneumonia, however. The inflammatory infiltrates were no longer visible in this case following bronchoalveolar lavage **(Fig. 144.1b)**.

Typical cases exhibit a positive air bronchogram (↗) caused by the increased density of the peribronchial lung tissue **(Fig. 144.2)**. CT **(Fig. 144.3)** shows fine nodular densities along with linear and reticular opacities caused by the inflammatory infiltrates, which in this case affect only the right lung.

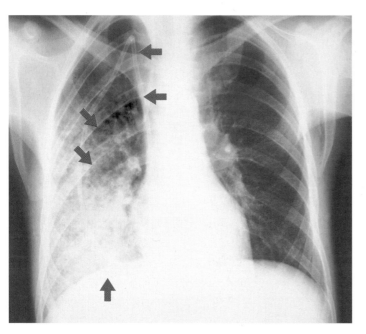

Fig. 144.1a

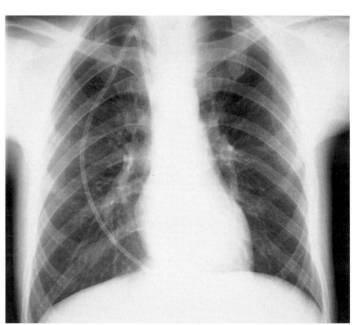

Fig. 144.1b

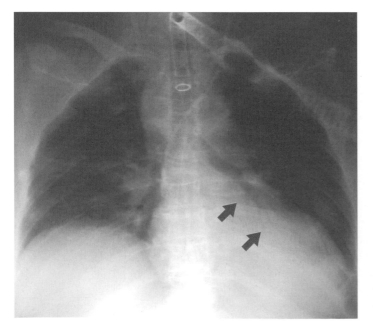

Fig. 144.2

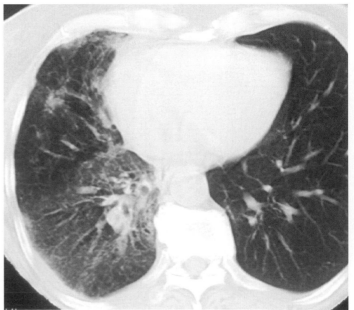

Fig. 144.3

Of course, pneumonia may also affect both lungs. In these cases and in patients with pulmonary emphysema **(Fig. 145.1)**, it is occasionally difficult to distinguish the pneumonia from infiltration due to pulmonary congestion (see p. 142-143). The diagnosis of these cases is often aided by the clinical presentation (fever, cough productive of purulent sputum) combined with laboratory findings (leukocytosis or eosino-philia in parasitic infections). In the case shown, infiltrates were visible in the left perihilar region (➴) and right retro-cardiac area (➡) **(Fig. 145.1a)** and progressed over time **(Fig. 145.1b)**. How can you tell that these infiltrates are located in the right lower lobe (LL) and not in the middle lobe (ML) (e.g., for planning bronchoscopic lavage)? If you do not remember how to do this, refer back to page 28.

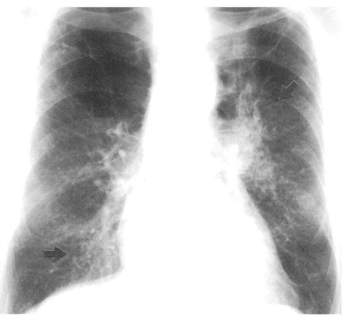

Fig. 145.1 a

Fig. 145.1 b

An abscess may occasionally develop as a possible compli-cation, especially in patients who are immunocompromised as a result of HIV infection or chemotherapy. An early-stage abscess can be recognized as an opacity with a central cavity that may or (as in this case) may not contain an air-fluid level. At the center of the retrocardiac pneumonic infiltrate in **Figure 145.2** is a subtle lucency (△) that can be seen only by careful scrutiny. Abscesses are not always as conspicuous as the one in **Figure 135.3**.

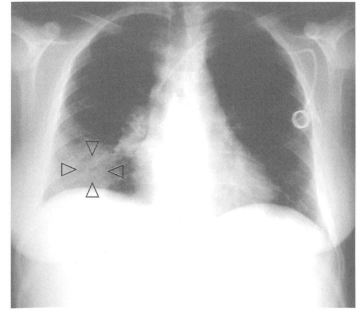

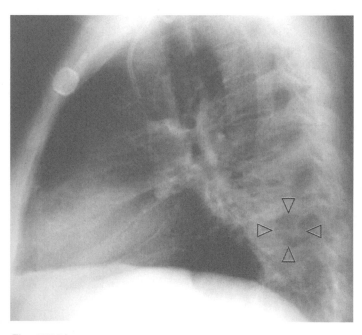

Fig. 145.2 a

Fig. 145.2 b

Pneumocystis carinii Pneumonia (PcP)

This organism is classified as a fungus based on its antigenic properties, but it does respond to antibiotics. It occurs in immunocompromised patients on corticosteroid therapy or chemotherapy and in HIV-infected patients and premature infants with impaired cellular immunity.

The organisms adhere to the alveolar walls and proliferate so avidly that masses of them can often be detected in bronchoalveolar washings. Many patients initially have no radiographic abnormalities or show only an elevated hemidiaphragm due to the decreased compliance of the lung.

Somewhat later, chest radiographs show an initially faint, bilateral, perihilar pattern of interstitial infiltration (**Fig. 146.1**) that spares the periphery of the lungs. CT scans show ground-glass opacity of the central parenchyma regions. A typical feature of PcP is the absence of accompanying pleural effusions and hilar lymph node enlargement.

Unless treatment is initiated early, the interstitial infiltration pattern increases over time (**Fig. 146.2**). This culminates in the appearance of focal and patchy opacities, while clinically the patient develops severe respiratory insufficiency and requires ventilation (**Fig. 146.3**).

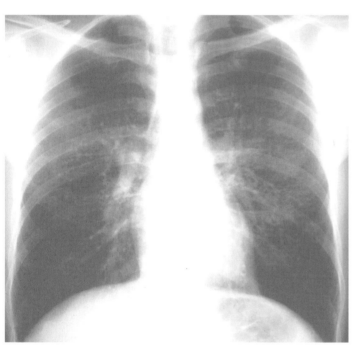

Fig. 146.1 a

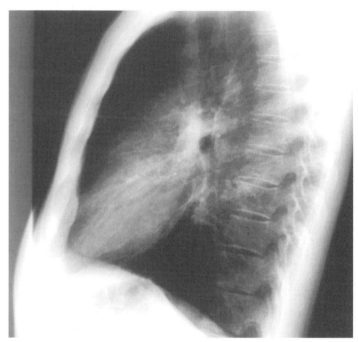

Fig. 146.1 b

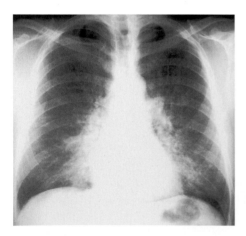

Fig. 146.2 a

Fig. 146.2 b

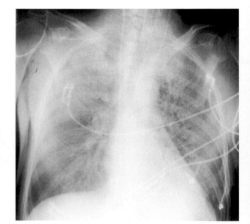

Fig. 146.3

Differential Diagnosis of Pneumonia

The dyselectasis of a lobe or segment (see p. 112-116) may cause a mottled pattern of opacity (↘ in **Fig. 147.1**) that resembles pneumonia. Aspergillosis most commonly presents as an aspergilloma in a preexisting cavity (see p. 136), but it may also incite an acute or chronic bronchopneumonia with numerous reticular or confluent focal opacities **(Fig. 147.2)**.

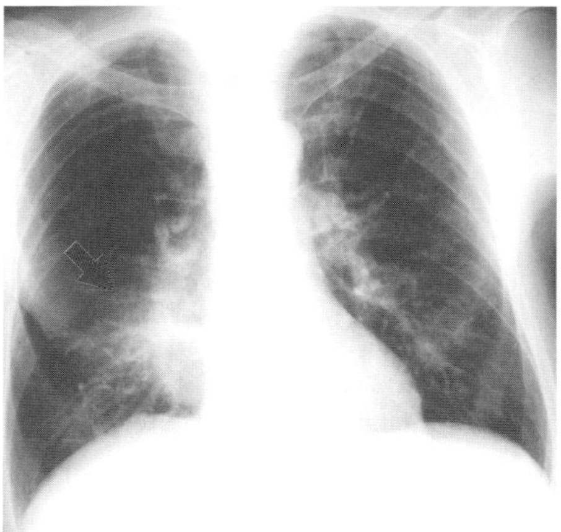

Fig. 147.1 a

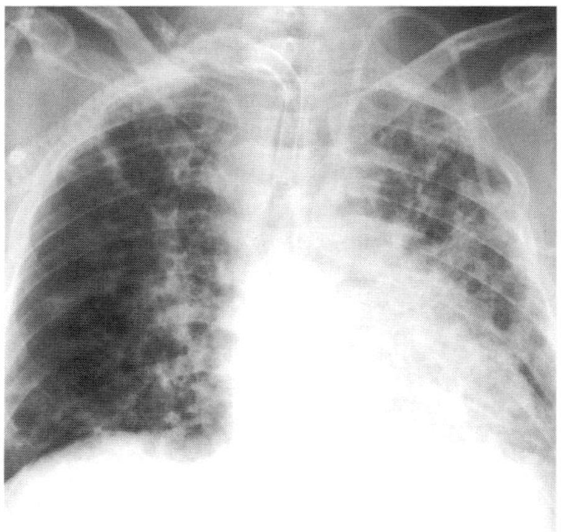

Fig. 147.2 a

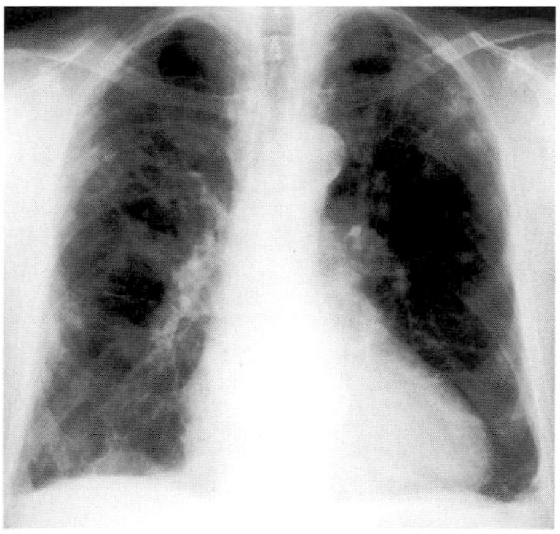

Fig. 147.3 a

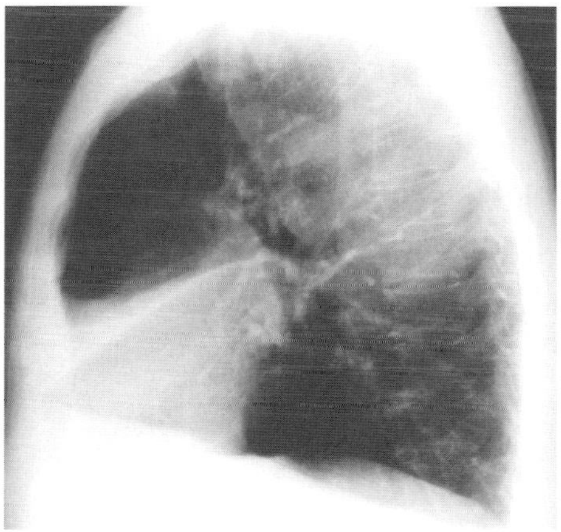

Fig. 147.1 b

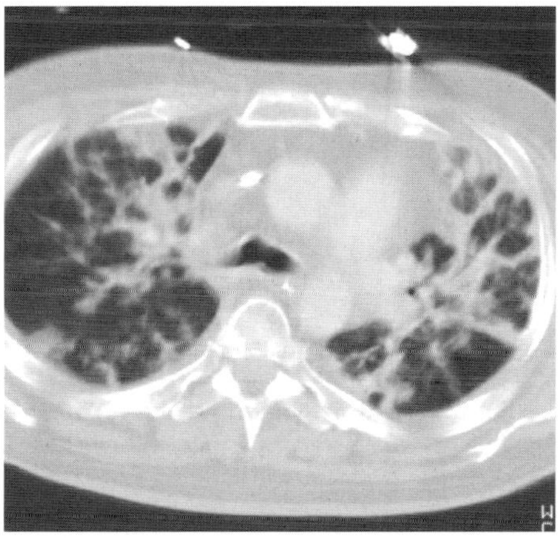

Fig. 147.2 b

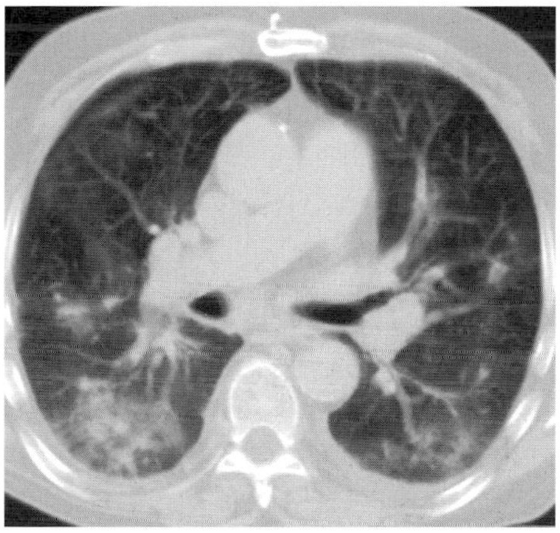

Fig. 147.3 b

Some cytostatic drugs (e.g., methotrexate, cyclophosphamide, bleomycin) can also incite a chronic, fibrosing alveolitis with lymphocytic infiltration of the lung. These changes are chronically progressive and culminate in pulmonary fibrosis or a honeycomb lung (see p. 150).

Many other drugs may evoke an allergic reaction in the lung of predisposed individuals, leading to eosinophilic infiltrates (see **Fig. 132.4**) or interstitial forms of pneumonia with asthmalike symptoms. **Figure 147.3** shows an example of an amiodarone-induced side effect, which is marked by the appearance of interstitial and fine confluent inflammatory foci in the lung. Generally these drug-induced changes are reversible and regress quickly after the offending drug is withdrawn. Thus, if you find these changes in a patient with no laboratory or microbiological evidence of infection, always consider the possibility of drug-induced pneumonitis.

Pulmonary involvement may also be found in autoimmune diseases such as antiglomerular basement membrane disease (hematuria + renal failure), ankylosing spondylitis (HLA B27), Sjögren syndrome, rheumatoid arthritis, Churg-Strauss syndrome, and Wegener granulomatosis (see p. 134).

Pneumoconiosis

Pneumoconiosis is a pulmonary silicosis that may develop in ceramic workers, sandblasters, and workers who mine quartz-rich stone. It may occur acutely due to massive inhalation, but generally it develops gradually following 10-20 years of exposure to inorganic quartz dust. Because particles of silicon dioxide (SiO_2) are only 2-5 μm in size, they can easily enter the alveoli where they are phagocytized by macrophages and transported to the interstitium. Fibroblasts and collagen fibers in the interstitium give rise to fibrotic zones that cause restrictive and obstructive ventilatory impairment. The chronic stage is characterized by vascular stenoses, pulmonary hypertension with progressive dyspnea, and eventual cor pulmonale.

Officially recognized as an occupational disease, pneumoconiosis-related lung changes have been classified as follows based on the criteria of the International Labor Office (ILO) [8.1, 8.2]:

ILO Classification of Pneumoconiosis

Film quality	Small round opacities (prevailing diameter)	Linear, reticular, and reticulonodular opacities
+ Good, with no loss of diagnostic information	**p** < 1.5 mm (micronodular)	**s** < 1.5 mm, fine, linear
+/- Technical deficiencies, but still no loss of diagnostic information	**q** 1.5 – 3 mm	**t** < 1.5 – 3 mm, moderately coarse
+/-- Limited ability to evaluate the lung and pleura	**r** 3 – 10 mm	**u** 3 – 10 mm, coarse
u Unreadable		

Profusion and location (determined by comparison with standard films)

These features are rated on a 0-3-point scale for four main categories and another 0-12-point scale (not shown here) within the main categories.

Large opacities

A One or more opacities > 1 cm, not exceeding a combined diameter of 5 cm

B One or more opacities with a combined diameter larger than **A** and with an equivalent area <u>not</u> exceeding the area of the right upper zone

C One or more opacities with a combined diameter larger than **B** and with an equivalent area exceeding the area of the right upper zone

Pleural abnormalities

Thickness
(measured from the inner border of the chest wall to the lung border):
a 3 – 5 mm
b > 5 – 10 mm
c > 10 mm

Maximum longitudinal extent
(distance from apex to sinus, measured separately for each side)
1 < 1/4 of this maximum distance (summation of all longitudinally imaged plaques)
2 1/4 - 1/2 of this maximum distance (summation of all longitudinally imaged plaques)
3 > 1/2 of this maximum distance (summation of all longitudinally imaged plaques)

Pleural calcifications
(summation of all calcified plaques, measured separately for each side)
1 One or more calcifications with a combined length < 2 cm
2 Same as **1**, with a combined length of 2–10 cm
3 Same as **2**, with a combined length > 10 cm

Additionally, a number of symbols are used to code abnormalities of cardiac shape, bullae, atelectases, aortic calcifications, emphysematous changes, etc. Please consult additional sources if you deal with disability examinations in occupationally exposed workers [8.1].

Silicosis

An advanced pulmonary silicosis may have various radiographic appearances, ranging from a generalized linear and reticular pattern (diffuse reticular fibrosis, **Fig. 149.1**) to multiple small, well-defined round opacities 1-10 mm in diameter (nodular fibrosis). The latter condition produces a "snowstorm" pattern **(Fig. 149.2)** that resembles the miliary form of tuberculosis (TB; see p. 133). A middle and upper zone predominance is occasionally seen. Eggshell calcifications in the perihilar lymph nodes (↘) are virtually pathognomonic

for silicosis **(Fig. 149.3)**. Some patients develop a massive, progressive fibrosis with zones of emphysema and plaque formation.

Silicosis is also associated with an increased incidence of lung cancer and predisposes to the reactivation of TB. Obstructive ventilatory impairment (chronic obstructive pulmonary disease , COPD) is more common than restrictive impairment on spirometric testing.

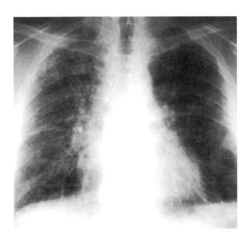

Fig. 149.1

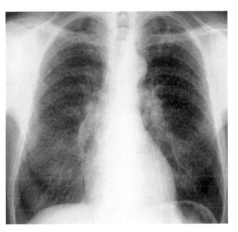

Fig. 149.2

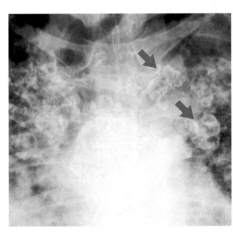

Fig. 149.3

Asbestosis

Inhaled silicate fibers from the production of insulating materials, textiles, paper, and plastic cause pulmonary fibrosis following a latent period of 15-30 years after initial exposure. They promote the development of pleural mesotheliomas and lung cancer. In contrast to silicosis, pleural changes are predominant and typically consist of pleural plaques on the anterolateral (↗) and diaphragmatic pleura **(Fig. 149.4b)**. These plaques frequently become calcified (↓ in **Fig. 149.5**). The pleural plaques (see p. 53, p. 56) often cause areas of

unsharpness in the cardiac borders (→) and diaphragm (↑) **(Fig. 149.4a)**. Radiographs also show fibrotic changes in the pulmonary interstitium with areas of bronchiectasis (see p. 151), paracicatricial emphysema, and eventual progression to a honeycomb pattern (see p. 150). These changes predominantly affect the basal lung zones.

Spirometry in asbestosis shows a predominance of restrictive ventilatory impairment over obstructive impairment. Additional causes of pneumoconiosis are listed on the next page.

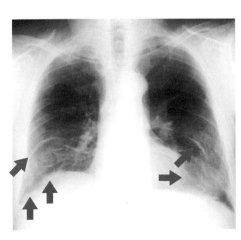

Fig. 149.4a

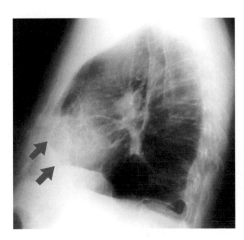

Fig. 149.4b

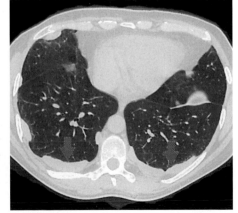

Fig. 149.5

Other types of inhaled particles besides quartz dust (see p. 148-149) can cause pneumoconiosis. The most frequent causes are listed in **Table 150.1**.

Additional Causes of Pneumoconiosis

Inorganic dusts	Organic dusts
• Anthracosis (coal dust) • Siderosis (iron oxide) • Bauxite (aluminum) • Hard metals (tin, tungsten, titanium, vanadium, cobalt, etc.) • Berylliosis (aircraft industry)	• Farmer's lung (damp hay) • Grain workers (weevils) • Bird breeders (proteins in bird droppings) • Cork and wood workers (mold) • Malt workers (moldy barley) • Cheese washers (mold)

Table 150.1

Pulmonary Fibrosis

Chronic diseases that may culminate in pulmonary fibrosis were reviewed on the previous pages. They include inflammatory processes, chronic pulmonary congestion, the end-stage of sarcoidosis (Boeck disease), and the inhaled dusts listed above. A linear and reticular pattern is often dominant on chest radiographs. This pattern may be combined with regional lucencies caused by postinflammatory scar emphysema **(Fig. 150.2)**. **Figure 150.3** shows a postpneumonic honeycomb pattern (↘) in which most of the right lung parenchyma has been lost and the mediastinum is shifted toward the right side (←).

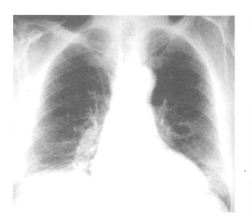

Fig. 150.2 a

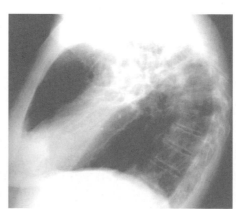

Fig. 150.3 a

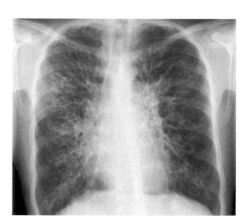

Fig. 150.4 a

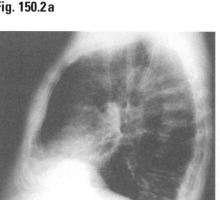

Fig. 150.2 b

Fig. 150.3 b

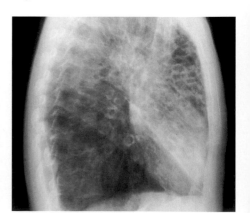

Fig. 150.4 b

The changes may progress to involve the entire lung, creating the radiographic appearance of a honeycomb lung **(Fig. 150.4)**. Eventually the clinical picture progresses to a hypoxemic state with exertional dyspnea followed by dyspnea at rest, clubbing of the fingers, and other clinical manifestations of cyanosis.

Bronchiectasis

Bronchiectasis is an abnormal, irreversible dilatation of medium-sized and smaller bronchi. Unlike the larger bronchi (segmental, lobar, mainstem), the walls of these smaller air passages are not stabilized by cartilage rings. Bronchiectasis usually shows a regional distribution pattern and is secondary to early childhood bronchiolitis, pneumonia, or pulmonary fibrosis. Less commonly, bronchiectasis occurs as a congenital anomaly or in the setting of cystic fibrosis (viscous mucus production, often with involvement of the pancreas and sweat glands) or an alpha-1-antitrypsin deficiency (often involving the basal lung in patients 30-40 years of age). Kartagener syndrome refers to a combination of chronic sinusitis and visceral transposition.

Three morphological types of bronchiectasis are distinguished: cylindrical (most common in adolescents), varicose (caused by fibrous strictures), and saccular (most common in elderly patients). All three forms are usually located in the posterobasal lung region (Fig. 151.1a-c). It is likely that the stasis of secretions in a chronically inflamed airway leads to dilatation of the bronchial walls. The disease predisposes to chronic recurring bouts of bronchopneumonia, often with copious purulent sputum.

The radiological findings range from parallel line shadows ("tramlines") and a regional distribution of increased, thickened linear densities to cylindrical or saccular cavities (✎ in Figs. 151.2, 151.3). A "signet ring" sign is seen in axial CT scans because the dilated bronchus presents a larger cross section than the companion artery that abuts the bronchus.

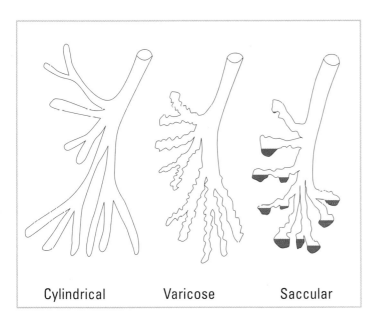

Cylindrical   Varicose   Saccular

Fig. 151.1

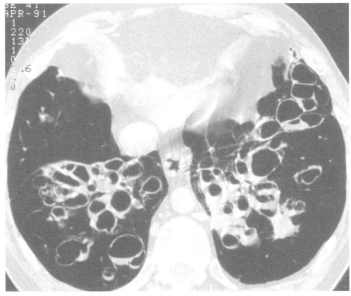

Fig. 151.3

8

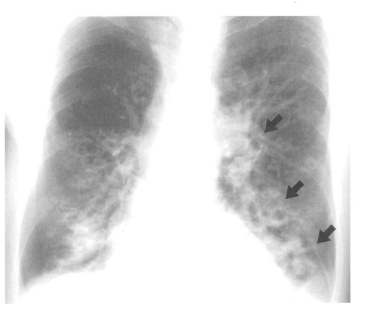

Fig. 151.2a

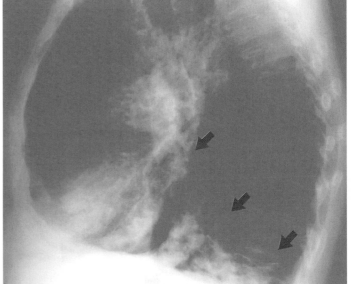

Fig. 151.2b

Carcinomatous Lymphangitis

In patients with bronchial carcinoma (BC), tumor cell dissemination may occur along lymphatic pathways as well as other routes, causing a regional increase in linear and reticular markings on the chest radiograph. In the patient with right hilar BC in **Figure 152.1a**, carcinomatous lymphangitis forms a pattern of linear markings (⤳) that radiate from the tumor site into the periphery of the lung. CT reveals thickened interlobular septa, which may have a string-of-beads appearance,

along with micronodular densities **(Fig. 152.1b)**.

A follow-up radiograph in another patient with left-sided BC **(Fig. 152.2b)** shows a marked increase in carcinomatous lymphangitis compared with the previous film **(Fig. 152.2a)**. The radiograph also shows possible infiltration of the right lung (↘) and apical cicatricial bullae (↓). Other examples of BC are shown on page 76 and page 129.

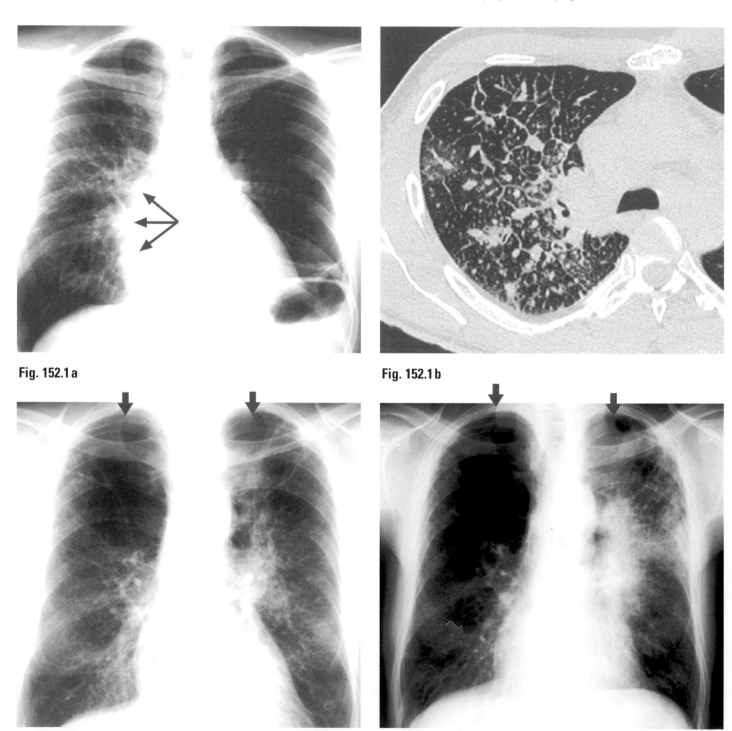

Fig. 152.1 a

Fig. 152.1 b

Fig. 152.2 a

Fig. 152.2 b

An increased incidence of carcinomatous lymphangitis is also found in patients with primary tumors of the stomach or breast. Though it occurs more frequently on the side of the affected breast **(Fig. 153.1)**, carcinomatous lymphangitis may develop in both lungs **(Fig. 153.2)**. If you see a Port-A-Cath system (←) on the radiograph (see p. 164), you may assume that the patient has received chemotherapy for a malignant underlying disease, as illustrated in both of the cases shown here.

A similar pattern may develop after an approximately one- to four-month latent period following radiotherapy at 20 Gray or more. The changes are confined to the radiation port and are sharply demarcated from the nonirradiated surroundings **(Fig. 153.3)**. The typical straight-edged, well-delineated pattern of radiation pneumonitis (↘ ↙) is also seen after radiation to the mediastinum. Initial changes usually consist of linear and stippled opacities, which gradually coalesce and often culminate in radiation fibrosis (see p. 150).

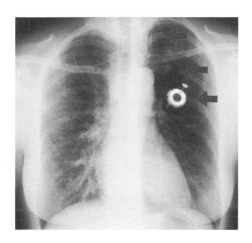

Fig. 153.1

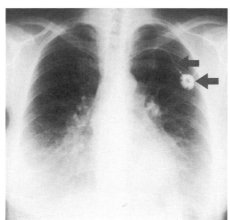

Fig. 153.2

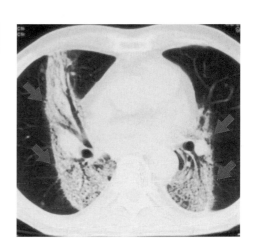

Fig. 153.3

When dyspnea occurs in a patient with cancer of the lung, breast, or stomach and conventional chest radiographs show no pulmonary abnormalities, radionuclide imaging (scintigraphy) may be helpful in early cases. The images may reveal early inhalation or perfusion defects before signs of carcinomatous lymphangitis become visible on radiographs **(Fig. 153.4)**. If an effusion also develops, in this case with a visible

fluid level (→ in **Fig. 153.5**), the collection may as sampled by percutaneous needle aspiration to check for malignant cells that would confirm the diagnosis.

In cases with bilateral lung involvement **(Fig. 153.2)** or even the diffuse involvement of an entire lung **(Fig. 153.6)**, the lymphangitis might be misinterpreted as pulmonary fibrosis (see p. 150).

8

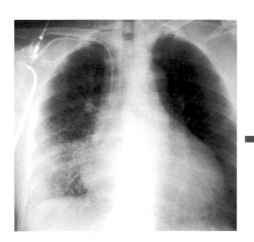

Fig. 153.4

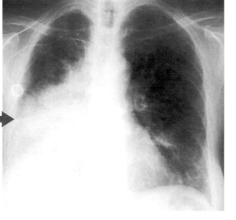

Fig. 153.5

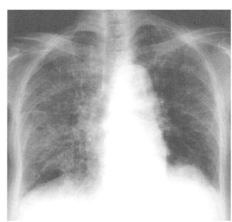

Fig. 153.6

Again, please complete the entire quiz before checking the answer key at the end of the book. Otherwise you might spot additional answers that would "spoil the suspense" and keep you from getting the most out of the quiz.

49 Do you remember the criteria that can help you differentiate between silicosis and asbestosis? Please write them in the boxes below:

Differentiating criteria	Silicosis	Asbestosis
Sites of predilection for fibrotic changes:		
Spirometric ventilation defects?		
Very typical features and their location:		

50 Write down from memory some typical signs that would distinguish pulmonary congestion from inflammatory infiltrates:

Checklist: Signs of Pulmonary Congestion

Direct signs	Indirect signs

51 What signs <u>are</u> consistent with inflammatory infiltration of the lung?

52 What is the difference between PcP and other forms of pneumonia? Why is the early detection of PcP so important?

53 Interpret this supine radiograph **(Fig. 155.1)** as completely and systematically as you can:

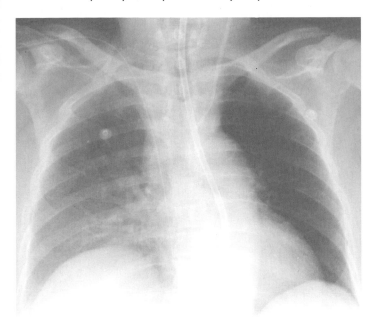

Fig. 155.1

54 This small child is referred to you with itching vesicles and pustules covering the skin and oral mucosa and with suspected otitis media. He has fever, severe lethargy, and some throat irritation **(Fig. 155.2)**.

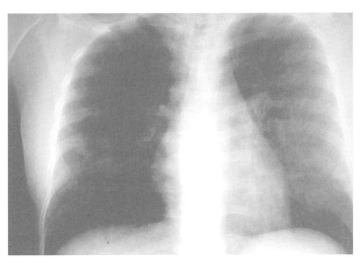

Fig. 155.2

55 Look at these two radiographs, which were taken one day apart in the same patient **(Fig. 155.3)**. What is your diagnosis?

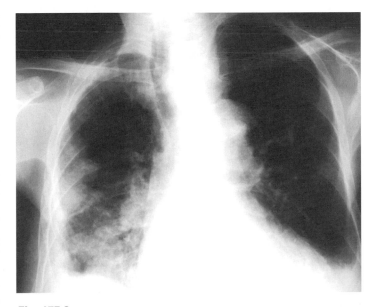

Fig. 155.3a

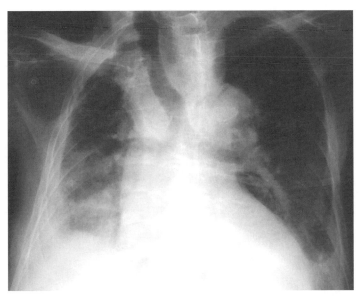

Fig. 155.3b (Next day)

8

Q

56 A 42-year-old woman presents for a routine chest radiograph **(Fig. 156.1)**. What do you see?

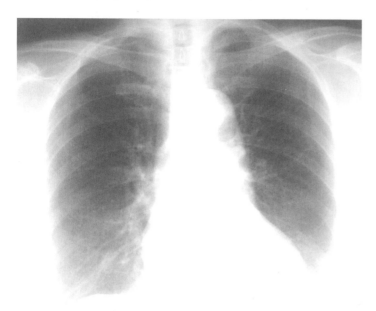

Fig. 156.1

57 Describe the abnormalities in **Figure 156.2**. What aspect of the patient's history would you like to learn more about, and what questions would you ask?

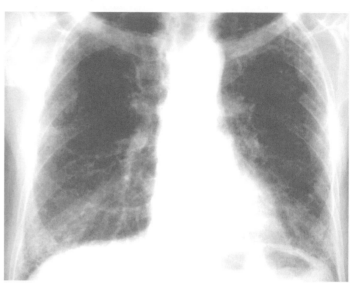

Fig. 156.2

58 As a final challenge, here are two radiographs from the same HIV patient **(Fig. 156.3)**. Please make a differential diagnosis. What diagnostic and therapeutic options would you consider for this patient?

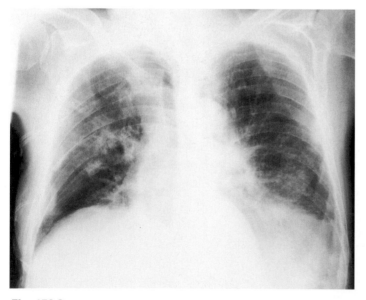

Fig. 156.3a

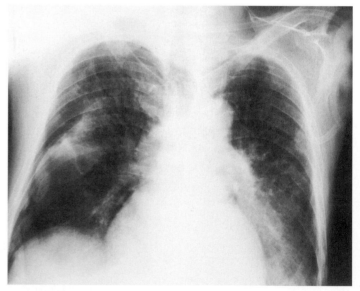

Fig. 156.3b   (Next day)

Lars Kamper
Matthias Hofer

Foreign Bodies

Chapter Goals:

This chapter deals with the most commonly encountered foreign materials, such as catheters, pacemaker systems, and various heart valves and tubes. Because these foreign materials are widely used in intensive care medicine, it is important to be able to recognize them on chest radiographs. On completing this chapter, you should be able to:

- know the steps involved in the placement of a central venous catheter (CVC) and recognize the most frequent complications on the chest radiograph;

- describe the correct position of various catheters on the chest radiograph;

- explain the functions of different catheter systems;

- be able to distinguish different cardiac pacemaker systems on the chest radiograph and know their different modes of operation;

- recognize different types of prosthetic heart valves on the chest radiograph;

- confirm the correct placement of an endotracheal tube.

9

Central Venous Catheters

Chest radiographs are taken after the placement of a central venous catheter (CVC) to check the catheter position and exclude complications relating to catheter insertion. The catheter tip should be positioned in the superior vena cava (SVC) approximately 2 cm proximal to the opening of the SVC into the right atrium **(Fig. 158.1)**. Published reports vary somewhat with regard to radiographic landmarks for positioning the catheter tip (➡). For practical reasons [9.1], we favor the termination of the azygos vein in the SVC at the level of the tracheal bifurcation (⬆ in **Fig. 158.2**) or slightly above the right main bronchus **(14a)**. Several different catheter types and their applications are reviewed in **Table 158.3**.

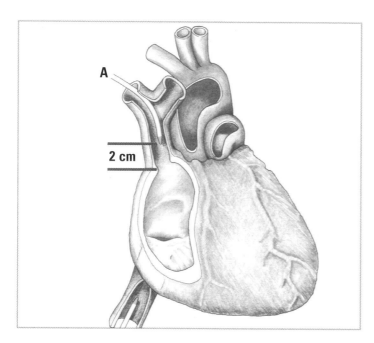

Fig. 158.1

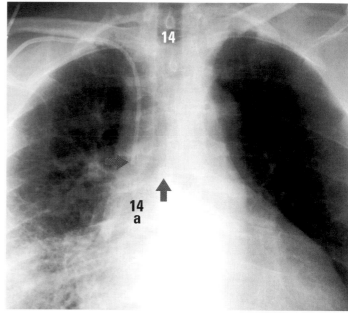

Fig. 158.2

Type of catheter	Applications
CVC (central venous catheter)	**Plastic catheter for the central administration of drugs with venotoxic and cardiotoxic properties** • Catheter is introduced into the venous system through a venipuncture site (usually in the upper half of the body) • Tip is advanced through the superior vena cava to the right atrium (see pp. 158–163)
Hickman	**Long-term CVC; applications include chemotherapy in children** • Introduced into the subclavian vein or internal jugular vein under radiographic control • Tip is advanced through the superior vena cava to the right atrium • Infection risk is reduced by using an antimicrobial cuff and tunneling the catheter through the subcutaneous tissue before exiting the skin • Retention is aided by a Dacron cuff that adheres to the skin
Shaldon	**Large-bore catheter for acute dialysis and volume-replacement therapy** • Advanced through the superior vena cava to the right atrium (see Fig. 165.2)
Demers	**Large-bore catheter for longer-term dialysis** • Used in patients without a dialysis fistula or shunt • Unlike the Shaldon catheter, is usually advanced into the right atrium through the subclavian vein (see Fig. 165.4) • Infection risk is reduced by using an antimicrobial cuff and tunneling the catheter through the subcutaneous tissue before exiting the skin
Subcutaneous port	**Subcutaneously implanted plastic reservoir (port system) for multiple chemotherapy cycles** • Port system consists of a central venous catheter and a subcutaneously placed injection port (see p. 164) • Advanced through the superior vena cava to the right atrium • Plastic reservoir accessible with special port needles

Table 158.3

Catheter Insertion

The sterile tray for catheter insertion **(Fig. 159.1)** should include the following:

- Several syringes with isotonic saline solution **(A)**
- One scalpel **(B)**
- One syringe with local anesthetic **(C)**
- One syringe with an introducer needle **(D)**
- One vessel dilator **(E)**
- One guidewire **(F)**
- Suture material **(G)** and clip **(H)**
- One CVC with three-way stopcocks **(K)**
- Sterile compresses and adhesive strips **(J)**

The catheter is inserted using the Seldinger technique. For a subclavian catheter, experience has shown that the best site for needle insertion is approximately 1-2 cm below the clavicle in the midclavicular line (MCL).

The area around the insertion site is swabbed with an alcohol solution using a swirling motion in an inside-to-outside spiral **(Fig. 159.2)**. The ipsilateral side of the chest is covered with a sterile fenestrated drape, and the insertion site is infiltrated subcutaneously with local anesthetic **(C)**. The needle is advanced to the clavicle with continuous a spiration, and anesthetic is injected all along the needle tract **(Fig. 159.3)**.

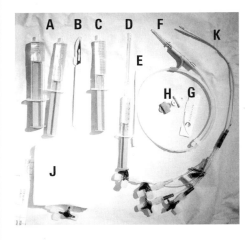

Fig. 159.1 Sterile catheter kit

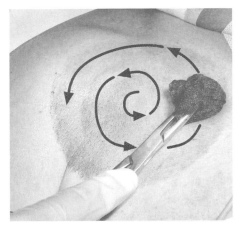

Fig. 159.2 Disinfection

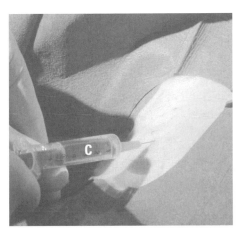

Fig. 159.3 Local anesthesia

Insertion of the introducer needle is done in two steps: First the needle **(D)** is inserted to the clavicle, directing it at a shallow angle to the skin **(Fig. 159.4)**, and it is passed beneath the bone. In a second step, the angle of the needle is adjusted so that the tip is directed toward the sternoclavicular joint or jugular fossa **(Fig. 159.5)**.

In the photograph, the middle finger indicates the direction of needle insertion. The needle is advanced further while drawing back the plunger until the sudden aspiration of blood (⬉) confirms that the needle has entered a vessel **(Fig. 159.6)**.

Pulsations of the blood column and the color of the blood may signify an inadvertent arterial puncture. In patients with a low arterial blood pressure or poor oxygenation, venous and arterial blood can be distinguished by obtaining a blood gas analysis or recording a pressure waveform.

In some cases, distal traction on the ipsilateral arm in line with the longitudinal body axis and slight external rotation of the arm may facilitate needle insertion. These maneuvers place maximum tension on the subclavian vein and move it forward.

9

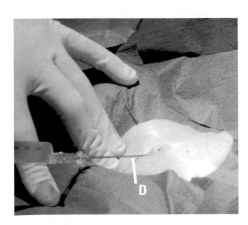

Fig. 159.4 Puncture towards clavicle

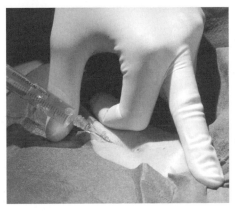

Fig. 159.5 Adjustment towards jugular fossa

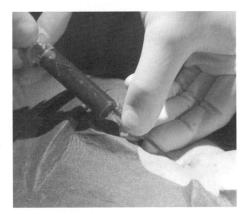

Fig. 159.6 Aspiration

When intravenous placement has been confirmed, the Seldinger wire **(F)** is introduced through the preplaced needle **(D)** (⬊) and advanced for a distance of approximately 20-25 cm **(Fig. 160.1)**. The needle is removed over the Seldinger wire, and the insertion site is incised with a scalpel **(B) (Fig. 160.2)**. The needle tract is then enlarged with a rigid plastic dilator **(E)** (⬊ in **Fig. 160.3**).

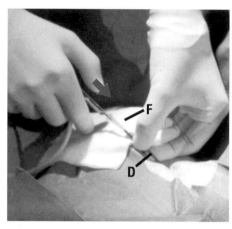

Fig. 160.1

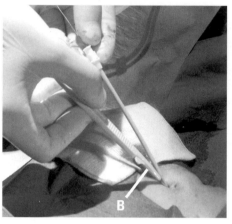

Fig. 160.2

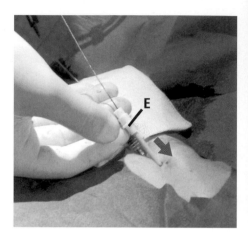

Fig. 160.3

Next the catheter **(K)** is threaded over the guidewire **(F)** **(Fig. 160.4)** and advanced approximately 16-18 cm along the vessel lumen **(Fig. 160.5)**. The CVC should be previously filled with isotonic saline solution as a precaution against air embolism. The catheter is advanced over the Seldinger wire until the end of the wire (⬈) protrudes from the catheter.

The guidewire should protrude from the distal limb of a multi-lumen system, and therefore the three-way stopcock should be opened on that limb!

Even in an emergency catheter insertion, always remember to secure the protruding free end of the wire (⬈) with your fingers (⬊ ⬉) as shown in **Figure 160.6**.

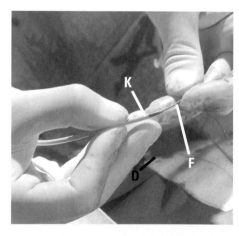

Fig. 160.4

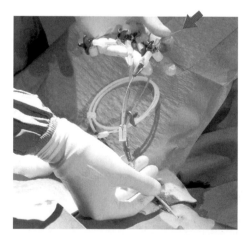

Fig. 160.5

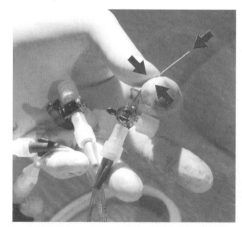

Fig. 160.6

After the guidewire is removed, the plunger is drawn back ( ) in **Fig. 161.1**) to aspirate blood ( ) and confirm intravascular placement of the CVC. The catheter is then flushed with iso-tonic saline solution (in **Fig. 161.2**). When a multilumen catheter is used, this process is repeated for each lumen (!). Before the syringe is removed, it is important to check for effective closure of the three-way stopcock **(Fig. 161.3)**. An

open stopcock might lead to an air embolism or bleeding from the catheter, depending on the central venous pressure.

The risk of air embolism can be reduced by positioning the patient in a head-down tilt. This position will raise the hydro-static CVP and increase the volume of blood in the upper neck veins.

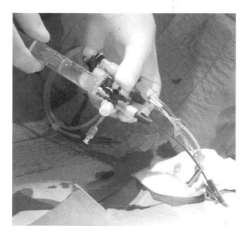

Fig. 161.1

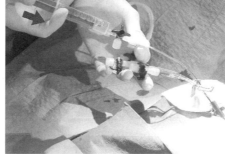

Fig. 161.2

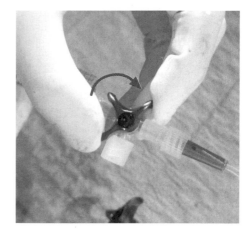

Fig. 161.3

For secure retention of the CVC, a plastic clip **(H)** is attached to the catheter and sutured to the skin on each side **(Figs. 161.4, 161.5)**. The entry site is dressed with sterile gauze **(J)** and adhesive tape **(Fig. 161.6)**. Especially in difficult or emergency insertions, a radiograph should be taken within an hour after catheter insertion to check the catheter position and rule out complications.

Catheter maintenance includes regular wound inspections and dressing changes. Generally a CVC is left in place for 10-14 days if the entry site appears normal. The CVC should be removed at once if local or systemic signs of infection are noted without an identifiable focus. If a catheter-associated infection is suspected, the catheter tip should be tested for pathogenic organisms and antibiotic resistance.

9

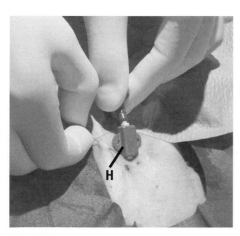

Fig. 161.4

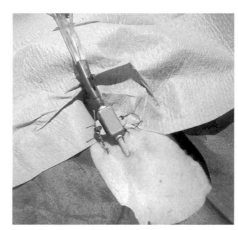

Fig. 161.5

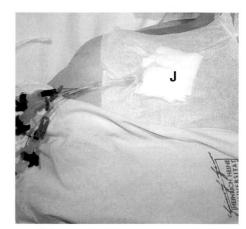

Fig. 161.6

Alternatively, the catheter can be positioned under electrocardiogram (ECG) guidance by recording a continuous ECG trace via the catheter tip (**Fig. 162.1**). While the catheter tip is in the venous system, a normal waveform (**A**) will be recorded as the catheter passes through the SVC. When the tip enters the right atrium, the p-wave (⬇) undergoes a characteristic change from a monophasic (single-peak) form (**B**) to a biphasic (**C**) deflection in the ECG (**Fig. 162.1**). When the tip passes the sinus node, the amplitude of the p-wave declines and finally becomes negative (**D**). It remains negative even if the catheter tip is inadvertently placed in the inferior vena cava (IVC) (**E**) (**Fig. 162.2**).

During the insertion, the catheter is advanced until the amplitude of the p-wave just increases (**C**). It is then retracted until the p-wave amplitude returns to normal (**B**).

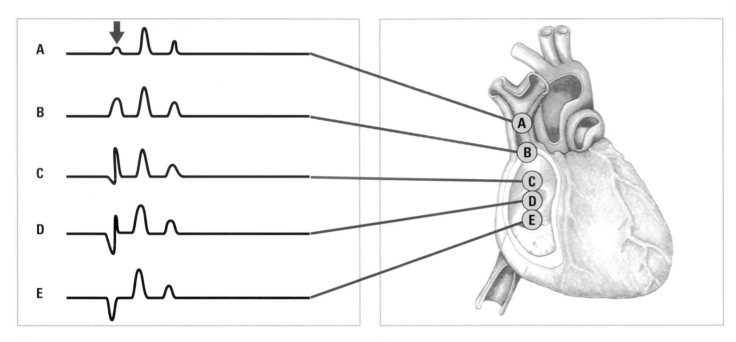

Fig. 162.1

Fig. 162.2

Finally, the catheter is withdrawn an additional 2 cm from that site, placing the catheter tip safely in the SVC (**Fig. 162.3**). **Figure 162.4** shows a radiograph of a CVC tip (➡) correctly positioned in the SVC (**1**). The radiograph is useful not only for checking catheter placement, but also for detecting complications relating to the catheter insertion (see p. 163).

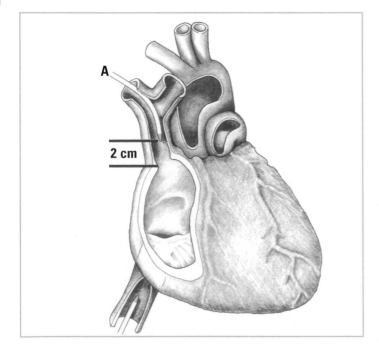

Fig. 162.3

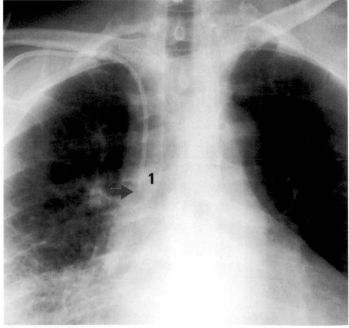

Fig. 162.4

Complications

If the catheter is advanced too far, the catheter tip (➡) may enter the right atrium **(Fig. 163.1)** and precipitate a cardiac arrhythmia. If the catheter has been placed too deeply, it should be withdrawn to a point just outside the atrium. In extreme cases the catheter may even extend into a hepatic vein, or it may be misdirected into other vessels **(Fig. 163.2)**. In **Figure 163.3**, the tip of a jugular CVC (➘) has passed from the jugular vein into the subclavian vein, missing the SVC altogether. The upper part of the catheter in **Figure 163.4** is looped (↲), although the tip (➡) could still be maneuvered into the SVC. If this occurs, the catheter should be removed and a new catheter inserted because the catheter is not sterile enough to be advanced further or repositioned. Pneumothorax is another possible complication, especially during the insertion of a subclavian CVC. Placement should therefore be checked on an expiratory radiograph, particularly after a complicated subclavian insertion (see p. 191). A rare but serious complication is pericardial tamponade caused by inadvertent entry of the catheter into the pericardial sac.

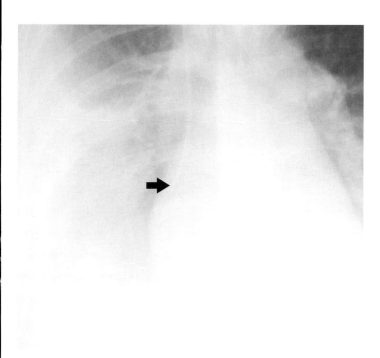

Fig. 163.1

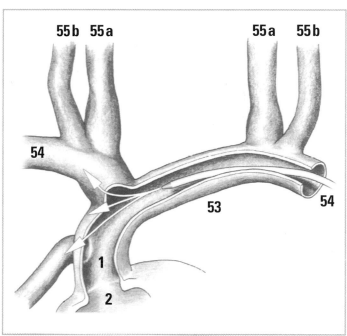

Fig. 163.2

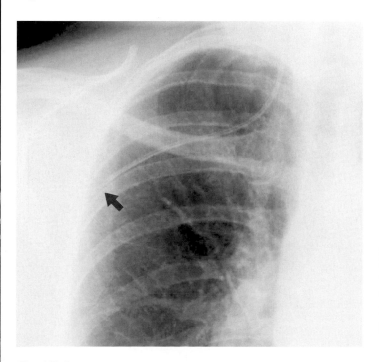

Fig. 163.3

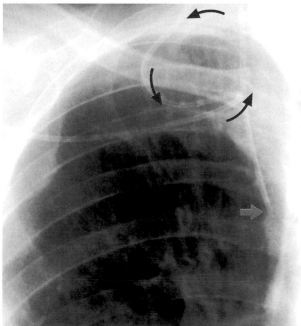

Fig. 163.4

Subcutaneous port systems are used for long-term ambulatory treatment with centrally administered venotoxic drugs (e.g., chemotherapy). The port is surgically implanted as follows: The catheter is introduced into the cephalic vein under fluoroscopic guidance, and the catheter tip is advanced through the subclavian vein into the SVC. Next the reservoir is implanted between the pectoralis muscle and body fascia. A postoperative radiograph is taken to exclude puncture-related complications. **Figure 164.1** shows the correct placement of a port system. The reservoir (↑) is projected below the clavicle **(23)**, and the catheter tip (→) is in the SVC **(1)** just above the entry to the right atrium **(2)**. The intravascular position of the port catheter can be confirmed by contrast administration, as shown in **Figure 164.2**: The course of the catheter and the spillage of contrast medium (▶) distal to the catheter tip (↗) are clearly visualized. Although the tip projects correctly into the SVC **(1)**, extravascular pooling of contrast medium (↙) can be seen in the tissue below the clavicle **(23)**. This signifies a leak in the proximal catheter system.

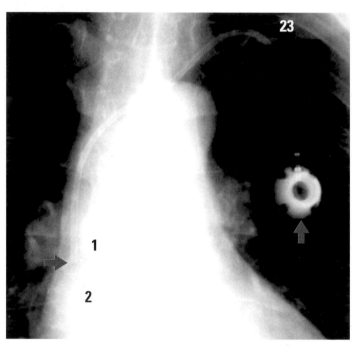

Fig. 164.1

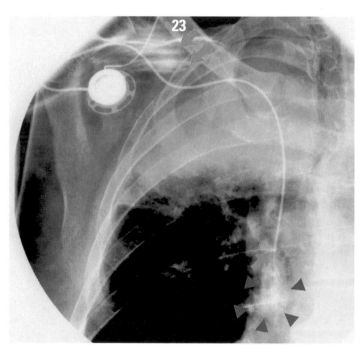

Fig. 164.2

The titanium housing of older port systems **(Fig. 164.5)** may cause artifacts on magnetic resonance (MR) images. In **Figure 164.4**, the housing has produced a conspicuous signal void (↓) on the anterior side of the left pectoralis muscle.

Newer generations of port systems **(Fig. 164.3)** are MRI-compatible, however, and do not cause troublesome artifacts (→ in **Fig. 164.4**).

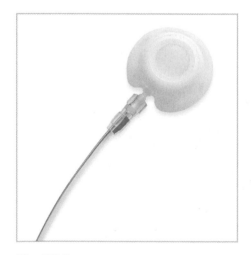

Fig. 164.3

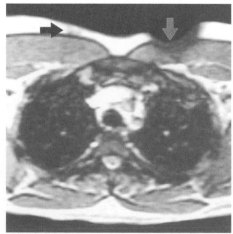

Fig. 164.4

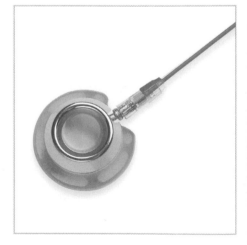

Fig. 164.5

Among the most widely used dialysis catheters at present are the Shaldon catheter (L) and Demers catheter (M) (Fig. 165.1). The Shaldon catheter is used for temporary vascular access in emergency situations such as acute renal failure or acute fistula thrombosis. The Shaldon catheter usually has a double lumen and is made of a harder material than the Demers catheter. It is used for no more than two to three weeks due to the greater risk of infection. As shown in **Figure 165.2**, it is introduced into the SVC (1) and occasionally into the inguinal vein. **Figure 165.3** shows the normal position of a Shaldon catheter in the chest radiograph. The tip (←) is in the SVC (1) at the entrance to the right atrium (2). The tracheal bifurcation (↑) can provide an additional landmark and normally should be projected above the catheter tip. If the Shaldon catheter is advanced too far, it should be withdrawn into the SVC to eliminate the risk of atrial perforation. The entire course (▶) of the catheter should be visualized.

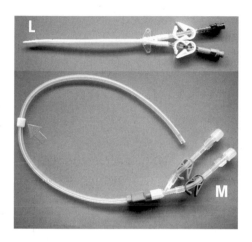

Fig. 165.1

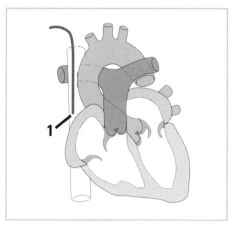

Fig. 165.2

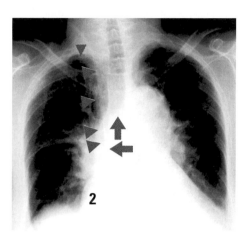

Fig. 165.3

The Demers catheter (M) (Fig. 165.1) is durable enough for one to two years of continuous service. It usually has a single lumen and is made of a flexible material. Unlike the Shaldon catheter, the tip of the Demers catheter is placed within the right atrium (2) because higher volumes are exchanged within the cardiac chamber (Fig. 165.4). Figure 165.5 shows an anteroposterior (AP) radiograph of a Demers catheter. The extracardiac portion of the catheter (▷) is clearly visualized, but the catheter tip cannot be positively distinguished from the cardiac shadow. Identification is aided by a lateral radiograph (Fig. 165.6), which confirms that the tip of the Demers catheter (→) is in the right atrium (2). Another advantage of this catheter is that it is usually tunneled through the subcutaneous tissue, thereby reducing the risk of infection. It also has a subcutaneous felt collar (↖ in Fig. 165.1) that functions as a germ barrier. Generally, the risk of infection is further reduced by covering the catheter exit site with sterile tape.

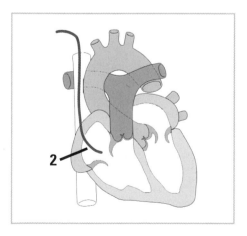

Fig. 165.4

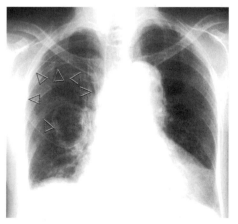

Fig. 165.5

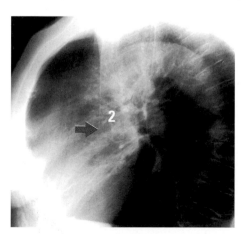

Fig. 165.6

Due to the increased risk of thrombosis and infection, central vascular access lines require particularly close attention from doctors and nurses. They should not be used for drawing blood samples or administering infusions. The lumen is filled with heparin solution to prevent catheter thrombosis between dialysis sessions.

Pulmonary Artery Catheter

Pulmonary artery catheters (Swan-Ganz [9.2, 9.3]) are used in the monitoring of hemodynamically unstable patients. They make it possible to measure the pressures in the pulmonary circulation. They are inserted by a central venous route, like CVCs, but an inflatable balloon at the catheter tip (→) allows the catheter to be carried by the blood flow from the SVC **(1)** through the right atrium **(2)** and ventricle and subsequently

into a pulmonary artery **(Fig. 166.1)**. A chest radiograph is taken to exclude insertion-related complications such as pneumothorax (see p. 191) and looping (↙) of the catheter **(Fig. 166.2)**. Moreover, the pulmonary artery may be injured due to penetration of the vessel wall by the catheter tip or overinflation of the balloon. This may cause intrapulmonary hemorrhage (see p. 130) and hemoptysis.

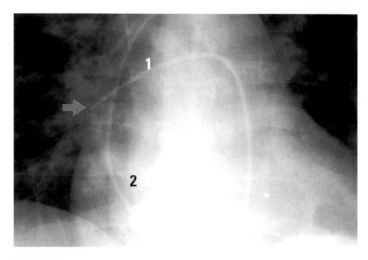

Fig. 166.1

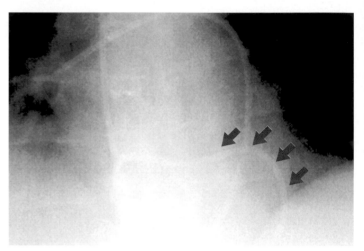

Fig. 166.2

While the catheter is being maneuvered into place, the instantaneous catheter position is monitored by recording a pressure waveform **(Fig. 166.3)**. When the catheter tip is in the vena cava or right atrium of a healthy patient, the waveform indicates a mean pressure of 2-6 mmHg **(RA)**. After the tip has passed through the tricuspid valve, the right ventricular pressure curve shows systolic pressures (↓) in the range of 15-30 mmHg **(RV)**. With entry into the pulmonary artery, the diastolic pressure (↑) rises abruptly to 6-12 mmHg while the systolic value (↓ ↓) shows little if any change **(PA)**. When

the inflated balloon reaches a branch of the pulmonary artery and becomes "wedged" in the vessel, occluding its lumen, the following takes place: The pressure curve shows a sudden drop in amplitude (↘) and the systolic pressure peaks disappear **(PCWP)**. The mean pressure at this level should be slightly below the diastolic pressure in the pulmonary artery. At this point the insertion is complete and the balloon is deflated, at which time the pulsatile waveform of the pulmonary artery reappears **(PA)**.

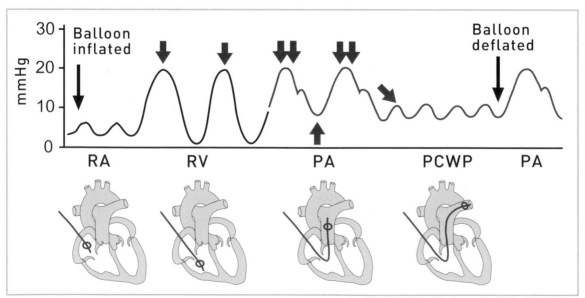

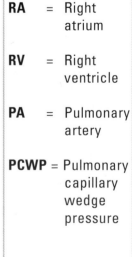

RA	= Right atrium
RV	= Right ventricle
PA	= Pulmonary artery
PCWP	= Pulmonary capillary wedge pressure

Fig. 166.3

Most pacemaker systems today are implanted in a subcutaneous pocket over the pectoralis muscle **(Fig. 167.1)**. The electrodes are advanced through a brachiocephalic vein into the right ventricle (↘) or atrium (↗) and secured there. Complications such as pneumothorax, electrode dislodgment, and fractures of pacemaker wires can be quickly and easily diagnosed on the chest radiograph **(Fig. 167.2)**.

In many cases it is possible to determine the pacing mode of the unit **(Tables 167.3, 167.4)** by noting the position and number of the pacemaker wires.

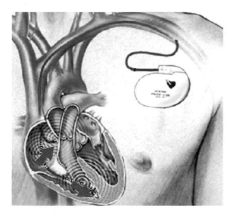

Fig. 167.1

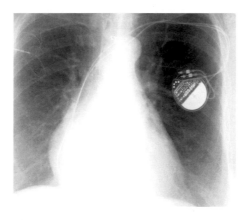

Fig. 167.2 a

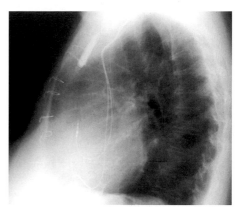

Fig. 167.2 b

Coding of pacemaker characteristics

Pacing	Sensing	Response mode	Rate adaptation
0 = none A = in the atrium V = in the ventricle D – dual (A + V)	0 = none A = in the atrium V = in the ventricle D = dual (A + V)	0 = none I = inhibited T = triggered D = dual (T + I)	0 = none R = rate-adaptive

Inhibited:	Pulse generation is inhibited by cardiac activity (most common response mode)
Triggered:	Pulses are generated in response to spontaneous cardiac activity (e.g., ventricular stimulation after sensing a spontaneous p wave)
Rate-adaptive:	Adaptation to various stress conditions, e.g. based on biological parameters (QT interval, respiratory rate, muscle impedance)

Table 167.3 [9.4]

Pacing mode	Function	Typical ECG trace
VVI (52%)	Ventricular pacing, ventricular sensing, pulse inhibition	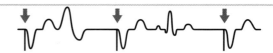 Ventricular pacing (↓) on demand with a deformed ventricular complex
DDD (41%)	Dual (A + V) pacing, dual (A + V) sensing, pulse inhibition and triggering	Atrial and ventricular pacing are triggered sequentially if needed (↓ ↓), but the atrium (←) and ventricle (→) can also be paced individually
AAI (2%)	Atrial pacing, atrial sensing, pulse inhibition	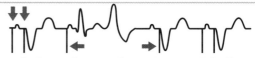 Atrial pacing (↓) on demand with a normal ventricular complex. **Caution:** use only with intact AV conduction

Table 167.4

The pacing modes that are most commonly used in modern pacemakers are designated VVI (approximately 52%), DDD (approximately 41%), AAI (approximately 2%), and VDD (approximately 5%) [9.4]. Other modes are strictly for diagnostic use and are almost never used for permanent pacemaker operation. VVI pacemakers (Fig. 168.1a-c) have only one electrode in the right ventricle (↗). They are inhibi-

ted by spontaneous ventricular activity and deliver pulses only when the ventricular rate falls below a preset value.

One disadvantage of this pacing mode is the unphysiological (retrograde) excitation of the atrium by way of the right ventricle. Thus, VVI pacemakers are used mainly for the control of bradyarrhythmias with atrial fibrillation.

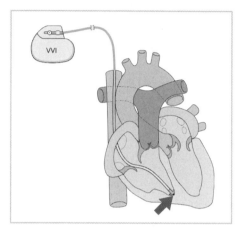

Fig. 168.1 a

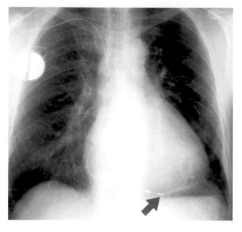

Fig. 168.1 b

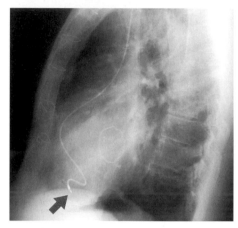

Fig. 168.1 c

DDD pacemakers (Fig. 168.2a-c) have one electrode in the right atrium (→) and one in the right ventricle (←). They are used in patients with arterioventricular (AV) block, for example. When the heart rate falls below a preset value, the atrium and ventricle are successively stimulated (sequential AV pacing). This time delay maintains a more physiological relationship between atrial and ventricular contraction, resulting in a better cardiac output. As in a VVI pacemaker,

the ventricular electrode (←) is implanted on the floor of the right ventricle close to the diaphragm (Fig. 168.2c). The wires are clearly displayed in this case because they are not obscured by the superimposed vertebral column or descending aorta (8). The atrial electrode (→) is clearly visible at the right cardiac border in the posteroanterior (PA) radiograph (Fig. 168.2b).

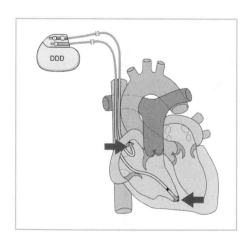

Fig. 168.2 a

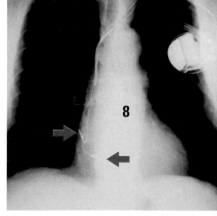

Fig. 168.2 b

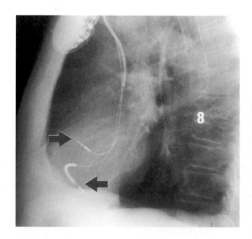

Fig. 168.2 c

The AAI pacemaker **(Fig. 169.1a)** has only one electrode (↓) in the right atrium and uses it for both sensing and pacing. The pacemaker is inhibited by spontaneous atrial activity and takes over only when the atrial rate falls below a preset minimum value. Of course, AAI pacing is appropriate only in cases where AV conduction is intact (e.g., in an isolated sinus node syndrome), since it cannot affect the ventricular rate in the presence of an AV block. It is not unusual for patients with a pacemaker to undergo open cardiac surgery. In this case the sternal cerclage wires **(52)** will be superimposed over the tip of the atrial electrode (←) in the PA radiograph **(Fig. 169.1b)**. The lateral radiograph provides a nonsuperimposed view that will clearly display any lead fractures **(Fig. 169.1c)**.

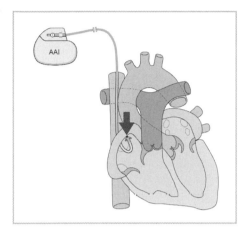

Fig. 169.1 a

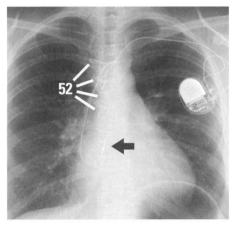

Fig. 169.1 b

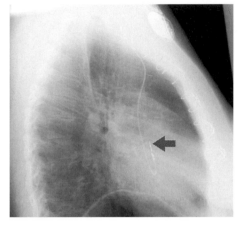

Fig. 169.1 c

The VDD pacemaker allows for sequential AV pacing without two separate electrodes. A single electrode is placed in the right ventricle (↗) and is used for both sensing and pacing. But the wire also bears two rings (↙) that float freely in the right atrium **(Fig. 169.2)**. Because the rings are not in contact with the atrial wall, they are used for sensing only. Unlike a DDD pacemaker, the VDD unit cannot perform atrial pacing.

Visualization of the atrial rings (→ in **Fig. 169.3a**) serves to distinguish this pacemaker from a VVI unit. The patient in this case had an implantable defibrillator (see **Fig. 170.2**), which can be recognized by the insulation (↓) on the ventricular lead.

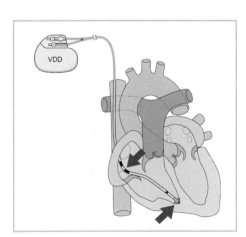

Fig. 169.2

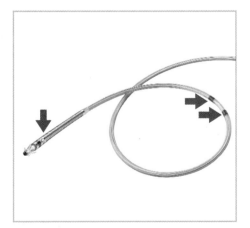

Fig. 169.3 a

Fig. 169.3 b

Biventricular pacemakers are used in patients with terminal heart failure, for example, or with a significant left bundle branch block. Besides the electrodes in the right atrium **(2)** and right ventricle **(4)**, these units have a third electrode for stimulating the left ventricular myocardium. This electrode is passed through the coronary sinus and placed in a coronary vein (← in **Fig. 170.1**).

The simultaneous biventricular pacing provides more rapid stimulation of the left ventricular myocardium than in pacemakers with only one right ventricular lead. In patients with a left bundle branch block, this pacing mode can improve the cardiac output by preventing asynchronous ventricular contractions.

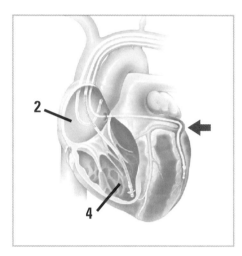

Fig. 170.1 a

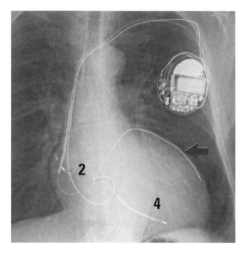

Fig. 170.1 b

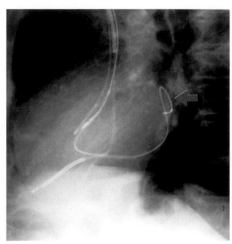

Fig. 170.1 c

Besides the antibradycardia function of the above pacemakers, **implantable cardioverter-defibrillators** (ICDs [9.5]) are also available that can interrupt life-threatening tachyarrhythmias. They have a specially insulated electrode (↓) that delivers a cardioversion or defibrillation pulse to the heart, depending on the nature of the arrhythmia. The ICD electrode can be identified on chest radiographs by its thicker insulation (↑ in **Fig. 170.2a, b**).

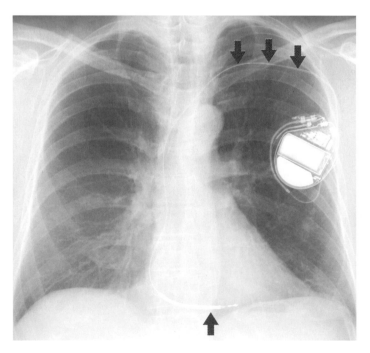

Fig. 170.2 a

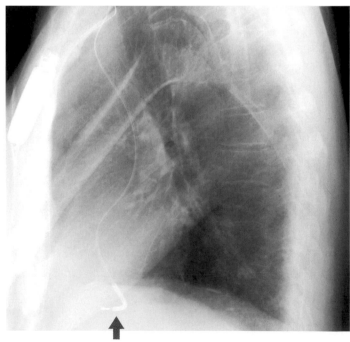

Fig. 170.2 b

Intra-Aortic Balloon Pump

Intra-aortic balloon counterpulsation (IABP [9.6]) is used in patients with cardiogenic shock, for example, or it may serve as a temporizing measure in terminal heart failure until cardiac surgery can be performed. It provides mechanical support for the heart. The intra-aortic balloon (◄) inflates during diastole **(Fig. 171.1)** to increase coronary perfusion and reduce myocardial oxygen consumption. It deflates during systole **(Fig. 171.2)** to permit unrestricted blood flow during the ejection phase of the cardiac cycle. Radiographs are obtained to check the position of the balloon. In **Figure 171.3**, the radiopaque marker can be seen at the upper end of the balloon (◄). When the balloon is correctly positioned, the marker should be distal to the origin (✎) of the left subclavian artery **(Fig. 171.2)**. If the balloon were placed too high, it could intermittently occlude the supra-aortic branches, leading to cerebral ischemia.

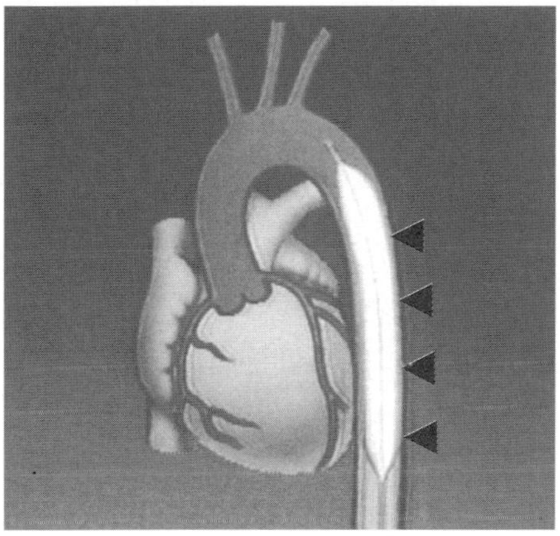

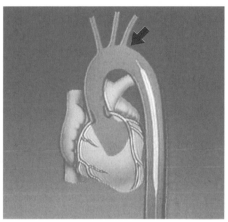

Fig. 171.1   Diastole

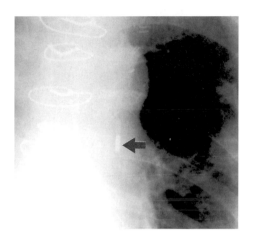

Fig. 171.2   Systole

Fig. 171.3   IABP Marker

Stent

Today the endovascular implantation of an aortic stent may be done as a minimally invasive alternative to operative treatment for thoracic aneurysms or dissections of the descending aorta **(Fig. 171.4a)** [9.7]. The stent (✎) is passed through the femoral artery and into the descending aorta with the aid of a catheter. In the lateral radiograph **(Fig. 171.4b)** the stent material is projected over the vertebral bodies **(26)**, thus demonstrating the paravertebral course of the descending aorta. Even intracoronary stent implants (✎) can sometimes be identified on conventional chest films **(Fig. 171.5)**.

Much as in the imaging of prosthetic heart valves, radiograph visualization depends on the metal content of the implants and on the heart rate. A stent can be defined without motion artifacts only in patients with a slow, bradyarrhythmic heart rate.

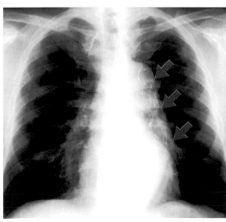

Fig. 171.4a

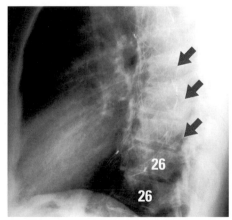

Fig. 171.4b

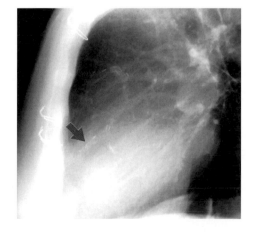

Fig. 171.5

Congenital or acquired valvular heart diseases lead to decreased exercise tolerance or even a shortened life expectancy. In most cases they necessitate surgical replacement of the affected valve. Surgery is indicated for almost every symptomatic patient and should be done at an early stage to prevent irreversible damage. The first-line option is valve repair. But if repair is not possible, a prosthetic heart valve should be implanted. Prosthetic valves are classified as mechanical or biological, each type having its advantages and disadvantages (**Table 172.2**). Mechanical heart valves can be differentiated into older and newer models (**Table 172.1**).

The first artificial heart valves were used in the 1960s. They include caged ball valves and tilting-disk or single-leaflet valves. Today, more modern designs like bileaflet valves (**Fig. 173.2a**) are used owing to their improved hemodynamic characteristics.

Mechanical prosthetic valves

Older models		Newer models
Caged ball	**Tilting disk**	**Bileaflet**
E.g., Starr-Edwards	E.g., Medtronic Hall and Bjork-Shiley	E.g., St. Jude Medical and Sorin Bicarbon

Table 172.1

Bioprosthetic valves

Advantages	• No need for life-long anticoagulation
Disadvantages	• Have limited longevity • Susceptible to deposits

Mechanical valves

Advantages	• Generally have unlimited longevity
Disadvantages	• Life-long anticoagulation • Alteration of blood flow

Table 172.2

Biological valves (bioprosthetic valves) are made either from porcine heart valves or bovine pericardium and function in much the same way as human heart valves. They are chemically treated to make them suitable for human valve replacement. Most patients who are treated with bioprosthetic valves do not require life-long oral anticoagulation and take only a temporary course of anticoagulants during the first three months after surgery. Also, unlike mechanical valves, biological valves function silently. One disadvantage of bioprosthetic valves is that they are less durable than mechanical valves, especially in diseases such as renal failure that may cause deposits to form on the valves.

Mechanical valves are made of metal or plastic and, in most cases, can function indefinitely in the body. The foreign material tends to alter the blood flow across the valve orifice, however, increasing the risk of thrombus formation. For this reason, patients with mechanical heart valves require life-long anticoagulation with a coumarin derivative. The principal complications are reviewed in **Table 172.3**.

Principal complications of prosthetic heart valves

Valve dysfunction	• Deterioration of bioprosthetic valves • Mechanical valve failure
Thrombosis and embolism	• Greater risk of embolism with mechanical valves • Mechanical valves require life-long anticoagulation
Prosthetic valve endocarditis	• Should be suspected if a change in valve sounds is noted • Valve replacement requires endocarditis prophylaxis
Heart failure	• Usually develops if surgery was delayed
Mechanical hemolysis	• Most common with older valve types

Table 172.3

Tilting-disk valves (e.g., Bjork-Shiley and Medtronic-Hall) were introduced in 1969. They consist of a disk (↓) that opens asymmetrically and is mounted in a circular frame (↙ in **Fig. 173.1a**). The function of the valve can be assessed by fluoroscopic observation.

The valve frame (→) and central tilting disk are also visible on chest radiographs **(Fig. 173.1b)**. In the case illustrated, the patient had undergone two valve replacements in the aortic and mitral valve positions (see **Fig. 182.2**). **Figure 173.1c** shows a lateral radiograph from a different patient who underwent mitral valve replacement (↗). Due to the different projection angles and valve compositions, this radiograph shows only the valve ring and the struts that hold the disk in place.

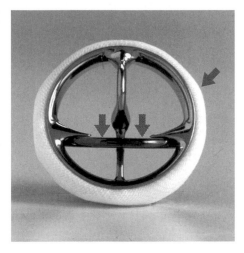
Fig. 173.1 a

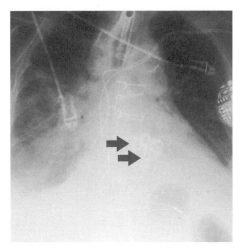
Fig. 173.1 b

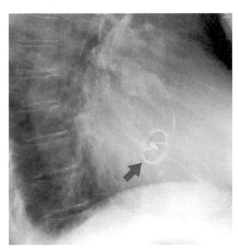
Fig. 173.1 c

Modern bileaflet valves (e.g., St. Jude Medical, Sorin-Bicarbon) have very favorable hemodynamic properties because the valve leaflets are directed parallel to the blood current when the valve is in the open position **(Fig. 173.2a)**. The two leaflets in the St. Jude Medical prosthesis contain a tungsten alloy that is easier to evaluate by fluoroscopy. Conventional chest radiographs may also demonstrate the paired leaflets without motion artifacts (← in **Fig. 173.2b**) at certain projection angles and in bradycardic patients with a slow cardiac cycle.

Given the relatively long exposure times of conventional radiographs, however, the images of prosthetic valves are often indistinct. A lateral radiograph in the same patient shows only the mounting ring (↑) of the aortic valve prosthesis **(Fig. 173.2c)**.

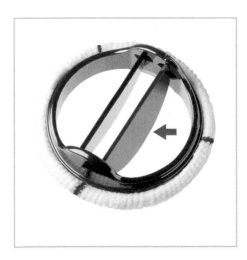
Fig. 173.2 a

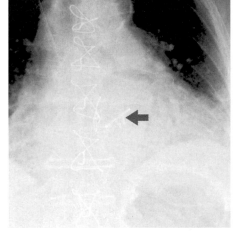
Fig. 173.2 b

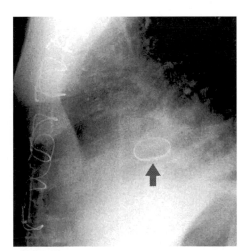
Fig. 173.2 c

Caged ball valves are the oldest type of artificial heart valve. The Star-Edwards valve **(Fig. 174.1)** was introduced in 1960 and was distinguished by its high reliability. It is no longer used today because of its unfavorable hemodynamic properties (high pressure gradient) and excessive risk of thromboembolism. Another disadvantage is the potential for mechanical hemolysis. The metal cage (➡) of an aortic valve consists of three struts **(Fig. 174.1b)**, while the cage of a mitral valve prosthesis (➚) has four struts **(Fig. 174.1c)**. The latter radiograph shows contrast medium in the esophagus (▶). The principle of the oral contrast examination is explained in the chapter on the mediastinum (see p. 84).

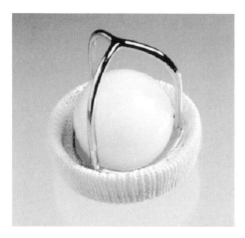

Fig. 174.1 a

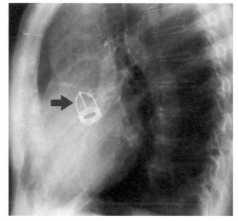

Fig. 174.1 b

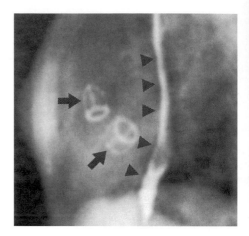

Fig. 174.1 c

Bioprosthetic valves include porcine and bovine xenografts, as well as human allografts **(Fig. 174.2a)**. While these valves eliminate the need for life-long anticoagulants, they are less durable than mechanical prostheses. Only bioprostheses with a metal frame (e.g., Carpentier Edwards) are visible on radiographs. Postoperative follow-up **(Fig. 174.2b, c)** in a patient with a biological mitral valve prosthesis (⬅) still shows a definite pneumopericardium (◀). Bioprosthetic valves implanted without a mounting frame are invisible on chest radiographs and may be suggested only by the presence of cerclage wires **(52)** from a previous sternotomy.

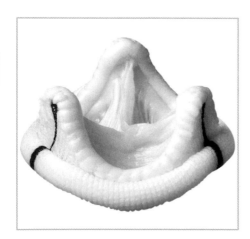

Fig. 174.2 a

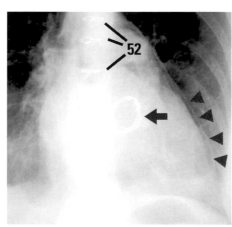

Fig. 174.2 b

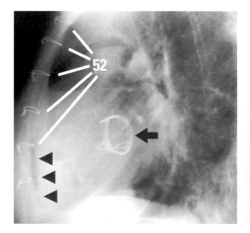

Fig. 174.2 c

In cases of isolated mitral valve insufficiency with dilatation of the valve ring, an annuloplasty can be performed using a flexible partial ring **(Fig. 175.1)** or a complete ring **(Fig. 175.2)** to restore tension to the valve cusps. This preserves the functional valve apparatus by tightening it with an annular prosthesis, thereby reducing the risk of thromboembolism and endocarditis. If the valve apparatus cannot be preserved, the valve should be replaced with a biological or mechanical prosthesis. The radiopaque mounting ring (➡) of a bioprosthetic valve **(Fig. 175.3)** can be distinguished from a partial annular prosthesis **(Fig. 175.1)** but not from a complete annuloplasty ring **(Fig. 175.2)**.

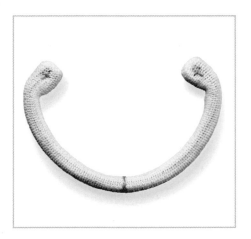

Fig. 175.1

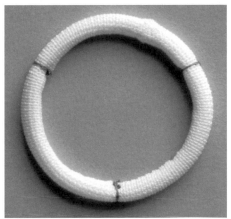

Fig. 175.2

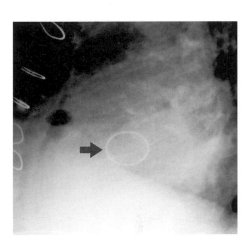

Fig. 175.3

The patient in **Figure 175.4a** had a prosthetic heart valve implanted for treatment of her mitral stenosis. Preoperative radiographs showed a definite mitral heart configuration with an obliterated cardiac waist (↙), dilatation of the right (◄) and left atria with splaying of the tracheal bifurcation (↖ ↗), and a double contour sign of atrial enlargement (▽) (see also **Fig. 82.1**). This finding and the pulmonary venous congestion showed significant improvement after surgery **(Fig. 175.4b)**. The cerclage wires **(52)** from the medial sternotomy are also visible.

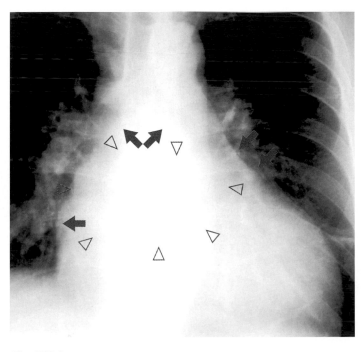

Fig. 175.4a

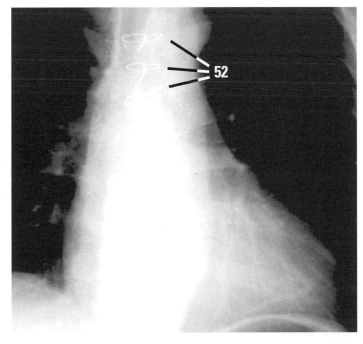

Fig. 175.4b

Echocardiography can be used for the functional evaluation of prosthetic heart valves and follow-up examinations **(Fig. 176.1)**. When the Bjork-Shiley mitral valve prosthesis (→ ←) is imaged in the four-chamber view, it produces conspicuous artifacts (⬈) in the underlying atrium **(2)**. The accelerated flow pattern (⬋) along the tilting disks from the atrium into the ventricle can also be seen. The titanium ring of artificial heart valves and the mounting ring of bioprosthetic valves frequently produce foreign-body artifacts (⬇) when imaged by CT. The scan in **Figure 176.2** shows a tricuspid valve replacement with prominent artifacts in the right atrium **(2)** and right ventricle **(4)**.

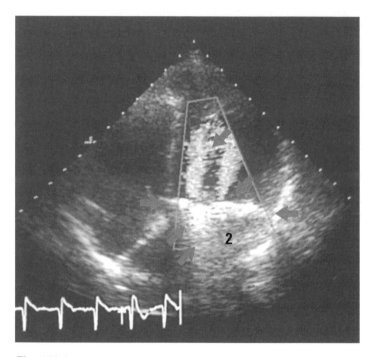

Fig. 176.1

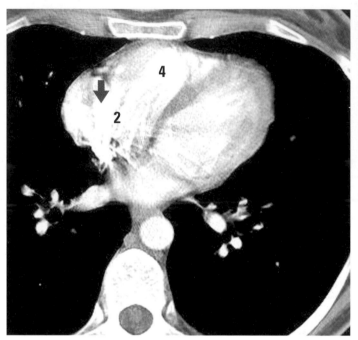

Fig. 176.2

Modern tilting disks and bileaflet valves are composed mainly of Pyrolite carbon. This material is only slightly radiopaque, and so most modern prosthetic valves can be identified only by their titanium frame on chest radiographs. The titanium ring and the carbon portions of the occluders within the frame have no magnetic properties. As a result, selected patients with modern prosthetic heart valves can safely undergo MRI after the valve material has been carefully checked **(Table 176.3)**.

Manufacturers have issued MRI safety warnings for certain older valve models such as the Starr-Edwards valves **(Fig. 174.1a)** produced by Baxter Healthcare (models 1000 and 6000) [9.11].

Type of valve	Name of valve	Occluder	Frame	MRI-compatible
Bioprosthetic	• Carpienter-Edwards • Hancock	Porcine heart valve	• Elgior® alloy, Dacron ring • Haynes® alloy, Dacron ring	Yes
Bileaflet	• Carbomedics • St. Jude Medical	• Pyrolite carbon • Pyrolite carbon with tungsten	• Titanium and nickel, Teflon suture ring • Pyrolite carbon, Dacron ring	Yes
Tilting disk	• Bjork-Shiley • Medtronic Hall	Pyrolite carbon	• Haynes® alloy • Titanium, Teflon suture ring	Yes
Caged ball	Starr Edwards (Baxter 1000 and 6000)	Silicone rubber ball	• Stellit® alloy, Teflon ring	No

Table 176.3

Endobronchial Tubes

Chest radiographs are considerably more reliable than physical examination for confirming the correct placement of an endobronchial tube, particularly after emergency intubation [9.7, 9.8]. The tip of a correctly positioned endobronchial tube (➜) should be projected several centimeters above the carina (⬆) in the PA radiograph **(Fig. 177.1)**. A tube that is advanced too deeply **(Fig. 177.2a)** may enter the right main bronchus **(14a)** because of its more vertical orientation, leading to complete atelectasis **(36)** of the left lung **(Fig. 177.2b)**.

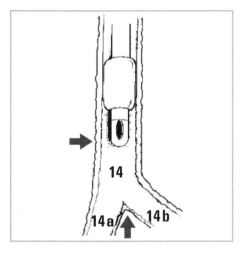

Fig. 177.1

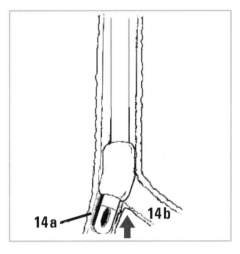

Fig. 177.2a

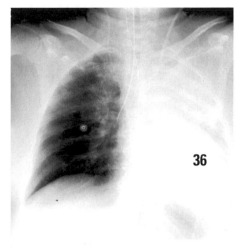

Fig. 177.2b

Esophageal intubation that is missed at physical examination can be detected on the chest radiograph **(Fig. 177.3)**. In the example shown, the endobronchial tube (⬅) can be identified to the left of the tracheal air column **(14)**.
For long-term ventilation (> 10 days), a tracheostomy tube (↘) is inserted to prevent vocal cord lesions and facilitate oropharyngeal care **(Fig. 177.4a, b)**. The fixation hooks (↙) on the tube are visible on the radiograph.

Radiographs are less important for checking tube placement immediately after a tracheotomy, because the tube is usually introduced under bronchoscopic guidance.

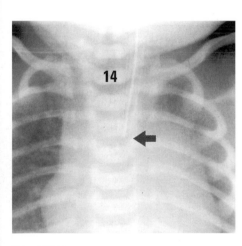

Fig. 177.3

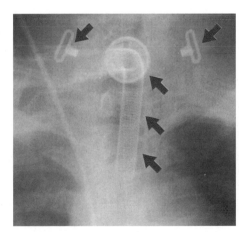

Fig. 177.4a

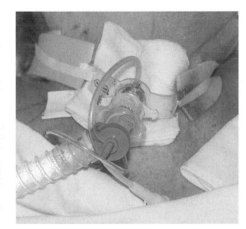

Fig. 177.4b

9

A transjugular intrahepatic portosystemic shunt (TIPSS) can be inserted in patients with portal hypertension and decompensated hepatic cirrhosis that have responded poorly to conservative therapy. This may be done for the decompression of esophageal varices, for example. The procedure creates an artificial connection between the portal venous system and a draining hepatic vein. **Figure 178.1** is a marked-ly rotated view in which the TIPSS (➡) can be identified within the liver shadow. The tip (⬅) of the right supraclavicular CVC is projected over the tracheal bifurcation (**14**), confirming that it is correctly positioned in the SVC.

An esophageal stent (↙) can be implanted for the palliative restoration of alimentary continuity in patients with inoperable esophageal cancer **(Fig. 178.2)**.

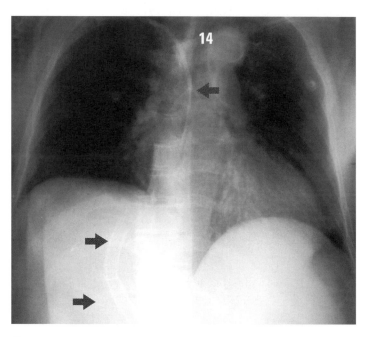

Fig. 178.1

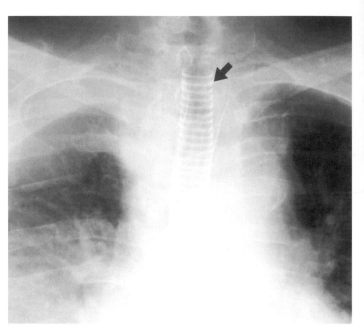

Fig. 178.2

Gastric tubes are passed down the esophagus and into the stomach by the transnasal or oropharyngeal route for aspirating gastric contents or introducing solutions. Their position can be assessed by physical examination and chest radiographs. **Figure 178.3** confirms the correct placement of the gastric tube (↘) by the position of the radiopaque marker. In **Figure 178.4**, however, the gastric tube (↗) has been inadvertently passed down the trachea (**14**) into the right main bronchus (**14a**). Prolonged intratracheal placement may obstruct a bronchial branch, leading to atelectasis.

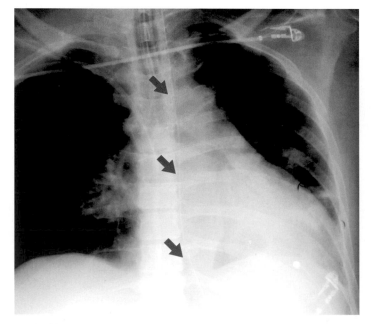

Fig. 178.3

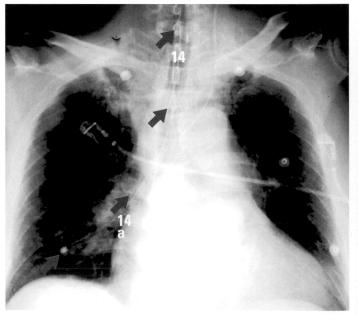

Fig. 178.4

Foreign-body aspiration is a common occurrence in small children, elderly invalids, and patients sedated for dental procedures. Larger radiopaque foreign bodies (→) may be found in the larynx **(Fig. 179.1)** or trachea **(14)**, while smaller objects **(48)** are typically projected onto the right main bronchus **(14a)** and right lower lung zone **(34) (Figs. 179.2, 179.3)**. Bronchitis and pneumonic infiltration **(37)** may develop after foreign-body aspiration as a result of local irritation or possible poststenotic dystelectasis **(Fig. 179.3)** [9.12].

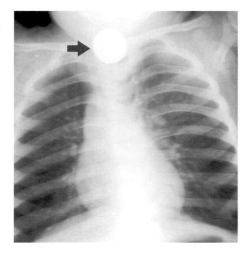

Fig. 179.1

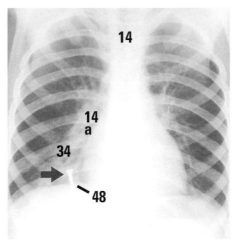

Fig. 179.2

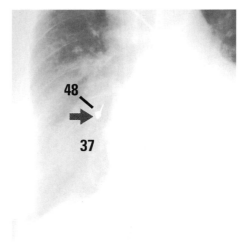

Fig. 179.3

In many cases a PA radiograph alone **(Fig. 179.4a)** is insufficient to define the precise location of a foreign body or determine whether it is in the esophagus or trachea. Often the situation is clarified by adding a lateral radiograph **(Fig. 179.4b)**, which in this case shows the broken fragment of a safety pin (↑) lodged in the trachea. The object is too far anterior to be located in the esophagus.

Figure 179.5 shows at least part of an incandescent light bulb that appears to be lodged in the esophagus.

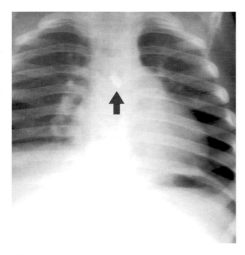

Fig. 179.4 a

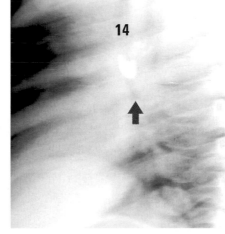

Fig. 179.4 b

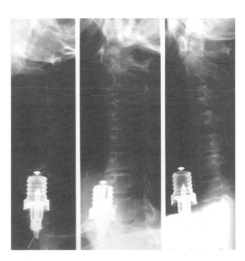

Fig. 179.5

9

Nonradiopaque foreign bodies (e.g., aspirated peanuts in children) can often be recognized by indirect signs. In 75% of cases they cause a ball-valve stenosis with decreased lucency in the affected lung region. Obstructive atelectasis develops in 15% of cases. Only about 10% of cases show no abnormalities on conventional chest radiographs. A unilateral ball-valve stenosis results in pulmonary hyperinflation with a mediastinal shift (←) toward the healthy side **(Fig. 180.1)**. In this case there was a ball-valve mechanism in the left main bronchus (less common), causing air trapping and increased lucency in the left lung.

If foreign-body aspiration is suspected in the absence of typical radiographic signs, the definitive diagnosis is established by bronchoscopy. Small children with suspected foreign-body aspiration often present with restlessness, anxiety, and respiratory distress, and so special care should be taken to position the child correctly for the radiograph. The child in **Figure 180.2** presented with hematemesis, and the superior thoracic aperture, for example, was not visualized in the PA radiograph **(Fig. 180.2a)**. Fortunately, however, the lateral radiograph demonstrated the cause of the clinical complaints: The child had swallowed the aerator from a water faucet (◀) **(Fig. 180.2b)**.

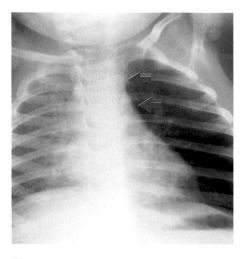

Fig. 180.1

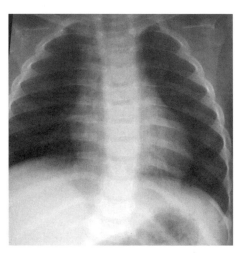

Fig. 180.2a

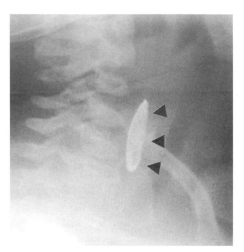

Fig. 180.2b

Injuries from bullets (↘ in **Fig. 180.3**) or shotgun pellets **(Fig. 180.4)** are diagnosed less frequently in Europe than in North America but are still a significant issue. In **Figure 180.4**, compare the two projections with each other to see which

pellets are in the lung and which ones have lodged in the soft tissues of the chest wall. (You will find the answer at the end of the book.)

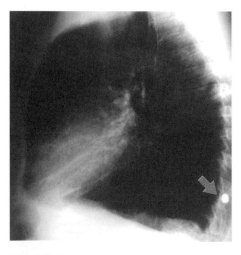

Fig. 180.3

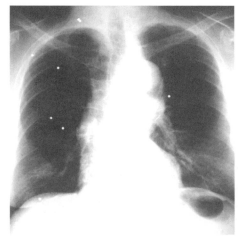

Fig. 180.4a

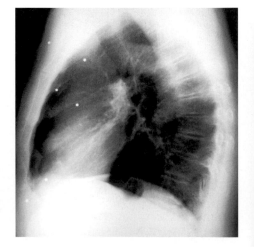

Fig. 180.4b

Checklist

The principal complications and correct positions of the various foreign materials reviewed in this chapter are summarized in the table below.

Type of catheter	Correct position	Complications
CVC	SVC at the level of the azygos termination	• Arrhythmias
Port systems	SVC at the level of the azygos termination	• Pericardial tamponade
Shaldon catheter	SVC at the level of the azygos termination	• Thrombosis
Atrial dialysis catheter	Right atrium	• Vascular injury
Pulmonary artery catheter	≤ 2 cm distally in the right or left main pulmonary artery trunk	**Same as CVC** • Rupture of the pulmonary artery • Pulmonary artery infarction
Pacemaker systems		
VVI	Lead in right ventricle	• Arrhythmias
DDD	Lead in right atrium and right ventricle	• Pericardial tamponade
AAI	Lead in right atrium	• Thrombosis
VDD	Lead in right ventricle	• Vascular injury • Pneumothorax
Biventricular	Leads in right atrium, right ventricle, and coronary vein	• Infections
Intra-aortic balloon pump (IABP)	Aortic arch, **distal** to the subclavian artery	• Vascular occlusion with ischemia • Gas embolism due to rupture
Endotracheal tube	5 - 7 cm above the carina	• Mucosal injury • Atelectasis • Pneumothorax • Vocal cord lesions
Feeding tubes	Distal to esophageal hiatus	• Reflux • Aspiration pneumonia • Esophageal perforation • Mediastinitis

Table 181.1

What findings can you recognize?

Write down your impressions of these radiographs in the boxes provided. (The answers are at the end of the book.)

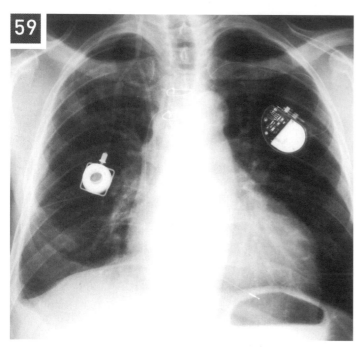

Fig. 182.1

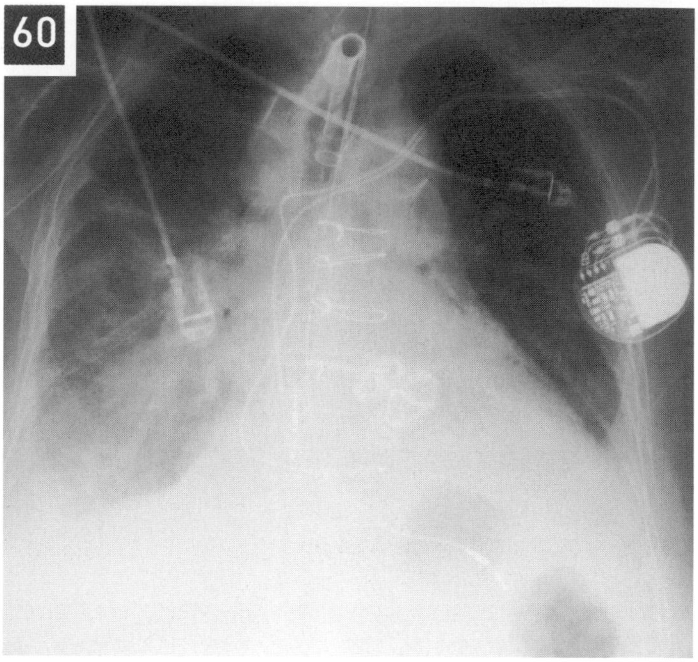

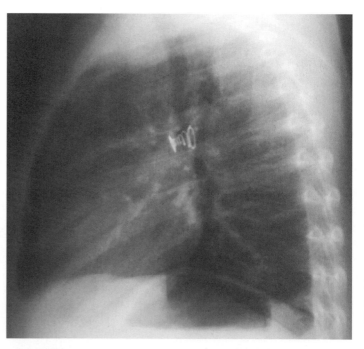

Fig. 182.2

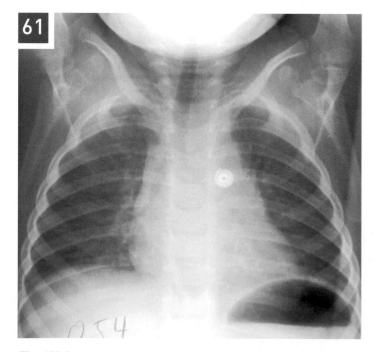

Fig. 182.3a

Fig. 182.3b

Henning Rattunde
Matthias Hofer

Thoracic Trauma

Chapter Goals:

This chapter deals with important changes that are associated with thoracic injuries. Thoracic trauma in Western Europe most commonly results from motor vehicle accidents, recreational injuries, and occupational accidents. Well-established trauma room algorithms include a primary ultrasound examination for the rapid detection or exclusion of free fluid. The chest and skeleton are evaluated with a series of conventional radiographs. Multislice computed tomography (CT) has become increasingly important in the primary workup of thoracic trauma, in some cases even eliminating the need for conventional radiographs. But because CT is not always immediately available in trauma and resuscitation rooms, conventional radiographs continue to be an essential study. After completing this chapter, you should be able to:

- diagnose fractures of the ribs, sternum, and vertebral bodies;

- recognize abnormal fluid collections in the pleural space and estimate their volume;

- recognize the different manifestations of parenchymal lung injuries;

- distinguish a simple mantle pneumothorax from a tension pneumothorax;

- detect traumatic air collections in the soft tissues;

- detect significant bleeding into serous cavities (pericardium, peritoneal and pleural cavities) on ultrasound images.

* FAST = Focussed assessment with sonography for trauma

10

The leading causes of multiple injuries vary from continent to continent. While traffic accidents account for 85% of multiple injury cases in Europe [10.1, 10.2], stab wounds and gunshot injuries are far more frequent causes of thoracic trauma in the U.S. and Africa, for example [10.3, 10.4]. These patterns of thoracic trauma are responsible for approximately 20 - 25% of deaths in patients with multiple injuries, underscoring the importance of their accurate diagnosis [10.5].

Rib Fractures and Hemothorax

Isolated rib fractures are easily missed in routine examinations of trauma patients **(Fig. 184.1a)** because of the priority given to the heart, mediastinum, and lung. Overall, it is estimated that only about 50% of all rib fractures can be detected on conventional posteroanterior (PA) radiographs [10.6, 10.7], especially when the fracture is located on the lateral chest wall and the fragments are minimally displaced. In doubtful cases, try turning the radiograph 90° **(Fig. 184.1b)** or 180° **(Fig. 184.1c)**. By looking at the film sideways or upside-down, you may find it easier to spot irregularities in the rib contours.

If you look closely at the radiograph in **Figure 184.1d**, you will see that the seventh rib is fractured (note the cortical discontinuity ←) and that there is also a subtle break in the continuity of the adjacent eighth rib (↘).

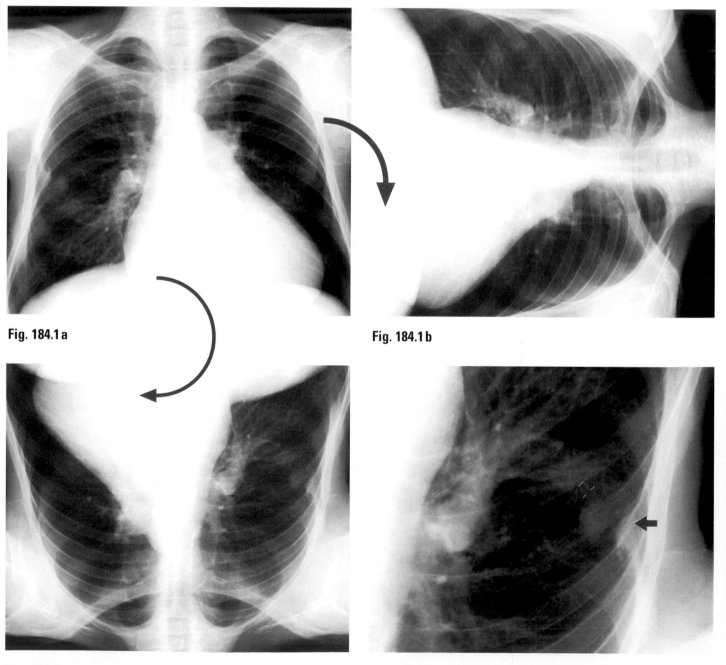

Fig. 184.1 a

Fig. 184.1 b

Fig. 184.1 c

Fig. 184.1 d

If the diagnosis is still in doubt, as in the case of a minimally displaced or lateral fracture, it may also be necessary to obtain 30° oblique radiographs **(Fig. 185.1a)**. These views may be taken in the upright or supine position. For a supine radio-

graph, a wedge (⬆) is placed beneath the side that is to be examined **(Fig. 185.1b)**. This "bony hemithorax" view **(Fig. 185.1c)** will reveal even subtle fracture signs (⬋) that may not be visible in the standard PA projection **(Fig. 185.1d)**.

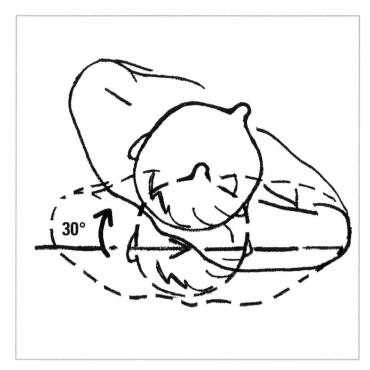

Fig. 185.1 a

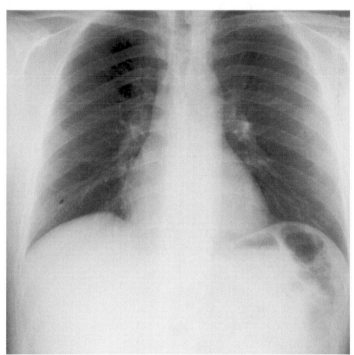

Fig. 185.1 b

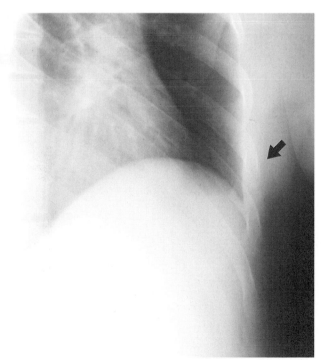

Fig. 185.1 c

Fig. 185.1 d

Rib fractures are commonly associated with focal extra-pleural hematomas, which appear radiographically as soft-tissue convexities (←) that displace the lung inward **(Fig. 186.1)**, possibly mimicking a pleural tumor. Ultrasound shows a discontinuity in the cortical rib outline (↑) that moves with respiratory excursions **(Fig. 186.2a)** plus a hypoechoic thickening of the surrounding soft tissue (↘ ↙) caused by the adjacent hematoma **(Fig. 186.2b)**.

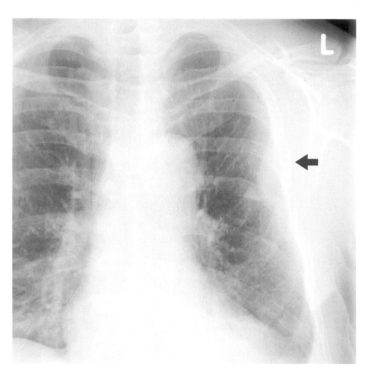

Fig. 186.1

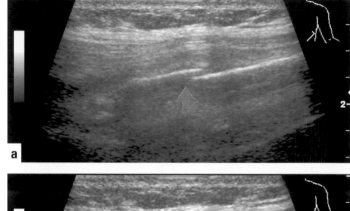
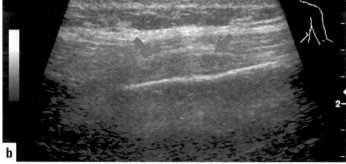

Fig. 186.2

Hemothorax

Hemothorax is particularly likely to occur as a complication of multiple rib fractures. It appears on radiographs as a crescent-shaped opacity that tapers superiorly (↙ in **Fig. 186.3a**). The opacity should show marked regression after percutaneous needle aspiration **(Fig. 186.3b)**. You should also consider possible traumatic lesions in the abdomen, however, and ultrasound should be used to exclude ruptures of the liver and spleen (see p. 194-195).

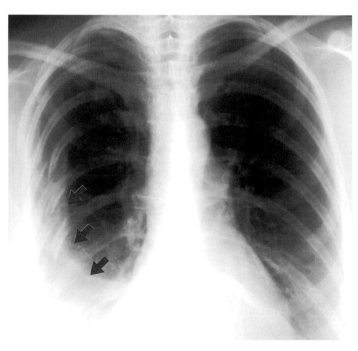

Fig. 186.3a

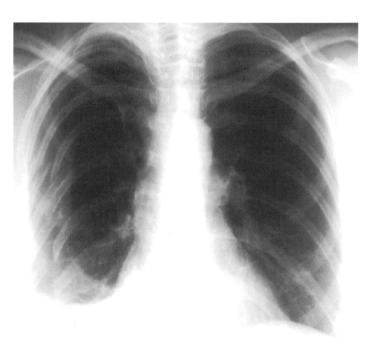

Fig. 186.3b

Multiple rib fractures (see **Fig. 187.3**) involve at least three ribs on one side of the chest. This injury may cause instability of the chest wall with paradoxical respirations, respiratory insufficiency, hemothorax, and pneumothorax (see **Figs. 190.2, 190.3**). Patients with significant chest-wall instability may require rigid internal fixation of the fractured ribs **(Fig. 187.1)**.

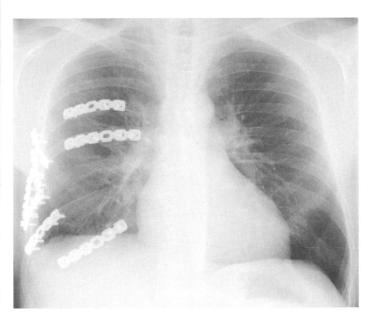

Fig. 187.1 a

Fig. 187.1 b

It may be advisable to supplement radiographs with CT scans **(Fig. 187.2b)** to exclude heart and lung contusions and a diaphragmatic rupture with associated enterothorax. In the case illustrated **(Fig. 187.2a)**, rib fractures have caused a left-sided hemothorax, and a vascular rupture has caused a mediastinal hematoma with widening of the mediastinal silhouette. If a bleeding site cannot be found, you should also consider the possibility of chylothorax following a surgical procedure, for example **(Fig. 187.3)**.

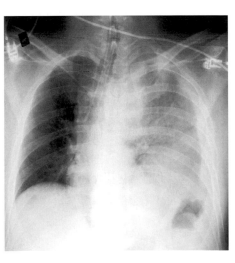
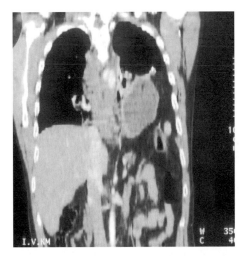
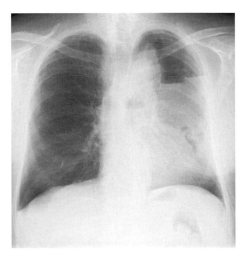

Fig. 187.2 a   **Fig. 187.2 b**   **Fig. 187.3**

Volume Estimation

The features of a hemothorax on supine radiographs depend largely on its volume. Standard radiographs permit only a rough estimation of the fluid volume. Pleural fluid collections of approximately 200 mL or more can be detected on upright radiographs, and collections of about 500 mL or more can be detected on supine radiographs (see p. 108). These volumes are sufficient to produce a visible fluid band located between the lung and chest wall and passing into the horizontal fissure. On supine radiographs, fluid volumes less than 250 mL cause only a slight haziness on the affected side. Fluid volumes of 150-500 mL obliterate the costophrenic angle and obscure the border of the diaphragm.

Sternal and Vertebral Body Fractures

Sternal fractures occur in 8-10% of all blunt thoracic injuries. Ordinarily they are easy to diagnose on lateral radiographs [10.8]. A site of predilection is the sternal angle (↘), approximately 2 cm below the junction of the sternal body with the manubrium **(Fig. 188.1a)**. Even fine fracture lines and minimal-ly displaced fractures (↓ in **Fig. 188.1b**) can be detected by spiral CT examination, aided if necessary by coronal reconstructions. CT can also detect cartilaginous rib fractures. In the case illustrated, CT shows an anterior pneumothorax **(38)** accompanying the rib fracture.

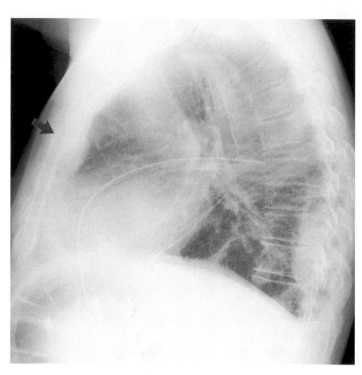

Fig. 188.1 a

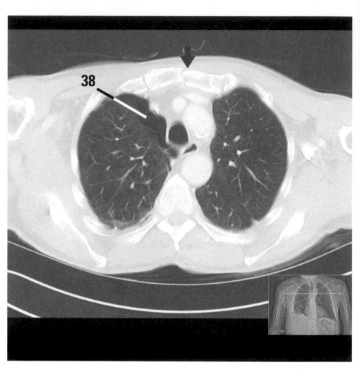

Fig. 188.1 b

Fractures of vertebral bodies are often missed on conventional radiographs, especially when they involve the lower thoracic spine. For this reason, standard radiographs in multiply injured patients are generally supplemented by special cervical, thoracic, and lumbar biplane views and, if necessary, by CT scans.

CT **(Fig. 188.2b, c)** is the best modality for diagnosing vertebral body fractures (↑ , →), which may appear as paraspinal opacities or mediastinal widening (←→) on conventional chest radiographs **(Fig. 188.2a)**.

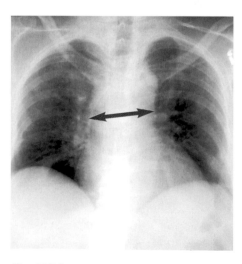

Fig. 188.2 a

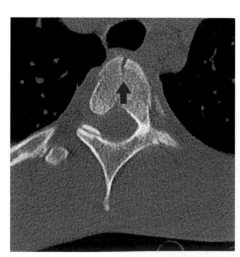

Fig. 188.2 b

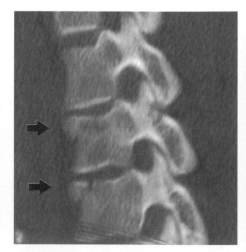

Fig. 188.2 c

Parenchymal Lung Injuries

Pulmonary contusions are among the most common severe lung injuries caused by blunt thoracic trauma. They are a major contributor to morbidity and posttraumatic mortality [10.9, 10.10]. Contusions are most likely to occur in lung areas that border on solid structures (vertebral bodies, ribs, liver, heart). Pulmonary contusions are generally manifested 6-24 hours after the trauma **(Figs. 189.1a, d, 189.2a)** and typically resolve in 7-10 days **(Fig. 189.1b, c)**. **Figure 189.1a-c** shows a series of radiographs from a patient injured in a motorcycle accident: The initial film in the trauma room **(Fig. 189.1a)**, 24 hours after admission **(Fig. 189.1b)**, and one week later **(Fig. 189.1c)**. In addition to the pulmonary contusion (★) and right clavicular fracture seen on conventional radiographs, CT **(Fig. 189.1d)** reveals a hemothorax (➡) and a mild bilateral pneumothorax (⬆).

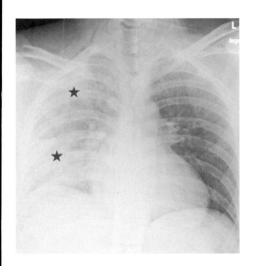

Fig. 189.1 a

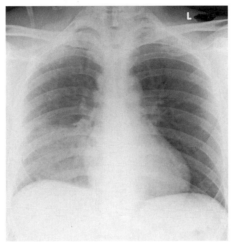

Fig. 189.1 b

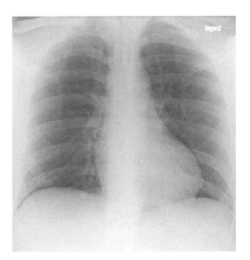

Fig. 189.1 c

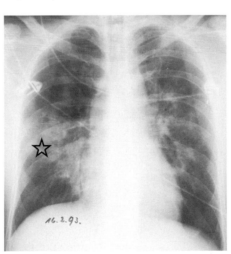

Fig. 189.1 d   Fig. 189.2 a

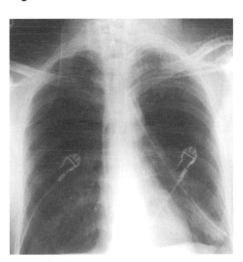

Fig. 189.2 b

Injuries to smaller vessels and the alveolar membrane lead to the extravasation of blood, causing interstitial and alveolar edema. Depending on the pattern of injury, this may lead to the appearance of unilateral or bilateral, focal or diffuse lung opacities on the chest radiograph (☆ in **Fig. 189.2a**). A positive air bronchogram may also develop if the hemorrhage has not caused bronchial obstruction. **Figure 189.2b** shows almost complete resolution of the changes at 10 days.

10

Opacity that persists longer than 10 days may be caused by atelectasis, pneumonia, or aspiration, or it may represent a hematoma from a pulmonary laceration, i.e., a slitlike or jagged tear in the lung parenchyma. Most of these injuries are caused by sharp trauma, in this case by a displaced rib fracture (↓ in **Fig. 190.1a**). Bleeding into this space produces opacities with lucent areas or fluid levels (↑). Hemoptysis and pleural hemorrhage may also be observed. Generally the changes will resolve in three to seven weeks **(Fig. 190.1b)**. Some cases may be complicated by the development of bronchopleural fistulas.

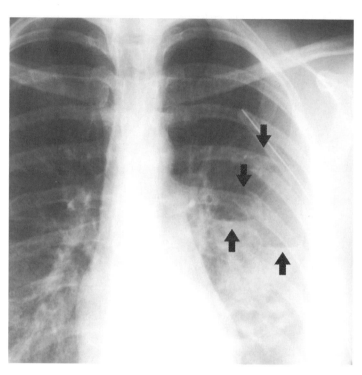

Fig. 190.1 a

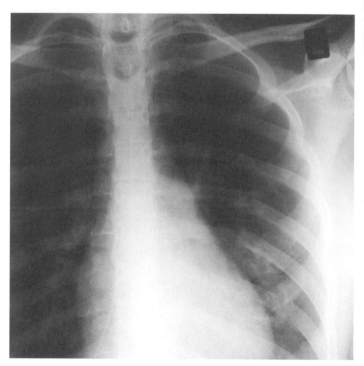

Fig. 190.1 b

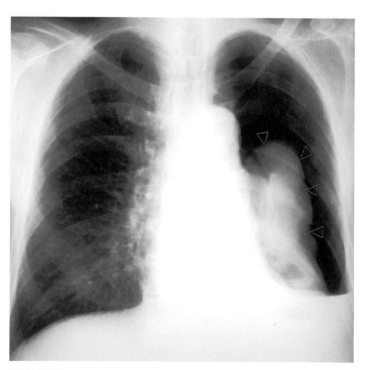

Fig. 190.2

Pneumothorax

Pneumothorax is a frequent complication of thoracic trauma. The injury allows air to enter the pleural space, creating a slightly positive pressure where a negative pressure normally prevails.

When the negative pressure is lost, elastic fibers retract the lung toward the hilum (▽) to which it is attached **(Fig. 190.2)**. A typical "mantle pneumothorax" can be recognized by an absence of peripheral pulmonary vascular markings and by the fine, thin boundary lines (↙) caused by the visceral pleura **(Fig. 191.1)**.

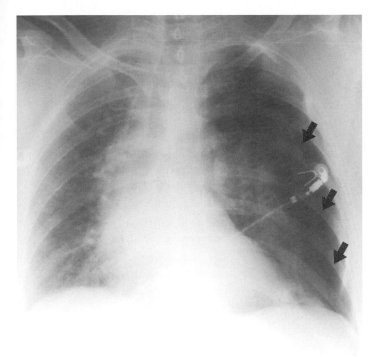

Fig. 191.1

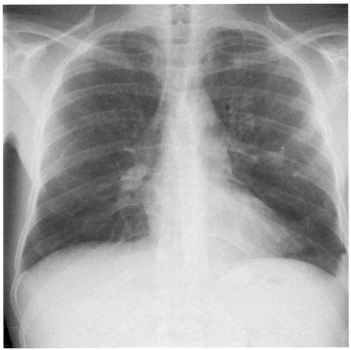

Fig. 191.2

In patients with a small pneumothorax, there is a danger that this important finding may be overlooked **(Fig. 191.2)**. If you are having difficulty locating the pleural boundaries, one criterion may be helpful: Check to see if pulmonary vessels are still visible lateral to the questionable lung boundary. If the findings are equivocal, it may be helpful to obtain a radio-graph with the lung in full expiration, as this position widens the pleural space and makes it easier to see than in the standard inspiratory view. Some authors have reported, however, that an expiratory radiograph does not improve the detection rate of pneumothorax in equivocal cases and may therefore be omitted [10.11, 10.12].

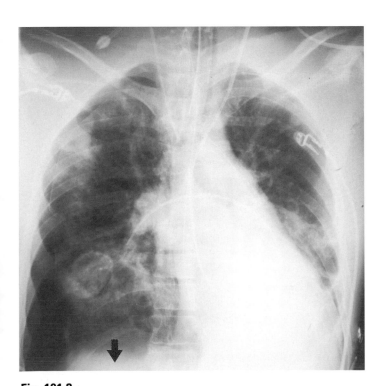

Fig. 191.3

The prompt diagnosis of even a small pneumothorax is important, because up to one third of patients with an untreated pneumothorax will subsequently develop a tension pneumothorax, with potentially life-threatening complications [10.13, 10.14].

In a tension pneumothorax, additional air enters the pleural space with each inspiration, like a valve that permits flow in one direction only (see p. 120). Because the air cannot escape during expiration, the pressure in the interpleural space rises and displaces the lung, heart, and mediastinum toward the opposite side **(Fig. 191.3)**. In addition to this "midline shift," radiographs generally show associated depression of the hemidiaphragm (↓) on the affected side (see also **Fig. 192.2**).

In an upright patient, the air tends to collect in the apical or lateral portions of the hemithorax. In the supine patient, however, the air tends to collect in the anterior costodiaphragmatic recess. Thus, a fine lucent stripe along the border of the cardiac silhouette or diaphragm (⬆) may be the only clue to the presence of a pneumothorax **(Fig. 192.1)**. It is estimated that 30-50% of all small pneumothoraces are undetected in the supine anteroposterior (AP) radiographs of trauma patients [10.15, 10.16]. If pleural adhesions are present (➡, ↗), the lung will remain partially expanded at the sites of the adhesions **(Fig. 192.2)**.

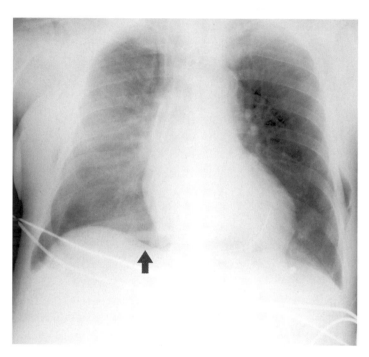

Fig. 192.1

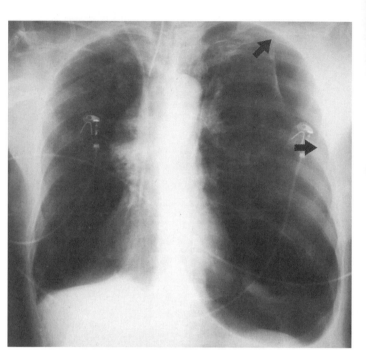

Fig. 192.2

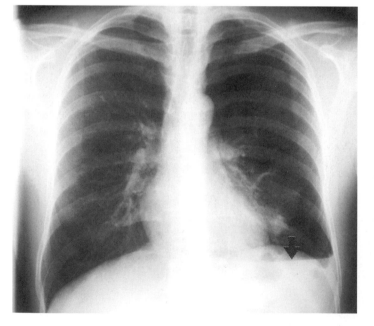

Fig. 192.3 a

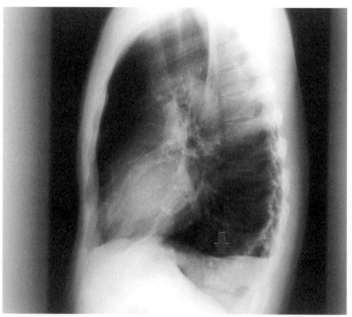

Fig. 192.3 b

It is common for a pneumothorax to coexist with a pleural effusion. In this case a horizontal air-fluid level (⬇) develops because the pleural fluid cannot layer out to form a meniscus in the pleural space due to the absence of a normal negative pressure **(Fig. 192.3)**. Another frequent result of blunt chest injuries is the entry of air into the mediastinal space.

A pneumomediastinum **(Fig. 193.1)** may result from rupture of the alveoli secondary to trauma or positive end-expiratory pressure **(PEEP)** ventilation. Other potential causes are injuries to the trachea, bronchi, or esophagus, as well as head and neck injuries. The air typically appears as vertical lucent streaks (◄) on the chest radiograph. Additional signs are cutaneous emphysema (▲) and an accentuation of the typical pennate pattern (▼) of the pectoralis muscles **(Fig. 193.2)**.

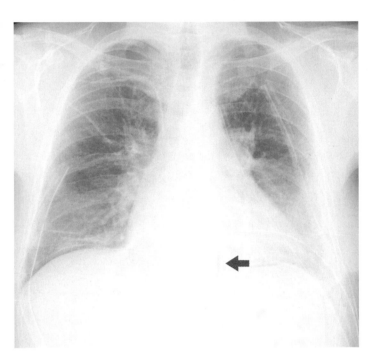

Fig. 193.1

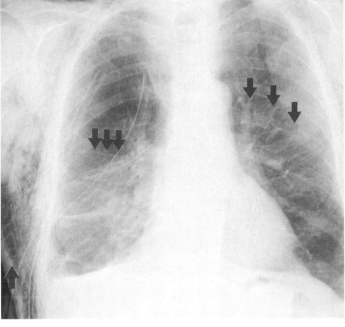

Fig. 193.2

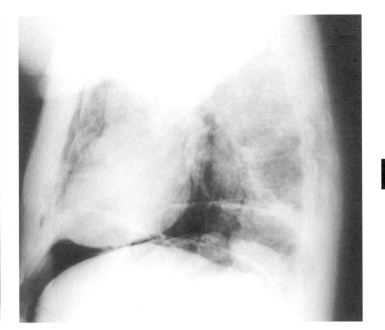

Fig. 193.3 a

Fig. 193.3 b

In pronounced cases air may also enter the pericardium (✎), dissect extraperitoneally along the anterior abdominal wall, or spread intraperitoneally (▲) as in a primary pneumoperitoneum **(Fig. 193.3)**. When findings are more subtle, it can sometimes be difficult to distinguish a pneumomediastinum from a pneumothorax or pneumopericardium. If doubt exists, it may be helpful to obtain an extra view in a different position: While the air collections in a pneumothorax and pneumopericardium move freely and easily in response to position changes, the air in a pneumomediastinum is "trapped" in the soft tissues and remains stationary even when the patient is repositioned.

Additional Tests

There is always a danger that significant thoracic injuries will be missed when the evaluation relies solely on clinical manifestations and conventional radiographs [10.5, 10.17, 10.18]. The primary adjunctive modality in emergency settings is spiral CT, which most traumatologists prefer over other, more time-consuming imaging procedures (angiography, magnetic resonance imaging [MRI]). But these studies can be used only if the patient is hemodynamically stable and, for example, the precise location of a bleeding site cannot be determined by CT for preoperative planning.

Focused assessment with sonography for trauma (FAST) is the term applied to a standardized, limited ultrasound examination that is used in trauma rooms [10.19]. It is a rapid screening test to detect free fluid that would indicate severe hemorrhage, as well as possible parenchymal tears in the liver and spleen. If free fluid is not detected, the examination should be repeated so that bleeding of delayed onset is not missed. With the FAST method, the most common sites of intrathoracic and intra-abdominal free fluid can be screened in a minimum amount of time. Four standard transducer placement sites are used (Fig. 194.1).

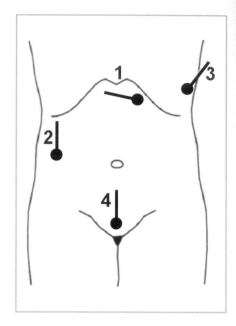

Fig. 194.1

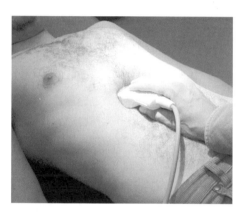 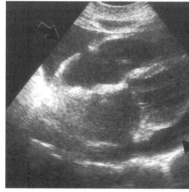 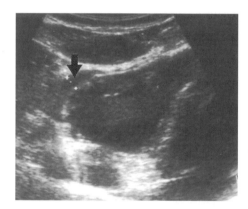

Fig. 194.2a   **Fig. 194.2b**   **Fig. 194.2c**

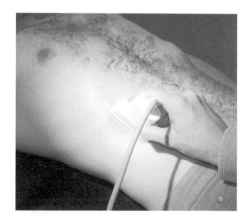 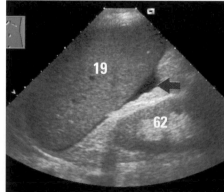 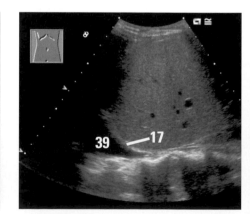

Fig. 194.3a   **Fig. 194.3b**   **Fig. 194.3c**

To evaluate the pericardium, the transducer is placed flat against the chest wall in the median plane **(Fig. 194.2a)**. If a hemopericardium is present, ultrasound will show an echo-free (= black) rim of fluid (↘ ↖) encircling the heart within the echogenic pericardial boundary line **(Fig. 194.2b)**. The differential diagnosis of this finding should include epicardial fat (↓), which also appears as an echo-free zone within the pericardial border **(Fig. 194.2c)**. Generally, however, epi-cardial fat is localized and does not move with changes of patient position. The transducer is placed in the right anterior axillary line **(Fig. 194.3a)** to check for bleeding into the free abdominal cavity. This hemorrhage appears as a hypoechoic (= dark) wedge-shaped area (←) spreading upward into Morison's pouch between the liver **(19)** and kidney **(62)** **(Fig. 194.3b)**.

Greater amounts of fluid may be found in the perihepatic area between the liver and diaphragm, as the intrinsic weight of the liver keeps it from displacing much fluid in that region. A hematoma in the pleural space **(39)** at this level appears cranial (= the left side of the image) to the diaphragm **(17)** in **Figure 194.3c**. The spleen is examined for hypoechoic blood collections **(39)** within the parenchyma and along its capsule **(Fig. 195.1b)**. First the transducer is angled upward and backward **(Fig. 195.1a)** to scan through the spleen **(44)**. Then it is angled forward (▲·ˑˑ in **Fig. 195.1d**) to scan the posterior part of the costodiaphragmatic recess, where a hemothorax tends to gravitate in the supine patient. The examiner should also exclude echo-free blood (←) in the space between the inferior pole of the spleen **(44)** and the kidney **(62)** (Koller's pouch, **Fig. 195.1c**).

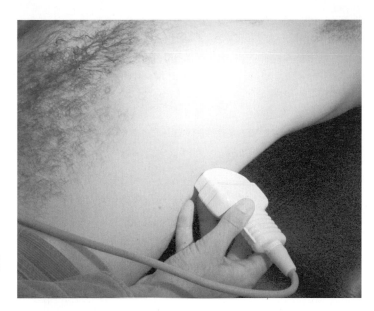

Fig. 195.1a

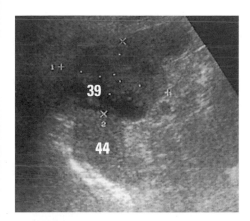

Fig. 195.1b

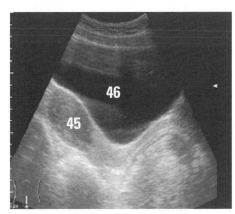

Fig. 195.1c

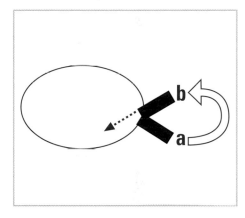

Fig. 195.1d

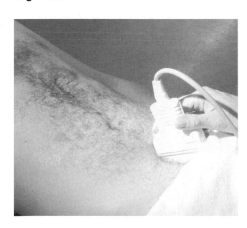

Fig. 195.2a

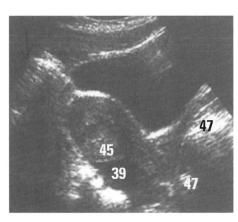

Fig. 195.2b

Fig. 195.2c

The FAST examination ends with a suprapubic longitudinal scan to demonstrate the Douglas pouch **(Fig. 195.2a, b)**, known as the cul-de-sac or rectouterine pouch in females and the rectovesical pouch in males. Free fluid **(39)** appears as an echo-free (= black) area between the rectum **(47)** and uterus **(45)** in the female **(Fig. 195.2c)** and between the rectum and bladder in the male. Fluid may also collect on the roof of the urinary bladder.

62 **Figure 196.1** shows the chest radiograph of a 29-year-old woman who was referred from the psychiatric unit. What abnormalities do you see? If you look closely, you will discover the cause of the pathology.

63 **Figure 196.2** is from a 78-year-old man who was taken to the emergency room by helicopter with "multiple injuries". What is your presumptive diagnosis based on the admission radiograph?

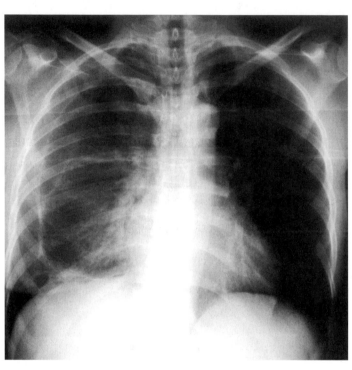

Fig. 196.1

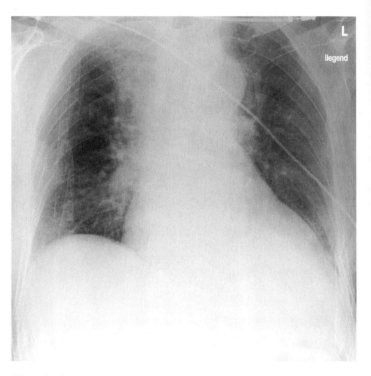

Fig. 196.2

Space For Your Notes

Matthias Hofer
Christian Zentai

Intensive Care Unit

Chapter Goals:

This chapter deals with clinical questions that are most commonly addressed in ventilated patients in an intensive care unit (ICU). Besides assessing the position of foreign materials, particular attention is given to problems such as infusion-induced over-hydration, inflammatory processes, and ventilation and expansion disorders of the lung. When you have finished this chapter, you should be able to:

- recognize ventilation and expansion disorders of the lung;

- diagnose a loculated or anterior pneumothorax on supine radiographs;

- describe the typical signs of an impending tension pneumothorax;

- differentiate a volume overload of the pulmonary circulation and pulmonary edema from a normal-appearing supine radiograph;

- describe the radiographic appearance and stages of infant respiratory distress syndrome (IRDS) and adult respiratory distress syndrome (ARDS);

- explain the typical changes associated with pulmonary embolism;

- explain the steps that are involved in inserting a chest tube.

11

Foreign Materials

Some radiographs of ventilated ICU patients are inherently difficult to interpret due to the presence of numerous electrocardiogram (ECG) leads, central catheters, endotracheal tubes, and gastric tubes. But it is particularly important to maintain close surveillance of these patients to ensure that all foreign objects that have been introduced into the patient are positioned correctly.

In **Figure 198.1**, note the (correct) position of both pacemaker lead wires in the trabecular meshwork of the right atrium (↓) and on the floor of the right ventricle (↗). Note also the (correct) position of the Tracheoflex tracheostomy tube **(48)** for ventilating the patient. Other foreign materials of interest are the ECG lead wires **(52)**, the postoperative sternal cerclage wires **(52)**, and two prosthetic heart valves (↖). While the inflammatory infiltrates **(37)** in the lower zone of the right lung (↘) are fairly easy to interpret, some observers may miss the fact that it is unclear whether the tip of the indwelling gastric tube **(65)** has been passed deep enough into the stomach (risk of aspiration).

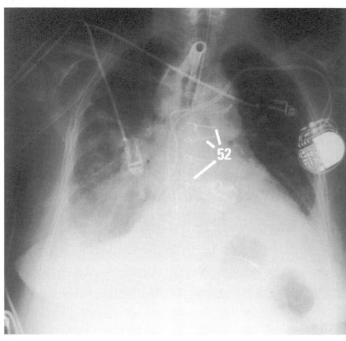

Fig. 198.1a

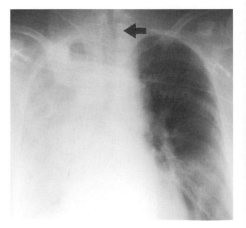

Fig. 198.1b

It is also important to note the tip of the endotracheal tube (↑ in **Fig. 198.2b**). It should not be advanced so far that it bypasses the left main bronchus **(43)**, causing atelectasis **(36)** of the left lung and right upper lobe **(32)**. Nor should the tube be positioned too high (← in **Fig. 198.3**), where it would be at risk of becoming dislodged.

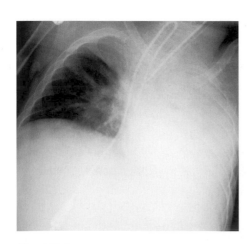

Fig. 198.2a

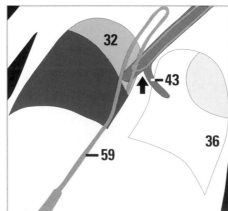

Fig. 198.2b

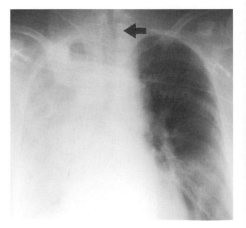

Fig. 198.3

When gastric tubes **(65)** are used in ventilated patients or children, whose throat irritation or subjective discomfort are not always easy to interpret, there are rare instances in which the tube is accidentally passed into the trachea or a mainstem bronchus **(Fig. 199.1a)**. **Figure 199.1b** shows the correct position of the gastric tube after it was withdrawn and reintroduced.

Close surveillance is recommended for a flow-directed pulmonary artery catheter, which in this case was introduced through the left subclavian artery (← in **Fig. 199.2b**; see also p. 130). The radiograph **(Fig. 199.2a)** shows that the catheter has been misdirected into the right atrium and that its tip is in the left internal jugular vein (↘) instead of a pulmonary artery. Note that a second central venous catheter (CVC) introduced through the right subclavian artery (↓)

is correctly positioned in the superior vena cava (SVC; →). If doubt exists, it is sometimes necessary to check the catheter position by fluoroscopy or repeat radiography after infusing contrast medium into the catheter (see p. 162). Immediately afterward, remember to flush the contrast medium from the catheter lumen with sterile saline and a dilute heparin solution to avoid clogging the CVC or pulmonary artery catheter.

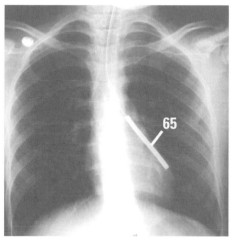

Fig. 199.1a

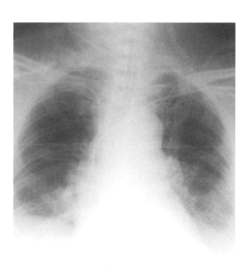

Fig. 199.2a

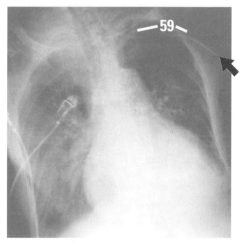

Fig. 199.3

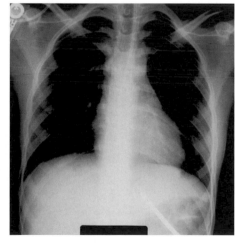

Fig. 199.1b

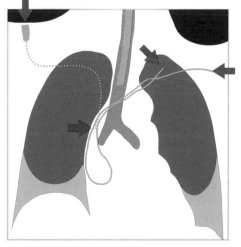

Fig. 199.2b

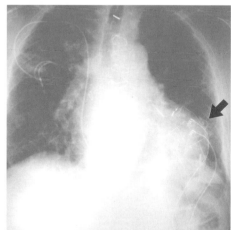

Fig. 199.4

Even with a "simple" CVC inserted by experienced personnel, the tip (↘) of a jugular vein catheter **(59)** may occasionally enter the subclavian vein **(Fig. 199.3)**.
In extensive heart operations and in patients with life-threatening arrhythmias, there may be cases in which intra-

corporeal pacemaker leads (↘) are temporarily left directly on the heart. The patches that transmit electrical impulses from the extracorporeal pacemaker unit to the heart can be identified radiographically by the square outline of their radiopaque margins **(Fig. 199.4)**.

Pulmonary Congestion and Edema

The balance between parenteral fluid administration and renal excretion may be so delicate, especially after cardiac surgery, that pulmonary overhydration can develop rapidly in patients with latent left-sided heart failure. **Figure 200.1** shows a freshly extubated patient after aortocoronary bypass surgery with a pleural drain (✎) in the left hemithorax and bilateral pleural effusions. The horizontal fissure of the right lung contains a loculated effusion (↑), which presents a typical lemon-shaped outline (see p. 125). The broadened cardiac silhouette plus the accentuated vascular markings indicate an early stage of pulmonary edema.

The pulmonary edema progresses rapidly over time (**Fig. 200.2a**) and naturally interferes with gas exchange, sometimes making it necessary to reintubate the patient. In the case shown, the edema quickly improved in response to treatment with loop diuretics (**Fig. 200.2b**)

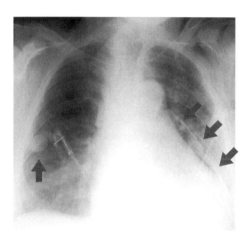

Fig. 200.1

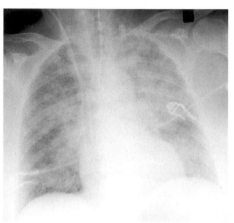

Fig. 200.2a

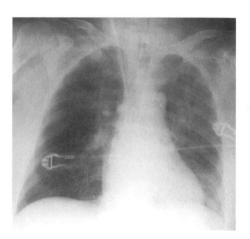

Fig. 200.2b

When the patient has just been moved from a lateral decubitus position to a supine position, the distribution pattern of edematous zones may be considerably altered in the supine radiograph. In this respect the distribution of the edema is position-dependent to a degree. A typical butterfly (perihilar) pattern of pulmonary edema (see **Fig. 142.1a**) is not always seen, and the frontal radiograph may show an irregular accentuation of both perihilar regions (**Fig. 200.3a**), associated in this case with inflammatory infiltration (↘) of the right middle zone (MZ). Unfortunately, this patient went into acute left-sided heart failure, accompanied by a marked deterioration of findings (**Fig. 200.3b**).

When a patient is intubated, the ventilation pressure will often cause increased pulmonary lucency that is misinterpreted as improvement. Conversely, the radiographs of freshly extubated patients will often show apparent lung congestion even though there has been no actual progression of left-sided heart failure.

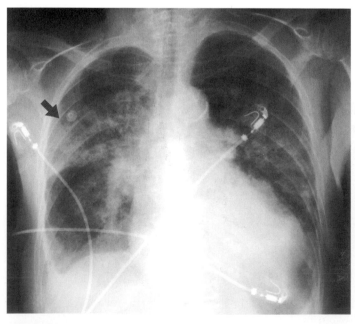

Fig. 200.3a

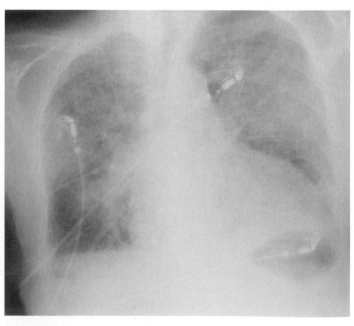

Fig. 200.3b

ARDS, IRDS

Adult respiratory distress syndrome (ARDS) may occur following a latent period of 12-24 hours after a pulmonary contusion, shock (hypotension), Disseminated intravascular coagulation (DIC), aspiration, or the inhalation of toxic fumes. Infant respiratory distress syndrome (IRDS) in premature babies is related mainly to pulmonary immaturity, barotrauma due to positive-pressure ventilation, and hyaline membrane formation.

The series of radiographs in **Figure 201.1** document the progression of findings in a newborn with IRDS. The infant required intubation immediately after birth **(Fig. 201.1a)**. After the initiation of positive-pressure ventilation **(Fig. 201.1b)**, we note an improvement of bronchial aeration, especially on the right side **(Fig. 201.1c)**. The positive-pressure ventilation in this case caused a right-sided pneumothorax (⬆ in **Fig. 201.1d**) that was especially pronounced along the mediastinum and enlarged over time **(Fig. 201.1e)**. Treatment with thoracentesis was attempted (⬇ in **Fig. 201.1f**), but respiratory failure persisted and the child died the same day. The various stages of ARDS are described in **Table 201.2**. **Figure 201.3** shows a stage II radiograph in which the findings are still mild **(Fig. 201.3)**

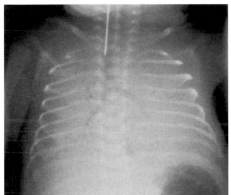

Fig. 201.1a

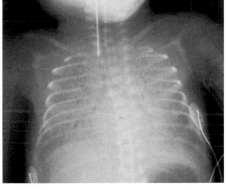

Fig. 201.1b

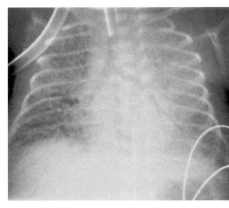

Fig. 201.1c

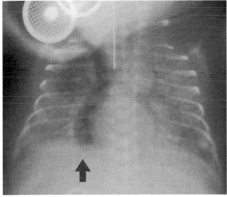

Fig. 201.1d

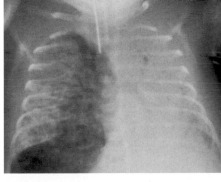

Fig. 201.1e

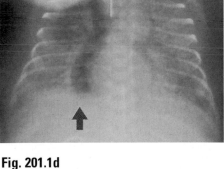

Fig. 201.1f

Stages of ARDS after Krug [11.1]

Stage	Timing	Cause	Radiographic Features
I	First hour	Interstitial edema	Vessels accentuated and indistinct. Loss of bronchial and hilar delineation
II	Hours 2-24	Progression to alveolar edema	Diffuse opacities, Later, confluent airspace consolidation
III	Days 2-7	Cellular proliferation, hyaline membranes, alveolar edema	Linear and reticular opacities. Focal or patchy opacities
IV	> 1 week	Incipient fibrosis	Signs of fibrosis (see p. 150)

Table 201.2

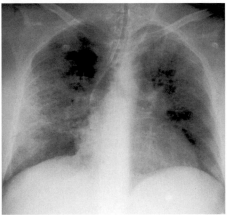

Fig. 201.3

Meconium aspiration in premature infants typically produces an infiltration pattern consisting of fine confluent and linear opacities **(Fig. 202.1)**.

Pneumothorax on Supine Radiographs

Pneumothorax in premature infants is usually a result of positive-pressure ventilation. **Figure 202.2** shows multiple pneumothoraces (▽) on both sides of the chest. Note in particular the anterior loculated pleural air collection (⬇) in the right basal zone, which is easily missed in a cursory viewing of the film. Pneumopericardium (⬋ ⬉ in **Fig. 202.3**) may also present as an initial finding. In this example, air collections **(38)** subsequently formed in both pleural cavities and had to be decompressed with chest tubes **(48)** **(Fig. 202.4)**.

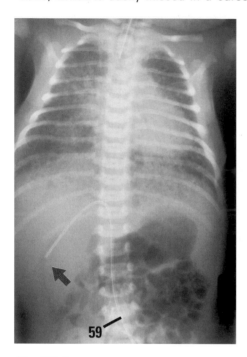

Fig. 202.1

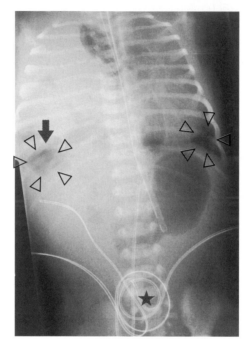

Fig. 202.2

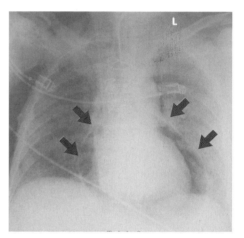

Fig. 202.3

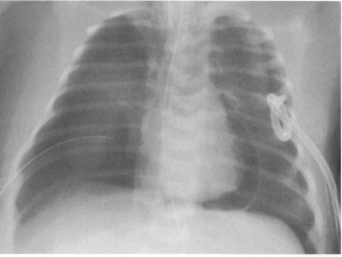

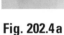

Fig. 202.4 a

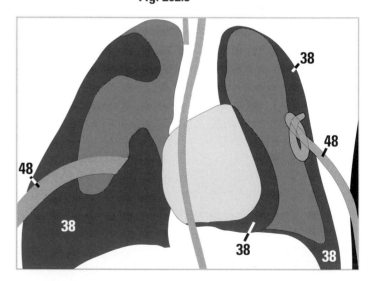

Fig. 202.4 b

In some premature infants that have been placed on a ventilator in an ICU, you may notice a catheter **(59)** in the lower part of the radiograph **(Fig. 202.1)**. In this case the tube is an umbilical vein catheter, which should run directly upward from the umbilicus through the umbilical vein, umbilical recess, and ductus venosus to the termination of the inferior vena cava (IVC) in the right atrium. In the case shown, however, the tip of the catheter (⬉) is in the portal vein, posing a danger of portal vein thrombosis (which is often missed clinically).

This device is distinguished from an umbilical artery catheter (★) by its course. A catheter introduced through the umbilical artery first runs obliquely along the lateral umbilical fold and then turns upward, passing through the internal iliac artery to the aorta **(Fig. 202.2)**. Its tip should be positioned either in the thoracic aorta at the level of the T6-T10 vertebral body or in the abdominal aorta at the L4 (L3-5) level just above the aortic bifurcation.

A pneumothorax in adults may also result from pulmonary hyperinflation, which causes depression of the diaphragm leaflets (↓ in **Fig. 203.1**). In the case shown, the chest tube (↙) has already been inserted (see p. 204-206) and the left lung has reexpanded.

64 For practice, determine the number and position of all the catheters that have been introduced in **Figure. 203.1**. Compare in particular the position of the pulmonary artery catheter with that in **Figure 203.2**.

You will notice that the tip of the second pulmonary catheter (↑ in **Fig. 203.2**) is in the descending part of the right lower lobe artery (see p. 130). This patient also has a mantle pneumothorax (▽) on the right side , multiple areas of bronchiectasis (↗) in the left lung (see p. 135), and an abscess (↘) in the right MZ. Note the CVC **(59)** that has been passed through the right jugular vein; its tip (↖) has been placed slightly too high in the brachiocephalic vein. The endotracheal tube (←) is correctly positioned.

Figure 203.3 shows a patient with multiple intrapulmonary hemorrhages **(39)** secondary to vasculitis. These lesions divert attention from a mantle pneumothorax (▽) on the right side and may be mistaken for inflammatory infiltrates. The pneumothorax in this case occurred during a catheter change. Can you distinguish the two CVCs **(59)** from each other? Notable signs of an impending tension pneumothorax are a mediastinal shift toward the opposite side and depression of the ipsilateral hemidiaphragm (see p. 191).

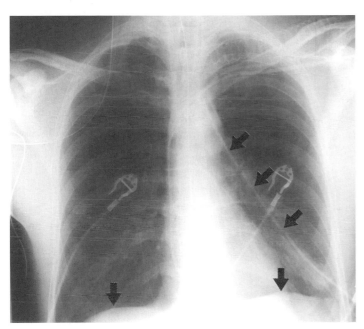

Fig. 203.1

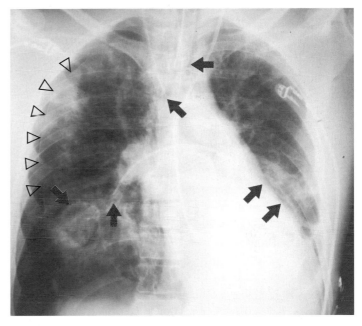

Fig. 203.2

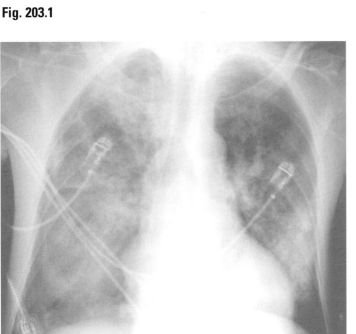

Fig. 203.3a

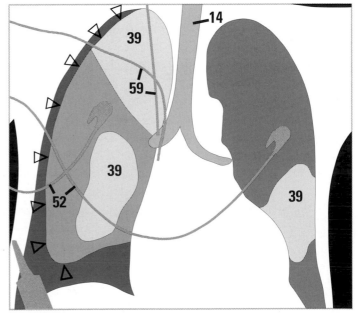

Fig. 203.3b

Insertion of a Chest Tube

A chest tube may be indicated for recurrent or malignant effusions, a hemothorax (see p. 186, p. 207), or an impending tension pneumothorax (see p. 191). Various access routes are available. The tube may be introduced from the anterior side in the fourth intercostal space (ICS) (midclavical line, MCL) or in the fifth or sixth ICS in the anterior axillary line (for a pneumothorax), or it may be introduced at a more posterolateral site in a lower ICS in the posterior axillary line (for an effusion or hemothorax). With an effusion, the tube should be inserted as low as possible to promote maximum drainage. For a pneumothorax, however, many colleagues favor a higher insertion site and recommend tunneling the tube in the soft tissues of the chest wall to create a better seal for when suction is attached to the drain.

The technique of chest tube insertion is described here for the elective drainage of a malignant pleural effusion (41). As this is **not** an emergency procedure, the insertion site can first be marked with a metal clip (⬇ in **Fig. 204.1**), and fluoroscopy **(Fig. 204.2)** can then be used to assess the location of the hyperlucent lung **(33, 34)** and diaphragm **(17a)** in relation to the marked site **(Fig. 204.3)**

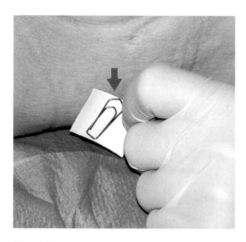

Fig. 204.1

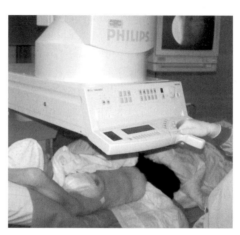

Fig. 204.2

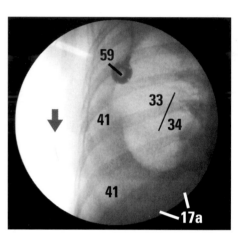

Fig. 204.3

Next, the course of the ribs and the proposed insertion site are marked on the skin **(Fig. 204.4)**, and the skin is sprayed with antiseptic solution prior to local anesthesia **(Fig. 204.5)**. Because the insertion of a chest tube can be quite painful, fully conscious patients should be premedicated and the insertion site should be liberally infiltrated with10-20 mL of local anesthetic (e.g., a 2% lidocaine solution), placing not just a subcutaneous depot (⬎ ⬏) but also infiltrating the needle track and especially the pleura. While infiltrating the site, keep the needle at the upper margin of the lower rib to avoid injury to intercostal nerves and vessels (see p. 60-61) **(Fig. 204.6)**. Also during the infiltration, carefully move the needle deeper with intermittent aspiration (⬅ in **Fig. 205.1**) until you draw air (with a pneumothorax) or a pale yellow effusion or reddish hematoma into the syringe. This will ensure that the entire needle tract has been anesthetized.

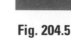

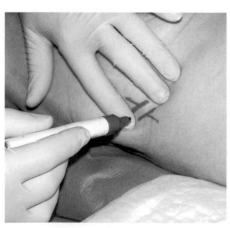

Fig. 204.4

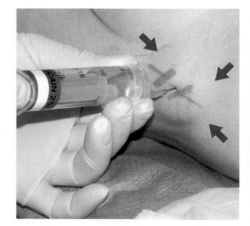

Fig. 204.5

Fig. 204.6

At this point you will need a sterile tray **(Fig. 205.2)** that includes antiseptic solution and swabs (↗), sterile drapes (↓), scalpels for making the skin incision (↑), several clamps (↘), the chest tube with stylet (↘), the valve (↙), and several compresses and suture material (★). After the area has been sterily draped and the antiseptic skin prep repeated **(Fig. 205.3)**, subsequent clogging of the drain by fibrin or blood clots can be prevented by cutting two or three extra holes at the distal end of the tube with the scalpel **(Fig. 205.4)**.

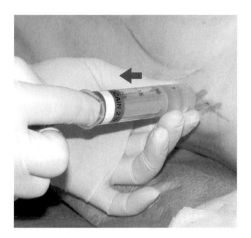

Fig. 205.1

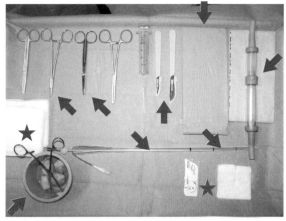

Fig. 205.2

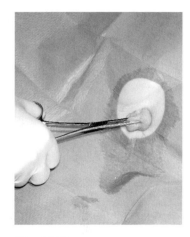

Fig. 205.3

Now the skin is incised with the scalpel (**Fig. 205.5**, and the drainage tube is inserted **Fig. 205.6**). If the tube is being inserted for the suction drainage of a pneumothorax rather than draining of an effusion, it may be advantageous to insert a clamp into the incision and open the jaws of the clamp several times to expand the drainage tract. You can avoid entering the pleural cavity by using the index finger of the free hand to control and direct the passage of the clamp through the skin.

If you want to develop a subcutaneous tunnel (not shown here), pass the tip of the closed (!) clamp to the **upper** margin of the next higher rib, and perforate the parietal pleura of the next higher ICS with the clamp. The moment you do this, you will notice a sudden rush of air (with a tension pneumothorax), effusion, or blood issuing from the pleural cavity (don't be alarmed).

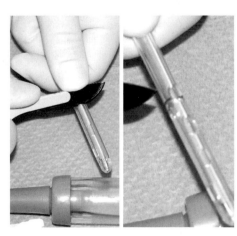

Fig. 205.4

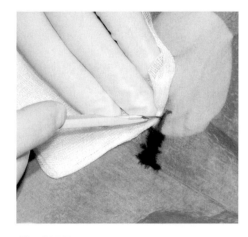

Fig. 205.5

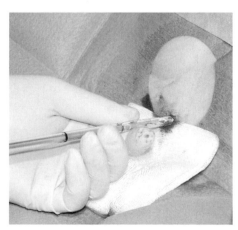

Fig. 205.6

When dealing with a large effusion, you should drain no more than 1000 mL of fluid in one sitting **(Fig. 206.7)**. This is done to prevent excessive protein losses and avoid sudden expansion trauma to the lung, which may lead to pulmonary edema. In all, you should drain no more than 1500 mL of effusion per day.

As the chest tube is advanced under pressure (→), demonstrated here by a right-handed operator using the dominant hand **(Fig. 206.1)**, the left hand (↘) acts as a "brake" to ensure that the tube will not plunge forcibly into the pleural cavity after passing through the parietal pleura **(Fig. 206.2)**. When the tube has been positioned on the floor of the pleural cavity under fluoroscopic guidance **(Fig. 206.2)**, the stylet is removed (↖ in **Fig. 206.3**) and the tube is clamped off (⌐ in **Fig. 206.4**). An adapter (↗ in **Fig. 206.5**) is then attached to the end of the tube, and the valve (↑) is connected **(Fig. 206.6)**. Make sure the correct symbol (↓) is toward the patient!

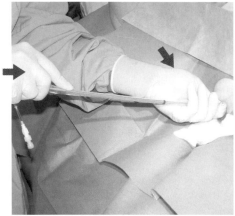
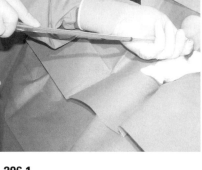

Fig. 206.1

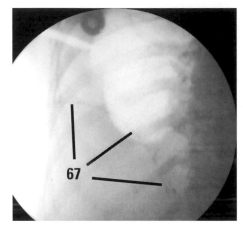

Fig. 206.2

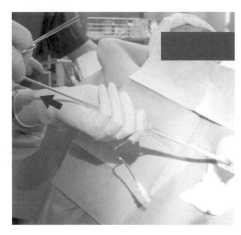

Fig. 206.3

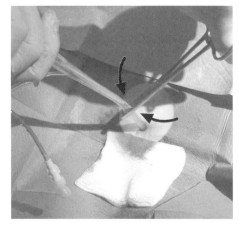

Fig. 206.4

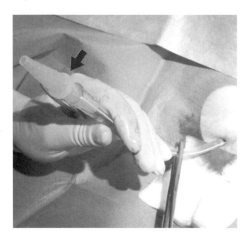

Fig. 206.5

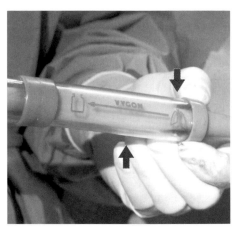

Fig. 206.6

Remember that the drainage of an effusion **(Fig. 206.7)** is limited to a maximum safe daily volume (see the bottom of p. 205). Finally, the drain is sutured to the skin **(Fig. 206.8)**, the suture having previously been wrapped tightly around the tube, and a sterile dressing is applied to protect the site and hold the tube in place **(Fig. 206.9)**.

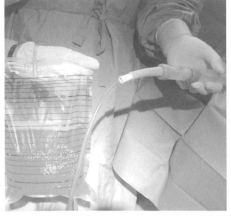

Fig. 206.7

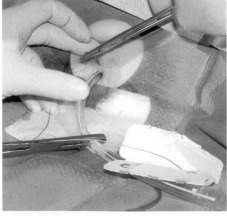
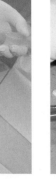

Fig. 206.8

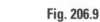

Fig. 206.9

Hemothorax

Especially after thoracic surgery or trauma (see p. 186), it is possible for hemodynamically significant blood volumes to enter one or both pleural cavities within a short time. **Figure 207.1** shows a large opacity in the right hemithorax, but in this case it was caused by a layered-out effusion accompanied by infiltrates. If a hemothorax is suspected, generally it can be excluded more quickly by sonography **(Fig. 207.2)** than radiography (see FAST, p. 194). The intrapleural blood **(39)** in this case appears as a uniformly echo-free (= black) collection between the parenchyma of the lower lobe (LL) **(34)**, which contains residual air **(38)**, and the diaphragm **(17)**, and liver **(19)**. A hemothorax may also show a nonhomogeneous echo pattern due to clotted blood, depending on the patient's coagulation status and the latent period between the hemorrhage and the examination.

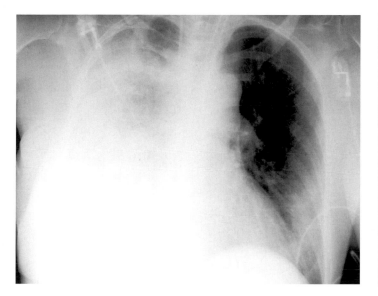

Fig. 207.1

Fig. 207.2

Pulmonary Embolism

A pulmonary embolism should be excluded in patients who experience an acute onset of dyspnea, chest pain, or circulatory symptoms and in ventilated patients who show a sudden deterioration of blood gas values. Frequently, a pulmonary embolism cannot be detected with conventional radiographs on the first day. In some cases, however, the chest radiograph may show "Westermark's sign" **(Table 207.3)** in the form of regional oligemia with increased lucency, as in the right lung in **Figure 207.4**. A pulmonary infarction or postinfarction pneumonia (↓) may develop 12–24 hours later, usually appearing as a wedge-shaped area of subpleural infiltration ("Hampton's sign", **37**). Scintigraphy can be performed in suspicious cases to check for a perfusion deficit, or transesophageal echocardiography (TEE) can be done to check for thrombi in the main trunks of the pulmonary arteries. Another option is spiral CT (see p. 19), which can detect thrombi even in the more distal pulmonary arterial branches. ECG reveals signs of cor pulmonale or acute right-heart overload, and laboratory tests show elevated D-dimers.

Signs of Pulmonary Embolus

- Westermark sign (see above)
- Abrupt caliber change in hilar vessels (centrally dilated, peripherally constricted)
- Peripheral pulmonary infarct or infarct pneumonia (after 12 h)
- Signs of cor pulmonale
- Ipsilaterally raised diaphragm
- Bands of focal atelectasis

Table 207.3

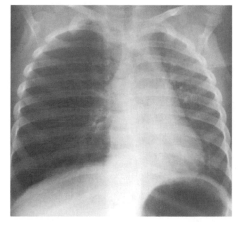

Fig. 207.4

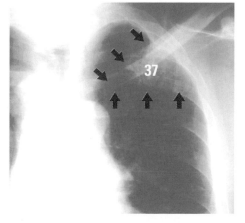

Fig. 207.5

65 What changes are often seen when a previously ventilated patient is extubated and you are reading the initial postextubation chest film? What is the basis for this phenomenon?

66 A ventilated patient with a Tracheoflex tracheostomy tube has developed a fever. What is your diagnosis based on the findings in **Figure 208.1**?

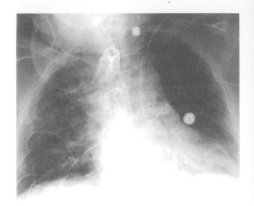
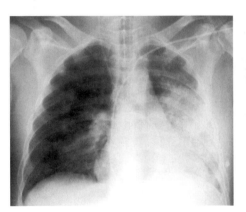

Fig. 208.1

67 Another ventilated patient underwent bronchial lavage for a high fever. **Figure 208.2** shows the radiograph taken after the lavage. What is your impression?

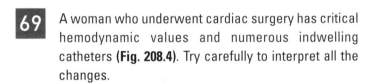

Fig. 208.2

68 A number of "tubes" have been placed in a young man with multiple injuries **(Fig. 208.3)**, and you want to check their position. What, in your opinion, is causing the right-sided opacity?

69 A woman who underwent cardiac surgery has critical hemodynamic values and numerous indwelling catheters **(Fig. 208.4)**. Try carefully to interpret all the changes.

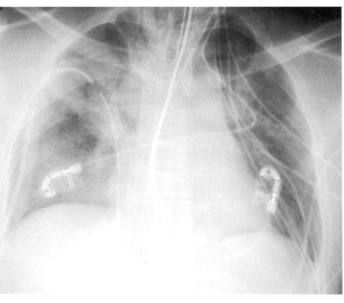

Fig. 208.3

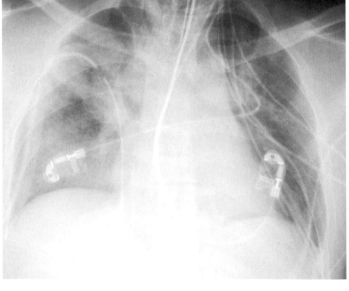

Fig. 208.4

1 – 3 Solution to p.32: The answers can be found on pages 10, 12-13, and 18.

4 Solution to p.33: The mediastinal contours are shown on page 20. Bulges or contour changes may have any of the causes (→) listed below:

a	(SVC)	→	Superior vena cava syndrome due to right-sided heart failure, mediastinal tumor, or hematoma
b	(Azygos vein)	→	Ditto in right-sided heart failure
c	(Right atrium)	→	Dilatation due to tricuspid valve disease, right-sided heart failure
d	(Usually only a fat pad, rarely IVC or atypical hepatic vein)	→	Right-sided heart failure
e	(Aortic arch)	→	Elongation due to chronic hypertension, aortic aneurysm
f	(Pulmonary trunk)	→	Poststenotic dilatation in pulmonary valve disease, congestion
g	(Left atrial appendage)	→	Left-sided heart failure, mitral valve disease, aortic valve disease
h	(Left ventricle)	→	Left-sided heart failure, aortic valve disease, myocardial aneurysm
i	(Fat pad, fibrous pleural thickening)	→	Generally of no significance; rarely, diaphragmatic hernia
j	(Ascending aorta)	→	Aortic aneurysm, dilatation due to aortic valve disease
k	(RSS)	→	Dilatation of the right ventricle (pulmonary valve disease, cor pulmonale)
l	(Anterior wall of right ventricle)	→	Same as RSS (**k**)
m	(Posterior wall of left atrium)	→	Mitral valve disease, left-sided heart failure
n	(RCS)	→	Narrowing as in **m**
o	(IVC)	→	Vena cava triangle disappears due to dilatation of the left ventricle (see **h**)

5 Solution to p.33: The four factors can be found in **Table 25.4** on page 24.

6 Solution to p.33: Remember the headstand? A detailed explanation is given on page 25.

7 Solution to p.34: The film on the left **(Fig. 34.1a)** is an upright PA radiograph with a CTR of 35:80 = 0.44. The film on the right **(Fig. 34.1b)** is a supine AP radiograph that shows slight elevation of the hemidiaphragm, causing a broadened cardiac silhouette with a CTR of 42:73 = 0.58 (both values are within normal limits). The correct method for determining the CTR is described on page 27.

8 Solution to p.34: **Description:** This supine radiograph shows a CVC introduced through the right jugular vein and a diffuse increase of opacity in the left lung. Pulmonary vascular markings are markedly diminished on the right side. There is no mediastinal shift or elevation of the hemidiaphragm; both diaphragm leaflets are sharply outlined. There is possible accentuation of the left hilum. **Differential diagnosis:** Layered-out effusion or hemothorax on the left side, right-sided pneumothorax after CVC insertion, angled scatter-reduction grid in a rotated projection (note the position of the clavicles). **Presumptive diagnosis:** Angled grid in a rotated projection (there are insufficient signs to support the other diagnoses). **Recommendation:** Straighten the grid, position the patient for a true AP projection, and repeat the exposure.

p.47 Answer to the question in the text: In addition to kyphosis, there is also aortic elongation (common in patients with long-standing hypertension), coronary artery sclerosis, and irregular ossification of the chondro-osseous junction.

9 Solution to p.48: The large calcified "mass" in the right LZ is a perifocal reaction to the insertion of an ipsilateral breast implant. The most significant changes, however, are the focal opacities in the left LZ. They are caused by skeletal metastases in the anterior segments of the fourth through sixth ribs. Doubtful cases can be resolved by radionuclide scanning.

10 Solution to p.48: The patient is an asthmatic woman with pneumonia in the right ML and left LL in addition to mediastinal emphysema, which has dissected into the soft tissues of the neck. The findings are suspicious for a ruptured subpleural bulla, allowing air to enter the mediastinum.

Q

11 Solution to p.48: These radiographs are from a woman with renal cell carcinoma. Besides the obvious intrapulmonary metastases, there is complete destruction of the T6 vertebral body (→) consistent with osteolytic metastasis.

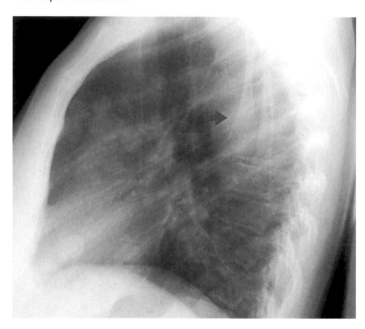

Solution to Fig. 49.3b

13 Solution to p.62:

- CT is indicated for unexplained pleural thickening > 3 mm.
- With pleural thickening > 1 cm, a tumor should be suspected.

14 Solution to p.62:

- Breast carcinoma and rib metastases
- Thyroid carcinoma and thymic neoplasm
- Central and peripheral bronchial carcinoma
- Gastric, pancreatic, and renal carcinoma
- Liver tumors
- Esophageal carcinoma

15 Solution to p.62:

Mit Hilfe der Lenk'schen Regel:
- Angle between the lateral chest wall and thoracic mass > 90° → Pleural mass
- Angle between lateral chest wall and thoracic mass < 90° → Intrapulmonary mass

12 Solution to p.62: The PA radiograph shows bilateral areas of basal pleural fibrosis (↓) following long-term asbestos exposure. There is also fibrosis in the right costophrenic angle (↙), which cannot be positively distinguished from an effusion. The linear opacity (←) projected over the left LZ is a typical fibrotic strand resulting from asbestos exposure.

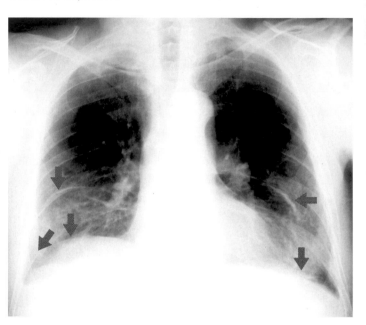

Solution to Fig. 62.1a

The lateral radiograph from the same patient clearly shows areas of hilar (→) and basal (↘) pleural fibrosis. Fibrotic changes are also visible in the anterobasal pericardium (↖) and in the posterior part of the costophrenic angle (↗).

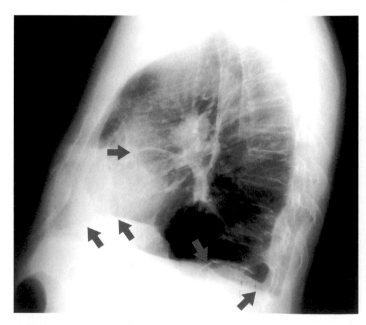

Solution to Fig. 62.1b

16 Solution to p.101:

- **Anterior mediastinum:**
  From the posterior wall of the sternum to the anterior wall of the heart
- **Middle mediastinum:**
  From the anterior to posterior wall of the heart
- **Posterior mediastinum:**
  From the posterior wall of the trachea and heart to the posterior chest wall (see also **Fig. 65.1**)

17 Solution to p.101:
- Retrosternal goiter
- Lymphoma
- Thymus (thymoma or reactive hyperplasia)

18 Solution to p.101:
- Cardiomegaly
- Lymph node enlargement

19 Solution to p.101: The superior mediastinum contains a nonhomogeneous mass (▷) that is particularly opaque in its upper portion (↖). On closer inspection of the PA radiograph **(Fig. 101.1a)**, you will notice (at least in retrospect) that the left shoulder region is generally more lucent than the right. The "mass" is a projection of the upper arm stump onto the superior mediastinum following an upper limb amputation. This also explains the linear opacity (↖) in the lateral radiograph **(Fig. 101.1b)**, which is a remaining segment of the upper humerus (compare with **Fig. 101.1a**).

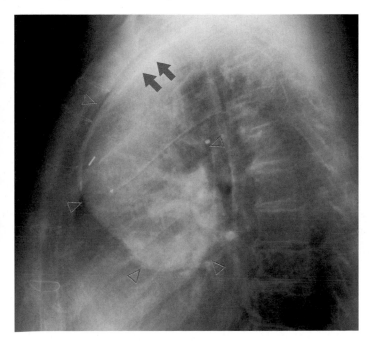

Solution to Fig. 101.1b

20 Solution to p.102: You probably noticed the prosthetic heart valve (↖) and cerclage wires **(52)** from a previous operation. The impression on the esophagus (➡) from the dilated left atrium (e.g., due to malfunction of the mitral valve prosthesis) is clearly appreciated after oral contrast administration. But the most important finding in this case is a pulmonary nodule (▷), which is metastatic to breast carcinoma.

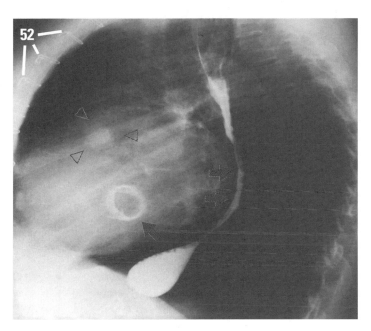

Solution to Fig. 102.1

21 Solution to p.102: In this example, you should notice the obliterated cardiac waist (←--→). The cause was an increased volume load on the pulmonary artery and right heart secondary to a VSD.

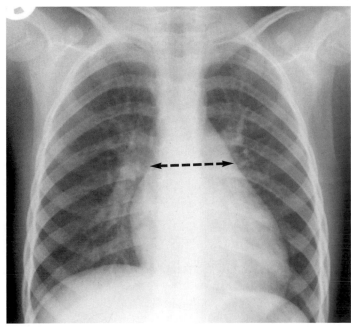

Solution to Fig. 102.2

Q

22 Solution to p.102: In the PA radiograph, the gastric bubble (▷) is projected onto the cardiac silhouette in a patient with a hiatal hernia. The air bubble (✔) is defined more clearly in the lateral radiograph. Incidental findings include an effusion in the right costophrenic angle (see **Fig. 102.3a**) and calcification of the aortic arch (**6**).

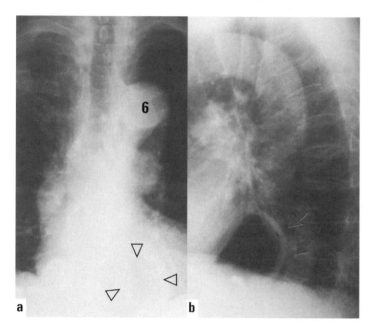

Solution to Fig. 102.3

23 Solution to p.103:
- Sarcoidosis
- Tuberculosis

24 Solution to p.103:

RA ⬆ = **PA radiograph:** Dilatation of the right cardiac border and expansion toward the right side

LA ⬆ = **PA radiograph:** Widening of the cardiac waist with a double contour sign and possible splaying of the tracheal bifurcation
Lateral radiograph: Narrowing of the RCS, posterior displacement of the esophagus

RV ⬆ = **Lateral radiograph:** Narrowing of the RSS

LV ⬆ = **PA radiograph:** Predominantly left-sided cardiomegaly with a normal cardiac waist
Lateral radiograph: Disappearance of the vena cava triangle

25 Solution to p.103:

RSR ⬇ = Pulmonary stenosis, pulmonary insufficiency

RCR ⬇ = Mitral insufficiency, mitral stenosis (may also occur secondarily in aortic insufficiency or in the late stage of aortic stenosis)

26 Solution to p.103:

The possible causes include:
- Viral and tubercular infections
- Rheumatological diseases
- Uremia
- Postmyocardial infarction syndrome or postcardiotomy syndrome
- Traumatic hemorrhage

Radiographic signs:
- Obliterated left cardiac border ("tent" configuration)
- Narrowing of the RSS and RCS
- Possible decrease in pulmonary vascular markings
- Prominence of the SVC at the right mediastinal border

27 Solution to p.103:

Lateral radiograph: $D_{AO} > 4.5$ cm
PA radiograph: $D_{TM} > 5.0$ cm, The ascending aorta forms the right border of the cardiovascular silhouette, the trachea is displaced to the right, and the left main bronchus is displaced downward.

28 Solution to p.103:

- Bilateral notching of the third through ninth ribs
- Dilated, prominent ascending aorta
- Prestenotic and poststenotic expansion of the descending aorta ("figure 3 sign")
- Possible widening of the superior mediastinal shadow due to dilatation of the subclavian artery

29 Solution to p.103: The answer is on page 213.

30 Solution to p.121: A straight-edged, homogeneous opacity is present in the right UZ, bounded by the horizontal fissure (important sign). There are confluent streaky opacities in the right pericardiac area that do not obscure the cardiac silhouette (i.e., they are located in the LL). There is no cardiomegaly and no evidence of pulmonary venous congestion. **Diagnosis:** Pneumonic infiltrates in the right UL <u>and</u> right LL.

31 Solution to p.121: A predominantly smooth-bordered mass with a fluid level is projected onto the upper mediastinum, creating the impression of mediastinal widening. Lateral radiograph shows a bandlike opacity in the middle to posterior mediastinum, which is continuous with the shadow of the aortic arch. **DD:** Mediastinal abscess (gravitated from the pharynx?), esophageal dilatation, or diverticulum. **Diagnosis:** Recurrent carcinoma of the cardia following gastric transposition.

29 Solution to p.121: The uniformly increased density of the right UZ is consistent with atelectasis **(36)**. The nonhomogeneous density in the left pericardiac area represents inflammatory infiltrate **(37)** in the left LL (the left cardiac border is well defined, indicating that the lesion is not in the UL or lingula). The correct diagnosis is suggested by the upward retraction of the hilum on the right side (↟) and the presence of the Port-A-Cath system **(59)**, which is used for chemotherapy. **DD:** Tumor or atelectasis in the right UL. **Diagnosis:** Atelectasis of the right UL secondary to bronchial obstruction by BC. Pneumonia is also present in the left LL.

32 Solution to p.122: At first glance, you might interpret the increased lucency at the periphery of the left lung as a mantle pneumothorax. But if you look more closely, you will see that pulmonary vessels are still visible lateral to the line. Also, there is no depression of the hemidiaphragm on the affected (left) side and no mediastinal shift toward the opposite (right) side. There is splaying of the tracheal bifurcation. **Diagnosis:** Thoracic aortic aneurysm (✔) with marked elongation of the aorta. Here is the lateral radiograph:

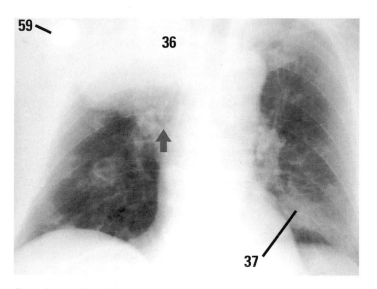

Solution to Fig. 121.1

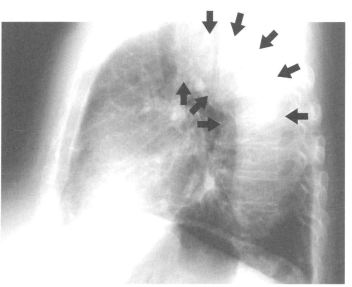

Solution to Fig. 122.1

33 Solution to p.122: Large opacity in the left MZ and LZ with a central lucency and air-fluid level (➡). The right MZ contains a round hyperlucent area with opaque horizontal streaks just below it. The heart presents a normal size and configuration. There is an abscess drain on the left side. The lateral radiograph **(Fig. 213.1)** shows the posterior

location of the opacity in the superior segment of the LL (no. 6). CT clearly demonstrates the perifocal infiltration (↘) and the correctly positioned drain (↖) **(Fig. 213.2)**. **Diagnosis:** Left pulmonary abscess secondary to a traumatic rupture of the diaphragm. Incidental finding: Large emphysematous bulla in the right lung with adjacent areas of dyselectasis.

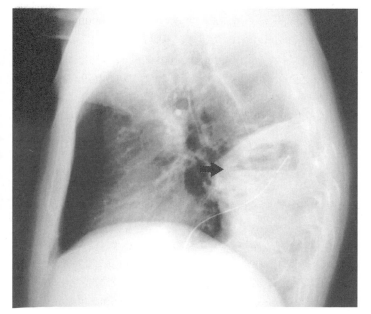

Fig. 213.1

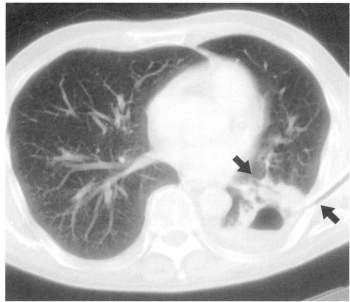

Fig. 213.2

Q

34   Solution to p.122: A rounded, nonhomogeneous area of confluent linear and focal opacities is visible on the right side and obscures the right cardiac border ("silhouette sign"). The right costophrenic angle is clear (important differentiating sign from pleural effusion). This radiograph is overexposed (pulmonary vessels are seen only in the retro-cardiac area).

DD: Pneumonia, left pneumothorax, emphysema (despite absence of flattened diaphragm leaflets on deep inspiration), atelectasis (although the opacity looks too nonhomogeneous for atelectasis).

Diagnosis: Pneumonia of the right ML. The lateral radiograph **(Fig. 214.1)** demonstrates the exact location.

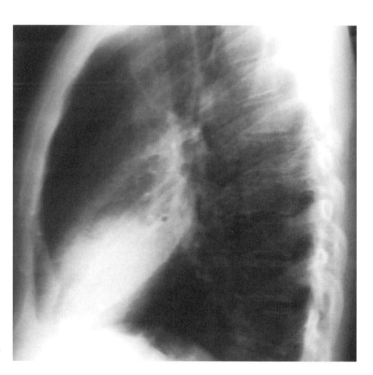

Fig. 214.1

35   Solution to p.122: Homogeneous opacity in the right LZ. Nodular masses on the right hilum. Opaque area with streaky, nodular, and confluent features in the right MZ. Peripheral opacity along the right chest wall with blunting of the costophrenic angle (also on the left side). Increased lucency on the left side. No signs of pulmonary congestion.

DD: Loculated subpulmonic effusion with cephalad extension. Pleural fibrosis. Prior radiotherapy. Enlargement of right hilar lymph nodes.

Diagnosis: BC of the right lung with hilar lymph node metastases and a concomitant malignant effusion. There is compensatory hyperinflation of the left lung.

36   Solution to p.137: A cursory look at this film may suggest an intrapulmonary mass in the left UZ. But the lobulated opacities on the right scapula are consistent with **chondromatosis** (chondroma formation in bones and joints), which also affects the left sternoclavicular joint. The lesion, then, is extrapulmonary. You are correct in thinking that we have not prepared you for a case of this kind. But please approach this challenge with an open mind. We just want to remind you: Always scrutinize the soft tissues of the chest wall so that you can avoid errors of interpretation.

Incidental finding: The right subclavian CVC is correctly positioned in the SVC. There is no evidence of pneumothorax.

37   Solution to p.137: The object of this problem was not to have you make an accurate diagnosis but to remind you of the options that should be considered in the differential diagnosis of multiple pulmonary nodules. If the patient were a newborn, you would also have to consider meconium aspiration (see **Fig. 133.4**). Miliary tuberculosis should also be considered, given the patient's history and possible weakened immune status.

Diagnosis: Multiple metastases from thyroid carcinoma, which has one peak age incidence in children and another in older adults. The patient is too young for stage II sarcoidosis, however.

38   Solution to p.137: This radiograph shows predominantly central dilatation of the pulmonary vascular calibers (↘ ↙) and moderate cardiomegaly (◄——►), although the radiograph was taken at only a moderate depth of inspiration (see p. 25 and **Fig. 215.1**). If you look closely, you will see sternal cerclage wires **(52)** at the right mediastinal border, indicating previous heart surgery. The horizontal fissure **(31)** is accentuated, and a biconvex opacity (↓) is projected over the fissure on the right lateral chest wall. Does the "lemon" shape sound familiar?

Diagnosis: Mild pulmonary venous congestion with predominantly left-sided cardiomegaly and bilateral pleural effusions, including a loculated effusion in the horizontal fissure of the left lung. If you would like to exclude a tumor, one way to do so is to reexamine the patient after cardiac recompensation (a little furosemide was adequate in this case).

Q

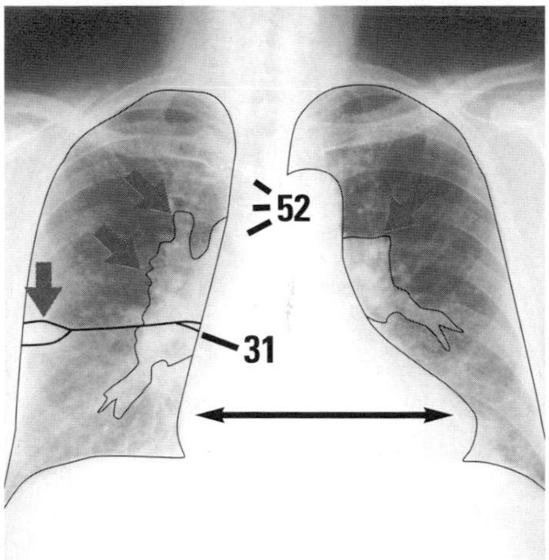

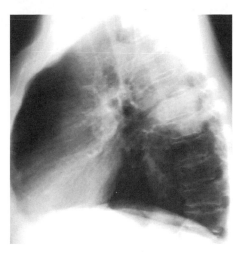

Fig. 215.1

Fig. 215.2a

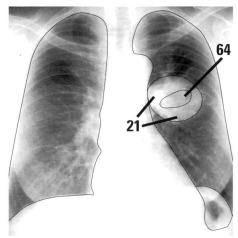

Fig. 215.2b

39 Solution to p.137: **Figure 215.2a** is a lateral radiograph of the same patient. In what segment is the large, globular density located? If you are not sure, refer back to page 12. The patient, incidentally, was a heavy smoker, and this accounted for her chronic bronchitis. The lucency at the center of the mass suggests the possibility of a lung abscess. But the fever in this case was the result of an ascending urinary tract infection.

Diagnosis: The pulmonary lesion was, unfortunately, a bronchial carcinoma **(21)** with central necrosis **(64) (Fig. 215.2b)**.

40 Solution to p.138: Admittedly, the quality of the radiograph is not very good. But if you look closely, you will notice that the left clavicle is obscuring a cavity located within an opacified area. The axial CT scan **(Fig. 215.3)** and positive tuberculin skin test in this case confirmed open pulmonary tuberculosis. You, the guards, and the prison inmates would have been at risk for infection – but you caught the problem in time.

41 Solution to p.138: Residual, bilateral enlargement of the hilar lymph nodes is still apparent, although the dominant finding is multiple focal opacities indicating pulmonary involvement by sarcoidosis. Clinically experienced readers will pardon us for giving obvious clues in the history (typical age of predilection and associated symptom), but it is important for less experienced readers to become familiar with this set of findings.

42 Solution to p.138: The radiograph shows multiple ring shadows with sharp inner margins and somewhat ill-defined outer margins, which are typical of abscess cavities. You saw the PA radiograph of this HIV- and HCV-infected patient earlier on page 135.

Q

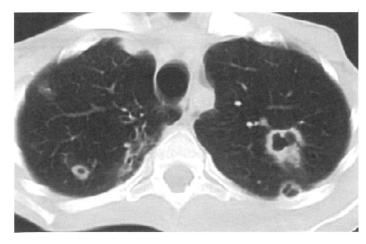

Fig. 215.3

43 Solution to p.138: A large hyperlucent cavity is present in the right apicolateral region, surrounded by an ill-defined area of increased density in the right UZ with upward retraction of the right hilum and a pronounced ipsilateral mediastinal shift. The focal opacities and pleural fibrosis are located mainly in the upper zones. The differential diagnosis would include an abscess following an upper lobectomy, a BC, or tuberculosis. The latter was the correct diagnosis in this case **(Fig. 216.1)**.

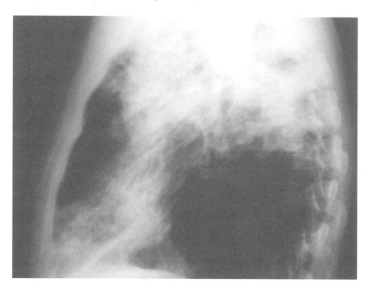

Fig. 216.1

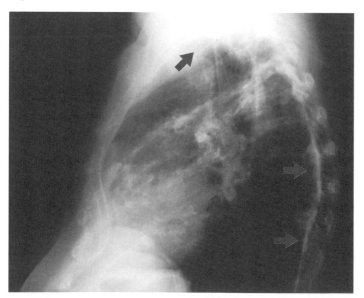

Fig. 216.2

44 Solution to p.138: This radiograph shows a complex pattern with a calcified pleural peel (➡) on the right side and numerous focal opacities in the lung. The area of increased density at the right apex also harbors a BC (➚), which was responsible for the sympathetic nerve lesion **(Fig. 216.2)**. Postinflammatory calcification is also noted in the left hilar lymph nodes.

45 Solution to p.138: Unfortunately, it is not unusual for radiograph request forms to contain scant information on the patient's history. (Try to avoid this in your own practice!) The radiograph shows bilateral hilar lymph node enlargement and calcifications (➘) **plus** unsharpness of the right cardiac border with right pericardiac opacity. The patient had resolving ML atelectasis **(36)** in a setting of sarcoidosis **(Fig. 216.3)**. Additionally, there are regional hyperlucencies consistent with pulmonary emphysema.

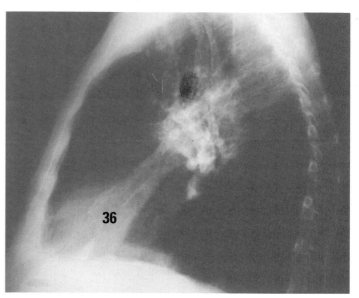

Fig. 216.3

46 Solution to p.140: The three vertical lucent bands are, from anterior to posterior, the trachea and the spaces between the scapulae. The relatively dense cortical lines of the scapulae create the appearance of intervening hyperlucent zones.

47 Solution to p.140: **Differentiating between a pneumothorax and the medial scapular border**. With a mantle pneumothorax, the area lateral to the pleural boundary line appears **hyper**lucent, or darker than the lung medial to it, and is avascular (see p. 120). With insufficient lateral rotation of the scapula (see p. 24), the area lateral to the scapular boundary line appears **hypo**lucent, or lighter than the area medial to it. This is the exact opposite of the relative densities that are seen with a pneumothorax.

48 Solution to p.140: **Companion shadow of the clavicle**. This line is horizontal and parallel to the clavicle and is caused by skin and subcutaneous tissue that are tangential to the roentgen ray beam (see p. 52).

49 Solution to p.154:

Table 217.1

Differentiating criteria	Silicosis	Asbestosis
Sites of predilection for fibrotic changes:	UZ, MZ	LZ, MZ
Spirometric ventilation defects?	Obstructive	Restrictive
Very typical features and their location:	Eggshell lymph node calcifications Bilateral, perihilar	Pleural plaques Usually basal and anterolateral

50 Solution to p.154:
You will find the signs of pulmonary congestion listed in **Table 143.3** (p. 143) and also on the pull-out sheet, which consists of four pocket-sized checklist cards.

51 Solution to p.154:
A pattern of fine confluent and linear opacities is always suspicious for inflammatory infiltration when it is unilateral or localized and there are no signs of cardiomegaly or pulmonary vascular dilatation (if evaluable, since vascular markings are often effaced within areas of pneumonia-unlike pleural effusions). A positive air bronchogram is typical of pneumonia, but occasionally it may occur in association with peribronchial edema due to congestion.

With an interstitial infiltration pattern, the differential diagnosis should also include fungi, viruses, parasites, and atypical pathogens. Equivocal cases should be investigated by microbiological analysis of sputum, bronchial secretions, or pleural aspirate and serological testing for elevated antibody titers, eosinophilia, etc.

52 Solution to p.154:
Pneumocystis carinii pneumonia (PcP) typically develops in immunocompromised patients (corticosteroids, HIV, chemotherapy). Other typical features are an interstitial pattern of markings and the absence of concomitant pleural effusions or hilar lymph node enlargement (see p. 116). Early detection is essential, as it may warrant the prompt discontinuation of chemotherapy, for example, and the initiation of antibiotics.

53 Solution to p.155:
A comparison of the two sides in **Figure 155.1** shows ground-glass opacity of the right lung with no signs of congestion (the left hilar vessels are not dilated, and there are no Kerley lines). The diaphragm leaflets are elevated on both sides (supine radiograph or poor depth of inspiration), but in themselves they cannot account for the increased linear and reticular markings in the right perihilar region or the unsharpness of the right cardiac border (silhouette sign, see p. 28). The left hilum appears normal.
Diagnosis: Right middle lobar pneumonia.
Associated findings: The catheter introduced through the left jugular vein is positioned slightly too high, and the catheter on the right side has been advanced too far into the right atrium and should be withdrawn by about 3-4 cm. The third catheter is a gastric tube.

54 Solution to p.155:
The child in **Figure 155.2** shows increased linear and reticular markings in the left lung and, to a lesser degree, in the right midzone with no cardiomegaly and no detectable pleural effusion. The clinical presentation is very helpful in making the correct interpretation.
Diagnosis: Varicella pneumonia, more pronounced on the left side than on the right.

55 Solution to p.155:
Both radiographs in **Figure. 155.3** are significantly rotated, as indicated by the displacement of the trachea toward the right side and the position of the clavicles. Because of this rotation, the left hilum is obscured by the cardiac silhouette in **Figure 155.3a** and there is apparent accentuation of the right hilum. The radiograph taken the next day show a marked progression of pleural effusions with pronounced cardiomegaly. Positive air bronchograms are not seen within the opacities. The rapid progression is not consistent with inflammatory infiltrates.
Diagnosis: Progressive pulmonary venous congestion.
Caution: With possible widening of the superior mediastinum, you should recommend a follow-up examination after cardiac recompensation. Mediastinal hematoma should be considered in postoperative cases.

Q

56 Solution to p.156: Despite the marginal quality of the radiograph, you can see faint linear markings in both basal lung regions and concomitant effusions. The cardiac size is borderline, and there are no signs of congestion. Malignant cells were detected in pleural aspirate.
Diagnosis: Carcinomatous lymphangitis in the lung due to metastatic breast cancer.

57 Solution to p.156: The radiograph in **Figure 156.2** shows a diffuse linear and reticular pattern of induration involving both lungs.
Diagnosis: Pulmonary fibrosis. In exploring the history, you would want to look for possible causes (exposure to organic or inorganic dusts, see p. 150) and ask about medications and previous infections. You should also try to exclude collagen diseases and metabolic defects (cystic fibrosis, alpha-1-antitrypsin deficiency, etc.).

58 Solution to p.156: Of course, the goal in this case was not to make a correct diagnosis. Both radiographs in **Figure 156.3** show linear and reticular opacities chiefly involving the left UZ and MZ, and the right MZ, the latter showing confluent small opacities. The second radiograph shows lateral hyperlucency on the right side with no residual pulmonary vascular markings. CT scans were also obtained and showed pleural thickening, enlarged mediastinal lymph nodes, and cavitating lesions in the left LL. The **differential diagnosis** includes pulmonary involvement by lymphoma, Kaposi sarcoma, atypical mycobacteria, and right-sided pneumothorax.
Recommendation: Microbiological or serological tests to identify the infecting organism and determine its antibiotic sensitivity, and closed pleural drainage on the right side.

p.180 Answer to the question in the text: The following shotgun pellets can be identified in the extrapulmonary soft tissues: (a) one in the right diaphragm leaflet, (b) one in the upper part of the right lateral chest wall, and (c, d) two closely adjacent pellets in the soft tissues of the right side of the neck. Three intrapulmonary pellets (e, f, g) are lodged in the right lung and one (h) is in the left lung close to the left mediastinal border (**Fig. 218.1a**).
The lateral radiograph (**Fig. 218.1b**) shows an additional pellet (i) close to the anterior diaphragm, which is easily missed in the PA radiograph. The pellet in the chest wall (b) and the intrapulmonary pellets (e-h) are also clearly visualized, but pellets c and d are obscured by the soft-tissue shadows of the neck and cannot be positively identified.

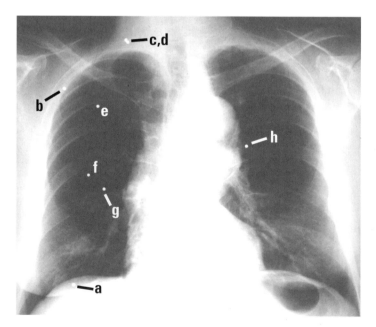

Fig. 218.1a

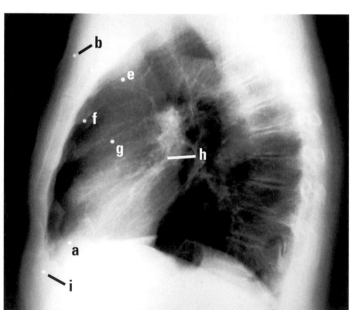

Fig. 218.1b

59 Solution to p.182: The PA radiograph (**Fig. 219.1**) shows a pacemaker (⬆) and also a port system for chemotherapy administration. The reservoir (⬈) of the port system and the catheter (▷) can be identified. The catheter tip (➡) is correctly positioned in the SVC.

This pacemaker is a VVI device with a cable whose tip (⬋) is on the floor of the right ventricle. The radiograph also shows cerclage wires (**52**) from a previous sternotomy. The gastric bubble (**18**) is clearly visible below the left hemidiaphragm.

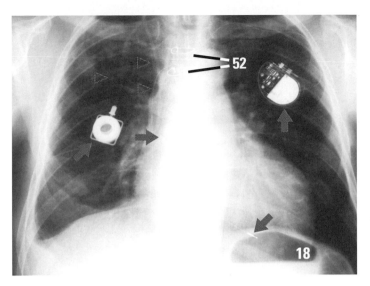

Fig. 219.1

60 Solution to p.182: A pacemaker unit with two electrodes, one in the right atrium (⬇) and one in the right ventricle (⬅), is projected over the left lung. Within the cardiac silhouette are two tilting-disk mechanical heart valves (▷) placed in the aortic and mitral valve positions. The cerclage wires (**52**) are also well defined. An ECG lead (▲) is projected over the right lung, and a tracheostomy tube (⬊) is correctly positioned with its tip above the carina. By looking closely, you can identify an indwelling gastric tube (⬉) to the left of the tracheostomy tube (**Fig. 219.2**).

61 Solution to p.182: The PA radiograph shows a PDA coil (▼) that was implanted to occlude a patent ductus arteriosus. The spiral shape of the device (▼) is seen more clearly on the lateral radiograph. The coil is correctly positioned in the patent ductus (**Fig. 219.3**).

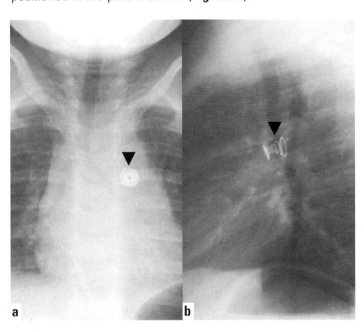

a   b

Fig. 219.3

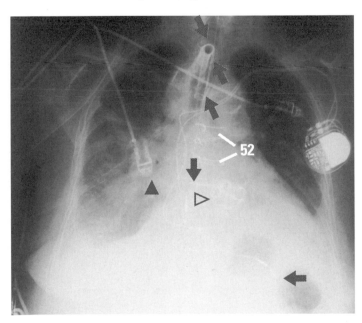

Fig. 219.2

62 Solution to p.196: The patient had a borderline personality disorder and a history of repeated self-inflicted injuries, some severe. Close scrutiny of this radiograph reveals that a fine needle has been passed into the right superior thoracic aperture, causing a significant pneumothorax and hemothorax on the right side. The "opacity" in the right pericardiac area is caused by bunched pulmonary vessels (an effect of elastic recoil toward the hilum).

63 Solution to p.196: The patient in **Figure 196.2** tumbled several meters down a steep slope while hiking in the Swiss Alps. The supine radiograph shows definite mediastinal widening consistent with a paravertebral and/or mediastinal hematoma. A CT examination was also performed **(Fig. 220.1a-c)**, confirming the suspected hematoma and also showing a longitudinal fracture of the manubrium sterni (↓) with a retrosternal hematoma (★), a comminuted fracture of the T3 vertebral body (→) with no paravertebral hematoma, fractures of the first through fourth ribs on the left side, and of the first and second ribs on the right side.

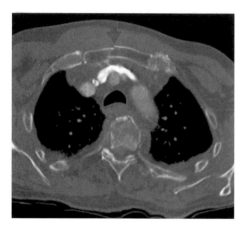

Fig. 220.1a

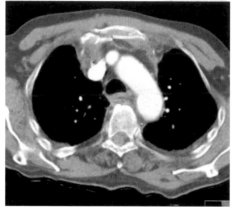

Fig. 220.1b

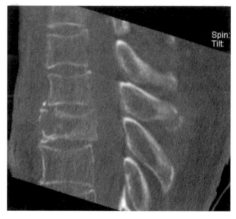

Fig. 220.1c

64 Solution to p.203: The tip of the endotracheal tube is projected onto the sternoclavicular joints and is an adequate distance from the carina. The chest tube is correctly positioned on the left side. The tip of the pulmonary artery catheter inserted by the left subclavicular route is correctly positioned in the right pulmonary artery. The tip of the CVC inserted by the left subclavicular route is correctly positioned in the SVC. The depth of the gastric tube cannot be assessed in this case because of the superimposed cardiac silhouette. Its extracorporeal portion is projected over the right UZ.

65 Solution to p.208: Because the ventilation pressure is lost when the patient is extubated, the chest radiographs of many freshly extubated patients appear slightly congested compared with the previous ventilated radiographs (see p. 200). Also, most extubated patients have a decreased depth of inspiration, leading to apparent widening of the cardiac silhouette and bilateral accentuation of the hilar vessels (all effects are increased by the supine position, see p. 24).

66 Solution to p.208: **Foreign material:** The radiograph shows a Tracheoflex tracheostomy tube in the correct position. The depth of the gastric tube is obscured by the cardiac silhouette and cannot be assessed.
Lung: An extensive positive air bronchogram (see p. 144) is visible in the left retrocardiac region. Multiple fine opacities are visible in the right lung. The left lung is generally more lucent than the right lung, probably the result of an angled scatter-reduction grid in a rotated projection.
Diagnosis: Left lower lobe pneumonia, possible right lower lobe pneumonia. Follow-up is recommended.

67 Solution to p.208: **Foreign material:** The endotracheal tube is correctly positioned. The pulmonary artery catheter was inserted by the left subclavicular route, and its tip is visible in the right pulmonary artery. The CVC was introduced through the right jugular vein, and its tip is projected at the junction of the right brachiocephalic vein with the SVC. **Lung:** Both lungs are fully expanded with no signs of pneumothorax. A pattern of confluent small and larger opacities is visible in the MZ and LZ (lingula + LL) of the left lung. The calibers of the pulmonary vessels are normal, at most showing a small degree of perihilar accentuation. **Heart:** Mild cardiomegaly predominantly affecting the left side. **Summary:** The increased density of the left lung may be caused by residual lavage fluid, and there is suspicion of residual inflammatory infiltrates in the lingula and left LL.

68 Solution to p.208: When you look closely at this expiratory (!) radiograph, you will observe posterolateral fracture lines **(29)** in at least three ribs (fifth through seventh) on the right side. These fractures are responsible for the hemothorax that is causing haziness on the right side. **Foreign material:** The tip of the endotracheal tube **(48)** is correctly positioned approximately 3 cm from the tracheal bifurcation **(14c)**. The pleural drain on the right side **(67)** extends posteriorly to the floor of the costodiaphragmatic recess; it appears too low only because of the poor depth of inspiration. The other lines represent ECG leads **(52)**. **Diagnosis:** Posterolateral fractures of the fifth through seventh ribs with a right hemothorax.

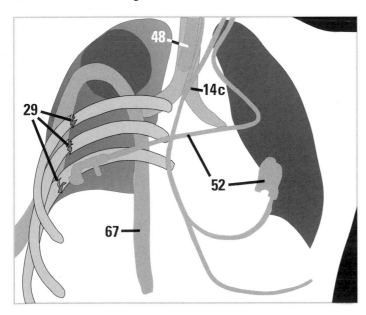

Fig. 221.1

69 Solution to p.208: **Foreign material:** The endotracheal tube **(48)** is correctly positioned. The tip of the pulmonary artery catheter is visible at the origin of the right pulmonary artery (➡). A Demers catheter (★) has been introduced by the left subclavicular route for hemodialysis (see p. 165). Its tip (⬆) is projected at the center of the right atrium. A CVC **(59)** has been passed through the right jugular vein, and its tip is also in the right atrium. A fourth CVC, introduced from the left side, is also in the right atrium and should be withdrawn by approximately 4 cm from its current position. The left pleural drain **(67)** is correctly positioned, and the sternal cerclage wires appear to be intact and undisplaced. The radiopaque marker on the IABP (✔) is projected onto the aortic arch or proximal descending aorta (a lateral radiograph is not available). **Lung:** The left lung is fully expanded (with possible slight residual pneumonia in the left apical lobe). Dilatation of perihilar vessels and Kerley B lines are noted in both lungs. There is no evidence of inflammatory infiltrates. **Heart:** The heart shows mild (for a supine radiograph), predominantly left-sided cardiomegaly with a subtle pneumopericardium **(38**, probably due to postoperative residual air). **Summary:** Signs of predominantly central pulmonary edema (left-sided heart failure? overhydration? renal function?). Three of the catheters are in the right atrium (see above).

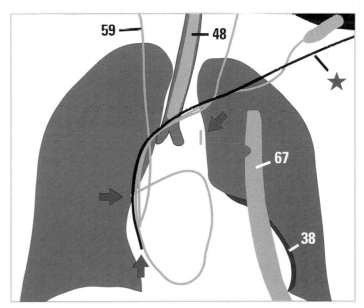

Fig. 221.2

70 If you would like to test your knowledge further, we suggest turning back to the Chapter Goals listed at the beginning of each chapter. Read through each of the learning points and provide detailed answers or descriptions to see how well you have accomplished the various goals. Good luck!

Radiation Safety

Always consider the ALARA principle ("as low as reasonably achievable") before exposing any patient to diagnostic radiation. The effective dose is the most useful parameter for assessing exposure, as it takes into account the individual radiosensitivities of different tissues. The unit of measurement for the effective dose is the millisievert (mSv). In the table below, the dose levels of conventional chest radiographs are compared with those of computed tomography (CT) scanning and with the average annual exposure to ionizing radiation.

Radiation Source	Effective Dose E	Percentage
Average total annual exposure in Germany	~ 4.20 mSv	100.0 %
Natural exposure (radon, terrestrial cosmic, etc.)	~ 2.40 mSv	57.0 %
Fallout from Chernobyl, nuclear weapons testing, etc.	~ 0.03 mSv	0.7 %
Ionizing radiation in medicine, average total	~ 1.50 mSv	35.7 %
Thoracic CT (breast, lung); dose depends on the examination technique	~ 5-10 mSv	120-240 %
Conventional chest radiographs in two planes	~ 0.20 mSv	5.0 %

The effective dose from a single posteroanterior (PA) radiograph without a lateral projection is substantially lower. These figures do not mean that the radiation dose from conventional chest radiographs is harmless, but they do allow a rational assessment of the exposure level, which is quite low in relation to other sources.

Technical Principles

The roentgen ray film itself is mounted in a **light-proof** cassette between two intensifying screens that are in direct contact with the film. These intensifying screens are made of substances that emit light when excited by roentgen rays. This secondary light emission produces up to 95% of film blackening; only about 5% is produced by the direct action of the roentgen rays themselves.

This secondary light is emitted in random directions, however, and so it could cause undesired blurring of the exposed film. To obtain a high-quality image, then, it is essential that the intensifying screen be pressed tightly against the film. This film-screen combination has made it possible to reduce the patient dose substantially below the levels required in earlier techniques (see below). As a rule, film-screen systems with a film speed of 400 are currently used for chest radiographs (a tradeoff between image resolution and intensification).

The film itself consists of a base material that is coated, usually on both sides, with a radiation-sensitive emulsion of silver bromide or silver chloride. Primary roentgen ray quanta or secondary light quanta incite a chemical reduction process that causes film blackening, and this effect is amplified when the film is processed. Thus, body areas that are more transparent to roentgen rays, such as aerated lung tissue, cause a greater degree of film blackening than less permeable structures such as bone (see p. 8). During fixation of the exposed film, nonreduced silver salts are removed from the emulsion. As a result, areas that receive little or no exposure to roentgen rays appear lighter on the image, while more heavily exposed areas appear dark. This gives the radiograph the appearance of a "negative" image.

Digital Systems

Increasingly, analog film-screen combinations (see above) are being replaced by digital systems, whose technical details are beyond our present scope. The main advantages of digital systems are the ability to postprocess the image data (brightness, contrast, etc.) and a reduced risk of overexposure or underexposure in very low or very high dose ranges. Lower doses result in a "nosier" image, but, unlike analog systems, provide just as much image information as higher doses. Moreover, digital images can be stored as computer files in hospital archives and can be quickly accessed by authorized colleagues for evaluation and consultation.

Quality Criteria
Technically acceptable chest radiographs should have the following characteristics:

PA radiographs:
- The scapulae are not superimposed over the upper lung zones (they are adequately rotated out of the field).
- The projection is not rotated, i.e., the spinous process of the T3 vertebra is centered and is equidistant from the clavicles.
- Coverage: The image encompasses both lateral costophrenic angles, all of the thoracic organs, and the soft tissues of the neck.
- Adequate depth of inspiration: The diaphragm is not superimposed over the posterior segments of the ninth ribs.

Additional rules for analog images:
- The image is not overexposed if peripheral pulmonary vessels can be seen.
- The image is not underexposed if the spinal column and large lower lobe vessels can be seen within the cardiac silhouette.

Lateral radiographs:
- Arms are elevated so that the (upper) arms are not superimposed over the lungs.
- The projection is not rotated, i.e., the right and left ribs are projected over one
- Sufficiently short exposure time: The heart, diaphragm, and great vessels are sharply outlined.
- Not overexposed: Pulmonary vessels are visible in the retrocardiac space (RCS).
- Not underexposed: Pulmonary vessels are projected over the cardiac silhouette.

For entries that appear on more than one page, the **boldfaced** numbers indicate page(s) on which the term is described in particular detail.